Contemporary Psychiatry

Edited by

Sidney Crown, PhD, FRCP, FRCPsych
Consultant Psychiatrist,
The London Hospital, Whitechapel, London

Butterworths
London   Boston   Durban   Singapore   Sydney   Toronto   Wellington

First published in *British Journal of Hospital Medicine* between October 1976 and November 1981. Revised and updated where necessary

© International Thomson Publishing Ltd and Butterworth & Co (Publishers) Ltd 1984 and published by Butterworth & Co (Publishers) Ltd by arrangement with International Thomson Publishing Ltd 1984

British Library Cataloguing in Publication Data

Contemporary psychiatry.
  1. Psychiatry
  I. Crown, Sidney
  616.89   RC454

ISBN 0–407–00293–6

Library of Congress Cataloging in Publication Data

Main entry under title:

Contemporary psychiatry.

  Bibliography: p.
  Includes index.
  1. Psychiatry–Addresses, essays, lectures.
I. Crown, Sidney. [DNLM: 1. Psychiatry–Collected works. WM 5 C7603]
RC458.C556 1983   616.89   83-23189
ISBN 0–407–00293–6

Typeset by Scribe Design Ltd, Gillingham, Kent
Printed in England at The University Press, Cambridge

Preface

Two previous collections of articles from the *British Journal of Hospital Medicine* have been published: *Contemporary Psychiatry* (Editors: Silverstone and Barra-clough, 1975) and *Practical Psychiatry* (Editor: Sidney Crown, 1982).

The present papers were selected by me, revised by their authors where necessary and reset by Butterworths as part of their Contemporary Series so that we have returned once again to the original title. We hope that the opportunity to reset the articles will answer the criticism of reviewers that large, double-column journal pages were awkward to hold and read when in book form.

Many people, the present Editor among them, consider the critical review particularly helpful for initiating new interests, for learning, or for revising for examinations. Critical reviews do not aspire to the narrow but inevitable specialism of the focused research study. Authors take a new and often lively look at a broad area they know well, synthesize their views and organize the material in a readable way.

The *British Journal of Hospital Medicine* is directed mainly at trainees' background reading for higher examinations. Thus for psychiatrists the MRCPsych, and equivalent examinations outside the UK, is the primary target. However it is genuinely hoped that consultants will find these reviews helpful. Certainly, editing them reminded me of how much I could learn a second time round!

Researchers from a medical, psychological or surgical background may find several aspects of psychiatry which impinge on their own areas of interest usefully reviewed.

We hope, therefore, to interest psychiatrists-in-training, senior psychiatrists, clinical psychologists and clinical or research-oriented social workers. We also hope that the price will bring the book within the range of the individual, as well as the library, buyer.

I am pleased to be able to express my thanks to Julian Marshall and Diana Briscoe of Northwood Books for publishing *Practical Psychiatry*; and to the staff of Butterworths for their enthusiasm and help with the present collection.

Sidney Crown

Contributors

M.O. Aveline MB, BS, MRCPsych, DPM
Mapperley Hospital, Nottingham

S. Bloch MB, PhD, MRCPsych, DPM
Warneford Hospital, Oxford

Professor **R.S. Bluglass** MD, FRCPsych, DPM
Midland Centre for Forensic Psychiatry, Birmingham

P. Bowden MPhil, MRCP, MRCPsych
The Maudsley Hospital, London

H. Brierley MA, DipEd, PhD
Newcastle Area Health Authority

J. Catalan MSc, MRCPsych, DPM
Warneford Hospital, Oxford

Professor **A.W. Clare** MB, MPhil, MRCPI, MRCPsych
Medical College of St Bartholomew's Hospital, London

J. Cobb BA, MRCP, MRCPsych
St George's Hospital, London

S. Crown PhD, FRCP, FRCPsych,
The London Hospital, Whitechapel, London

M.H. Davies MA, MD, FRCPsych
Midland Nerve Hospital, Birmingham

K. Davison MB, FRCP, FRCPsych, DPM
Newcastle General Hospital
Royal Victoria Infirmary, Newcastle upon Tyne

C. Fairburn MA, MPhil, MRCPsych
Warneford Hospital, Oxford

J.L. Fluker MD, FRCP
Charing Cross Hospital, London
Hammersmith Hospital, London

E. Fottrell MD, MRCPsych, DPM
Tooting Bec Hospital, London

H.L. Freeman MSc, FRCPsych, DPM
Hope Hospital, Salford, Manchester

J.J. Gayford MD, MRCPsych, DPM
Warlingham Park Hospital, Surrey

K. Hawton DM, MRCPsych
Warneford Hospital, Oxford

H. Merskey DM, FRCP(C), FRCPsych
University of Western Ontario
London Psychiatric Hospital, Ontario

E.M. Mitchell MA, DCP
St George's Hospital, London

Professor **P.E. Mullen** MB, BS, MPhil, MRCPsych
Otago Medical School, Dunedin, New Zealand

A. Munro MD
Camp Hill Hospital, Halifax, Nova Scotia

R.M. Murray MD, MPhil, MRCP, MRCPsych
Institute of Psychiatry, London

J.M. Pfeffer BSc, MB, MRCP, MRCPsych
The London Hospital, Whitechapel, London

B. Pitt MD, FRCPsych
The London Hospital, Whitechapel, London

A. Reveley MB, MRCPsych
Institute of Psychiatry, London

G. Rooth MD, MPhil, MRCPsych
Barrow Hospital, Bristol

K. Schapira MD, FRCP, FRCPsych, DPM
Royal Victoria Infirmary, Newcastle upon Tyne

D.F. Scott MB, FRCP, DPM
The London Hospital, Whitechapel, London

Professor **M.A. Simpson** MB, BS, MRCPsych, DPM
Temple University, Philadelphia

I. Smith BSc, FRCPath
The Middlesex Hospital Medical School, London

M. Swan MB, MRCPsych
Winterton Hospital, Cleveland

R.W. Tibbetts MA, BM, FRCPsych, DPM
United Birmingham Hospitals and Midland Centre for Neurosurgery

L. Wing MD, FRCPsych
MRC Social Psychiatry Unit, London

Contents

Introduction

I found it interesting, when selecting articles to republish, to try and understand principles guiding my choice. Obviously articles vary in basic qualtiy so that the weaker ones can be eliminated. There is also, with articles published in the *British Journal of Hospital Medicine* as distinct from other learned journals, a potential interest-and-unusualness component which may be somewhat outside the mainstream, such as the articles on fire raisers, monosymptomatic hypochondriacal psychosis or rape. These articles deal with topics which, though relatively uncommon, are common enough to be part of the ordinary clinician's work and so merit a review that might not be acceptable elsewhere. In general, articles are conventionally classified (clinical, social, psychotherapeutic, etc.) but underlying themes are discernible around which it is appropriate to introduce them.

Clinical psychiatry is based more and more on Units located within District General Hospitals. Pfeffer's contribution stresses this clearly in its attempt to define groups of acutely disturbed patients presenting on general medical wards and to outline the principles of their management. This is the case with toxic confusional or delirious states, alcohol-related confusion, parasuicide, acute anxiety or aggressive behaviour. There are two other topics related to liaison psychiatry. Davison, in an article or remarkable clarity and comprehensiveness, gives an account of organic mental disorders caused by drugs and poisons. The clinical pictures include drowsiness, delirious states, affective and paranoid reactions, dementia and pseudodementia. Care with the planning of prescribed drugs is especially advised. Fottrell considers violent behaviour by psychotic patients. The majority of psychotic patients are not violent; underlying personality is more relevant than diagnosed clinical disorder. However, an appreciation that a minority of such patients does become violent is timely, relating as it does to a topic not covered in this book—the mentally abnormal offender.

Another general ward problem relating to violence, but this time to violence turned on the self, is the management of the attempted-suicide patient. Hawton and Catalan cover the assessment of the risk of successful suicide and the repetition of parasuicide; the relation to psychiatric disorder and current problems; and after-hospital help and support. Before leaving the general ward we should remember that hysteria (Merskey) is the great mimic. The problem of nineteenth-century neurologists such as Charcot in differentiating the organically disturbed patient from the psychologically motivated, remains. Hysteria, although periodically banished by the academic, still baffles us. Merskey also emphasizes a point of current interest, namely that there are possible relations, in certain circumstances, between hysteria and organic brain disease.

It is, of course, a platitude to say that all behaviour is genetically based but that its expression depends on the psychological and social-cultural environment. However it might be argued that the emphasis on the psychosocial, as distinct from the genetic, is being overplayed at the present time and that a balance needs to be restored. In this sense the two articles summarizing the genetic contribution to psychosis (Reveley and Murray) and to neurosis (Murray and Reveley) are timely. With schizophrenic patients methodologically sophisticated adoption studies have been particularly fruitful.

More than many other areas of psychiatry, psychogeriatrics reflects the balance between the inborn and the acquired. Brice Pitt illustrates how the clinical picture varies not only with the psychosocial stress but also with the basic genetic material upon which the stresses of the aged are acting. His article is focused upon management problems: 25 per cent of the elderly suffer from psychiatric symptoms or disabilities. These may include confusion, mania, depression, as well as neurotic symptoms. Such patients should be assessed at home if possible. The practical problem then is who treats them? Unfortunately the "community" as such does not yet really care enough.

If the unholy alliance between psychoanalysis, ethology and developmental psychology is correct and the alignment of these groups is justified, then human aggression is at least as important as sexuality and more dangerous to our survival. While aggression turned outwards is dramatic it is no more so than aggression turned towards the self. Suicidology has become a clinical and research industry. Hawton and Catalan's article on parasuicide is practical in its emphasis on the management and aftercare of these patients. Simpson deals with another aspect of self-damage, self-mutilation. The main group of persons are wrist-cutters, mostly young women with a variety of psychosexual, identity and other personality problems. The venerable theory of "focal suicide" against part of the self still helps to conceptualise this group.

Organic psychiatry has, since the publication of Lishman's classic text (*Organic Psychiatry*, 1978), become a defined area in its own right. A sub-area of a not-so-rare group of disorders that are nevertheless not often studied by contemporary psychiatrists is that of tics and spasms. Tibbetts' article is particularly helpful for the assessment of these conditions and for understanding their underlying neuropsychiatry. Tics occur mainly in children who are more obsessional than matched non-tiqueurs. Their outlook is basically benign. Spasms consist of less sharply circumscribed movements: spasmodic torticollis is the most frequent clinical presentation. Again the basic personality in half these patients is obsessional. Tibbetts especially warns against the diagnosis of hysteria in these conditions although it may be justified if made for positive rather than for negative reasons.

Several areas of psychotherapy are considered, none of which has been adequately covered in short articles elsewhere. Bloch demonstrates an important clinical truth: that supportive psychotherapy has a framework of theory and clinical practice and is far more systematic than "what every good doctor does", a cry so often heard. Aveline brings another psychotherapeutic fringe area into clearer focus with his account of action techniques. These have their origins in psychodrama and the T-group and emphasize structured exercises in an attempt to induce personal fulfilment and growth. In this sense, these techniques are part of the Human Growth movement, the third arm of the psychotherapies, together with the psychodynamic and the behavioural psychotherapies. All psychotherapies involve both cognition (thought) and behavioural modification (action); only their emphases differ. An important application of this principal is illustrated by Mitchell's article on the treatment of obesity. She emphasizes the psychological aspects of management, external triggers, internal control, emotional arousal and its relation to eating, the personality characteristics of the obese, the problems of poor long-term therapy results. In my article, "Psychotherapy research today", I have attempted to introduce readers to some contemporary, intriguing approaches to psychotherapy research, especially those coming from the USA which are possibly not as well known as they should be in the UK. Such methods include the analysis of psychotherapy successes and failures in apparently similar patients treated by the same therapist.

One topic has been chosen to represent social psychiatry. Even with the improved drug therapy of schizophrenia and with greater interest in community management there is still a problem of coping with schizophrenia. Freeman presents an unusually complete and concise picture directed towards those that have to do the coping: relatives, hospitals, rehabilitation and community services.

Substance abuse overlaps with clinical, social, psychodynamic, behavioural and community psychiatry. Clare attempts to elucidate the most relevant factors in the multiple causes of alcohol dependence. He draws together contributions from biological, metabolic, genetic, psychological, psychoanalytical and sociocultural viewpoints and considers availability factors such as occupation which can make a client potentially vulnerable. Many contemporary psychiatrists and psychotherapists find themselves working with middle-class, professional persons who are alcohol-dependent. Murray deals with the difficult area of medical practitioners who abuse alcohol. Doctors' mental health in general is poor compared to matched groups from the general population. Drug and alcohol dependence is "disturbingly common". A problem in all high-level professional groups—doctors, academics, lawyers, businessmen—is the reluctance of colleagues to refer them for treatment. Part of the outcome of this reluctance is that doctors who are alcohol abusers stand a raised risk of suicide.

Psychosexual problems have, in the last ten years or so, been artificially separated from other areas of psychiatry and psychotherapy. These problems are ubiquitous and are found in primary care (general practice) as well as in all areas of hospital medicine. As with other psychological problems the causes of sexual dysfunction may be genetic (e.g. low sex drive), psychological or social. A sub-area of significant importance to general medicine deals with the sexual problems of persons with diabetes mellitus. These are discussed by Fairburn. Neither the assumption that all sexual dysfunction in diabetics is organic nor the assumption that it is functional can be sustained blindly. It seems likely that with the majority of proven diabetics, male sexual dysfunction, especially erectile impotency, is psychogenic. Fairburn directs attention particularly to the differentiation of organic and psychogenic erectile impotence. Organic impotence is gradual; it becomes complete but the retention of sexual interest remains. Disorders of ejaculation are much less common. Fairburn directs the reader's attention towards modified sex therapy and counselling methods of management. An area of current interest in the psychosexual field is the relationship of sexual deviance, especially male homosexuality, to sexually transmitted diseases and hence to important issues in social and community medicine. Fluker's article comes from a London clinic with extensive experience of this topic. Penile–anal sexual expression is particularly dangerous in terms of spread of disease especially with multiple partners. Syphilis, gonorrhoea, non-specific urethritis, genital warts, herpes genitalis, hepatitis B, and bowel infections may all be involved. Too recent for our collection is the problem of "Acquired Immune Deficiency Syndrome". However, knowledge of this condition is as yet too meagre and the mysteries are many. Why, for example, has the condition surfaced, and why now?

Transsexuality and exhibitionism may both provide depressingly difficult clinical and management problems. Rooth takes an eclectic approach to the management of exhibitionists using drugs, symptom control techniques, self-monitoring and self-discipline, psychotherapy and education of the individual and his family. Transsexuality is the more agonizing problem because of the possible involvement of surgery which is, by definition, irreversible. Schapira et al discuss the possible organic and psychological background to this condition as well as aspects of training in female skills and hormone management which should precede surgery and possibly render this unnecessary.

Child psychiatry is represented by a single article, but one in a core area and by a leading researcher. Wing emphasizes the basically educational rather than the medical–psychiatric aspect of management. Early diagnosis is helpful to parents, together with full explanation of the knowns and unknowns of the condition. There is no treatment for the underlying impairment but there is considerable scope for teaching parents skills in managing behaviour problems and teaching the child new skills where possible.

In the area of psychosomatic medicine and the application of this in general hospital (liaison) psychiatry, I have chosen two topics: a core area (Davies) is the relation between stress, personality and coronary artery disease. Is there a "coronary personality"—the so-called Type A personality: conscientious, striving for achievement, impatient and hostile? What is the influence of life events on precipitation of disease? These are major current preoccupations. At the other extreme to that of immediate clinical relevance is Mullen's look into the future search for the soul in the pineal gland, an endocrine organ active throughout life and perhaps involved in biorhythms connected with puberty, the menstrual cycle and reproduction.

Legal and forensic psychiatry is a rapidly growing area. Certain articles in other sections overlap with it, i.e. Fottrell's article on violent behaviour in psychotic patients and Cobb's on morbid jealousy. Cobb considers the classification and psychopathology of this condition and its occurrence in a background of organic, psychotic and depressive conditions: in neurosis and personality disorders; in alcoholism; and in sexual dysfunction. The forensic relevance of the condition, especially in terms of violence or possible homicide, is obvious. Similarly in Scott's unique study of fire raising, a condition which may have forensic implications and occur in a motivated background (e.g. political) or may appear motiveless, organic or psychiatric disorder may also be involved. A similar overlap with forensic psychiatry is possible through the monosymptomatic hypochondriacal psychoses (Munro) where the patient shows a single, long-sustained paranoid or hypochondriacal delusion.

Of more direct forensic importance are the articles on rape, incest and battered wives. Bowden discusses a possible classification of rapists. Some categories are descriptive (e.g. explosive, aggressive-sadistic) and others have a psychodynamic implication (e.g. latent homosexual). How far can victims be said to collude in some way? Perhaps 20 per cent. What are the after-effects of rape? Should rape be subsumed under the general laws of assault? Incest (Bluglass) is undoubtedly more prevalent than official statistics would suggest. Incest between sibs and between father and daughter are the common manifestations. Obviously, harmful effects may spread from the victim to the family and back to the father-rapist. Battered wives (Gayford) is another socially involved and currently emotive topic. The background may be psychiatric disturbance, morbid jealousy, alcohol abuse, incest or poor social conditions. Interest also centres on the classification of battered wives themselves. These may be surprisingly various. Obvious candidates are the inadequate, the abuser of alcohol or drugs, or those with a psychiatric history. Less obvious are the provocative, or even the highly competent—perhaps too competent—wife.

Swan considers an important medicolegal topic: fitness to plead. This is a topic involving complex nuances. The author examines these and also usefully discusses how to examine an accused person psychiatrically.

I hope I have whetted the potential reader's appetite to sample not only topics he knows well but also those which are outside his usual work practice but potentially within his general interest.

SIDNEY CROWN

Chapter 1

The genetic contribution to the neuroses

Robin M Murray/Adrianne Reveley, Institute of Psychiatry, London

One of the difficulties involved in studying the genetic contribution to nonpsychotic psychiatric illnesses is that many such illnesses fall on a continuum with normality. As with height or skin colour, the genetic component of human personality and neurosis is almost certainly the result of many genes—polygenic inheritance—interacting with the environment. As part of the background to this article, we shall therefore first review genetic investigations into normal personality.

Most such studies have used the twin method, comparing either monozygotic (MZ) with dizygotic (DZ) twins or MZ twins reared apart (MZA) with those brought up together (MZT). In the former case, comparing the twins on various measures gives an assessment of the effect of sharing 100 per cent of the genes (MZ) and that of sharing 50 per cent (DZ), assuming that the environment is similar for both. In the latter case, comparing MZAs with MZTs gives an indication of the effect of the environment. Vandenberg (1967) reviewed all available studies of personality in twins involving a total of 785 MZ and 908 DZ pairs and found that MZ twins were more alike in all but eight of the 101 variables investigated and the differences were statistically significant at the one per cent level for 29 variables.

Such studies have consistently shown a hereditary contribution to introversion–extroversion and many have demonstrated a similar contribution to neuroticism. In a study of normal adolescent twins Gottesman (1963) found heritability loadings ranging from zero per cent for hysteria to 71 per cent for social introversion. On the other hand Loehlin and Nichols (1976), who studied the responses of 850 sets of twins to the California psychological inventory test, came to the conclusion that all dimensions of personality as measured by questionnaire appear to be equally heritable, with about half the variation in personality being due to genetic factors. This study and others have concurred in finding no evidence that a common family environment contributes significantly to personality similarities in twins. Thus, although environment carries substantial weight in determining personality—it appears to account for at least half the variance—the salient environmental influences are not those due to having a family in common, which psychologists have traditionally presumed to be important. Instead, the environmental effect appears to come from the almost random action of specific events and influences.

Studies of MZA twins are, of course, designed to avoid any possible effect of a common home environment. Shields (1962) compared 44 pairs of MZAs with a control group of MZTs. In this and two smaller studies (Newman et al, 1937;

Juel-Nielsen, 1980) the degree of resemblance between the MZAs was very similar to that between the MZTs. Indeed, for some variables such as extroversion and neuroticism the MZAs were more similar. Shields (1962) explained this by suggesting that competitive effects might exaggerate any differences between twins reared together. He pointed out that family environment can vary dramatically without obscuring the basic similarity of genetically identical twins. There has recently been a resurgence of interest in MZAs and studies currently being carried out in Finland and Minneapolis appear to be confirming many of Shields' (1962) findings.

Although human personality traits are almost certainly polygenic, there are occasional hints that specific genetic variations may cause deviance from the norm. This parallels the inheritance of height which generally reflects quantitative genetic variation but sometimes dwarfism may result from specific inherited defects. Genetic disorders, especially those that cause mental retardation, may also lead to particular behaviour patterns. For instance, children with trisomy 21 (Down's syndrome) not only suffer from some degree of mental retardation but also are remarkable for their affectionate and sociable natures. On the other hand, the Lesch–Nyhan syndrome, which is caused by a defective gene on the X chromosome, is invariably associated with both subnormality and self-mutilation.

The possession by males of an extra X chromosome (Klinefelter's syndrome) tends to increase the risk of psychiatric problems (Theilgaard et al, 1971) but women with Turner's syndrome (XO) show no defect in intelligence or psychological stability; one study even found them to be more feminine than their sisters in behaviour and style of dress (Nielsen et al, 1977). It is, of course, well known that some prison populations contain an excess of tall men with an extra Y chromosome, and that evidence that a defendant has this XYY syndrome has been accepted in a court of law as a mitigating factor for his criminal behaviour (Pitcher, 1975). It is less well known that there is also an increased prevalence of XYY among subnormal individuals, and that many men with this karyotype lead blameless lives. Thus, although the 47,XYY karyotype tends to increase the likelihood of tall stature, lower IQ, and aggression, the majority of such men remain responsible members of society.

Anxiety neurosis

Interest in a possible genetic contribution to pathological anxiety goes back to Beard (1869) who wrote "hereditary descent terribly predisposes to neurasthenia". Subsequently Oppenheimer and Rothschild (1918) found a family history of nervousness in 45 per cent of 100 World War I soldiers with Da Costa's syndrome, while Wood (1941) described a family history of "probable cardiac neurosis" in 25 per cent of 84 World War II soldiers with this syndrome.

McInnes (1937) and Brown (1942) examined the parents and siblings of anxiety neurotics, while Cohen et al (1951) investigated the relatives of patients with what they termed "neurocirculatory asthenia (anxiety neurosis, effort syndrome)". All three studies reported rates of about 15 per cent among the relatives; comparative rates in the general population would be of the order of 3 per cent of men and 6 per cent of women (Helgason, 1978). Brown's (1942) study which was part of a wider inquiry suggested that the neuroses tend to "breed true". Although there was some overlap, anxiety states were diagnosed most frequently in the relatives of anxiety neurotics, obsessional states in the relatives of obsessionals, and hysterical states in the relatives of hysterics. Of course, Brown (1942) may have overestimated the consonance between probands and relatives by diagnosing the latter in the knowledge of the former's condition.

More recently Noyes et al (1978) used a structured history schedule to interview 112 anxiety neurotics and 110 surgical controls about their relatives. Although this method underestimates the psychopathology of relatives, the study had the merit that the interviews were carried out blind to the probands' diagnoses. Once again about 15 per cent of the combined parents and siblings were diagnosed as anxiety neurotics, compared with 2.7 per cent of control relatives. The risk for female relatives was twice that for male relatives, a ratio similar to that in most patient populations studied.

Six twin studies have included anxiety neurotics, but of those published only that of Slater and Shields (1969) stands up to critical examination. Out of 142 consecutive neurotic twins seen at the Maudsley Hospital, London, these authors identified 17 MZ and 28 DZ co-twins with an anxiety state. Some form of psychiatric disorder was found in 47 per cent of the MZ co-twins and 18 per cent of the DZ co-twins. When the same diagnosis was taken as the criterion of concordance, the MZ rate decreased only slightly to 41 per cent but the DZ rate fell to 4 per cent. Slater and Shields (1969) then re-examined their series in terms of marked anxiety rather than a primary diagnosis of anxiety state. The concordance rate for MZ twins rose to 65 per cent and that for DZ twins to 13 per cent. Clearly these findings argue in favour of not only a general neurotic predisposition but also some genetic specificity for anxiety. Torgersen (1980) has recently completed a similar twin study and concurs with Slater and Shields (1969) that the genetic predisposition is greater in anxiety states than in other neuroses.

Obsessional neurosis

Brown (1942) and Rüdin (1953) reported, respectively, that 7.5 per cent and 4.8 per cent of the parents of obsessional neurotics also suffered from obsessional illness. Rosenberg (1967) found lower rates, but even his figures were some eight times the prevalence in the general population. Estimates of the frequency of obsessional personality in parents have ranged from 3.3 per cent (Rüdin, 1953) to 37 per cent (Lewis, 1936), but tell us more of the differing breadths of the investigators' concepts of obsessional personality than of the true prevalence. There can be no doubt, however, that a high proportion of relatives show some psychological abnormality. Carey (1978) found that 48 per cent of parents, 39 per cent of siblings, and 16 per cent of children had some form of noteworthy psychological abnormality. This increased liability did not extend to psychotic conditions.

Obsessional neurotics are less likely to marry than the general population and within marriage their fertility is low. Hare et al (1972) noted that "the proportion of childless marriages in obsessional neurosis is greater than in all the neuroses or in affective psychosis, and for females the proportion exceeds that in schizophrenia". Nevertheless, Cowie (1961) observed a higher incidence of neurosis among the offspring of obsessionals than among those of neurotic patients while Rutter (1966) found that four out of nine children of obsessional neurotics had obsessional symptoms themselves.

The presence of obsessions among relatives could, of course, be evidence for transmission via a particular type of upbringing. In favour of this hypothesis is the evidence that male obsessional neurotics tend to be first-born or only children (Snowden, 1975) and that the children of more obsessional mothers tend to have a rather solitary restricted childhood with few easy-going, unstructured, and peer-orientated days (Cooper and McNeill, 1968).

Twins with obsessional neurosis are hard to come by. Nevertheless, Carey (1978) noted that 30 concordant and 13 discordant MZ pairs and no concordant but 14 discordant DZ pairs had been reported. Unfortunately, most reports have concerned only a few cases and it is well known that twins collected in an unsystematic way tend towards the MZ and concordant. Furthermore, in many cases the diagnosis was in doubt. Indeed, Black (1974) concluded that in only three cases had both the zygosity and the diagnosis been firmly established.

Two twin studies have recently been reported. Carey (1978) has given some preliminary details from a consecutive series of twin probands with obsessional neurosis presenting to the Maudsley Hospital. Six of the 12 MZ co-twins had had treatment for nervous complaints—three had definite and a further two had possible obsessional features. Only one of the 12 DZ co-twins was obsessional.

Murray et al (1980) administered the Leyton obsessional inventory test to 404 pairs of normal twins. The responses revealed that heredity accounted for 44 per cent and 47 per cent of the variance in obsessional traits and symptoms, respectively. There was a high genotypic correlation between obsessional symptom scores and neuroticism scores. This suggests that heredity may contribute to obsessional neurosis both through influencing the development of obsessional personality characteristics and through the transmission of a general neurotic tendency which predisposes to the manifestation of obsessional symptoms.

Hysteria

In 1931 Kraulis reported the results of a family study involving 106 probands who had been diagnosed as having hysteria in Kraepelin's clinic: 9.4 per cent of their parents and 6.25 per cent of siblings had also been hospitalized with a "hysterical reaction". Subsequently, Brown (1942) classified 11 per cent of the 107 parents and siblings of patients with hysteria as also having hysteria (more than in other neurotic and control families). Ey and Henric (1959) examined the families of 27 "randomly selected" hysterics and found that 21 relatives were abnormal; personality disorder was most common followed by depression, but there were also three cases of hysteria.

One should not read too much into these studies because of the vagueness of the diagnosis of hysteria. However, Ljungberg (1957) carried out a careful investigation into the first-degree relatives of 381 Swedish probands. All had been treated for hysterical conversion symptoms of which disturbances of gait (47 per cent) and fits (20 per cent) were the commonest. The risk of hysteria was 2.4 per cent for male relatives and 6.4 per cent for female relatives, rates well above the prevalence in the general population. Ljungberg (1957) concluded that hysteria was probably under some degree of polygenic control.

Slater (1961) set out to confirm what he originally thought was the hereditary nature of hysteria by studying 12 MZ and 12 DZ pairs of twins in whom the proband had been diagnosed as having hysteria. To his amazement he found that none had any close relatives with hysteria. As a result of this and a follow-up study which revealed no consistent outcome in cases diagnosed as hysteria, Slater and Glithero (1965) became convinced not only that hysteria had no genetic basis but also that it was merely a label that doctors attached to patients they neither liked nor understood. Their views were very influential and for a time it seemed that, in the UK at least, the term hysteria would be superseded.

However, as Lewis (1975) pointed out, "hysteria tends to outlive its obituarists". The year after Slater published his negative twin study (Slater, 1961) the St Louis school began to develop a radically different notion of hysteria as a genetic disease affecting women with a histrionic nature (Arkonac and Guze, 1963; Cloninger et al, 1975). These workers rejected such traditional diagnostic criteria as dissociation and conversion symptoms. Instead, they defined St Louis hysteria (or Briquet's syndrome) as a disease characterized by the early onset of multiple somatic complaints which generally leads to frequent hospitalization and surgery.

They noted an increased rate of sociopathy in the male relatives of such patients and postulated that hysteria and sociopathy were the sex-modified manifestations of the same underlying disorder. They assumed (Cloninger et al, 1975) that liability to the disorder has a normal distribution in the general population, but that as one moves towards the abnormal side of this distribution there are three cutoff points related to sex and severity. At the first threshold a man becomes sociopathic (3.3 per cent of men), past the second a women suffers from hysteria (2.4 per cent of women), and overstepping the third produces a sociopathic woman (0.9 per cent of women). The St Louis group have re-analyzed previously collected data and shown that it fits their multifactorial model, but it remains to be seen whether their findings will be confirmed in other centres.

Thus, the picture remains very confused, with family and twin studies seeming both to demolish and to validate the concept of hysteria as a genetic entity. But as Shields (1981) states, "Considering the diversity of opinion about what hysteria is, it is hardly surprising that there should still be different views about its genetics". His parsimonious explanation is that mechanisms such as conversion and dissociation are within the repertoire of us all but heredity contributes more to the development of sociopathic and hysterical personalities.

Neurotic depression

In a previous review on functional psychosis (Reveley and Murray, 1980) we concluded that there is a significant genetic component in affective psychosis. However, for neurotic depression the evidence is less compelling. There have been few studies and those show only a small and less specific genetic effect.

Stenstedt (1966) found a 4.8 per cent rate of affective disorder in the relatives of patients with neurotic depression, that is scarcely higher than in the general population. Shapiro (1970) used the Danish twin register to identify a small series of twins with nonendogenous affective disorder and concluded that the genetic effect seemed to operate on personality structure rather than on the depression itself. Torgersen (1980) found no evidence in his twin study that genetic factors contributed significantly to neurotic depression. Robins and Guze (1972) have advocated the classification of depression by the presence or absence of another pre-existing psychiatric disorder, and it may be that depression occurs either as a symptomatic manifestation of neurotic illness or personality disorder or as a primary illness itself. Distinguishing specific categories for example on this basis or on that of biochemical abnormalities such as response to the cortisol suppression test, may be the best way of isolating homogeneous subgroups which can then be investigated for any possible genetic effect.

Criminality and psychopathy

Criminality was one of the earliest behaviours to be studied genetically. Lange (1929) found very high concordance rates in twins, but these were not wholly confirmed by later workers perhaps because his ascertainment was not systematic. Nevertheless, Christiansen (1974) who studied the records of all Danish twins born between 1870 and 1920 reported concordance rates for criminality of 52 per cent and 22 per cent for male MZ and DZ twins, respectively. Female concordance rates were lower but the MZ:DZ difference and the contrast with the prevalence in the general population were even greater, suggesting that biological factors are more important in female than male crime.

Adoption studies support the view that genetic factors contribute to criminality. Hutchings and Mednick (1974) checked 1145 males on the Copenhagen adoption register against the criminal register. They found that 10 per cent of the control adoptees and a similar proportion of those who only had a criminal adoptive father had criminal records, but when only the biological father was a criminal, 21 per cent of the adopted-away sons had criminal records. There appeared to be an interaction effect because when both fathers were criminal the rate in the sons increased to 36 per cent. Adoptees with a noncriminal father who were brought up by a criminal were less likely to turn to crime than those with a criminal biological father who were raised by a noncriminal. The same authors identified 143 criminal adoptees and found that 49 per cent of their biological fathers had criminal records compared with 28 per cent of the biological fathers of noncriminal adoptees; the corresponding figures for adoptive fathers were 23 per cent and 10 per cent.

There have also been adoptive studies of psychopathy. Crowe (1974) compared 52 adoptee probands born to female offenders with a control group of adoptees. Six of the probands had antisocial personalities and 11 had committed a criminal offence. None of the controls had that diagnosis and only four had committed a crime. Unfortunately nothing was known of the fathers. Schulsinger (1972) used the Danish register to identify the biological relatives of 57 psychopathic adoptees and matched controls. He grouped together cases of psychopathy, doubtful psychopathy, criminality, alcoholism and hysterical character disorder in the families as psychopathic spectrum disorder and found the rate to be twice as high in the biological relatives of the psychopathic adoptees. When restricting the analysis to fathers the rate was 9.3 per cent compared with 1.9 per cent.

Alcoholism

No informed student of alcoholism would doubt that environmental factors are of major importance in determining the prevalence of alcohol-related problems in any society. But why is it that every study, irrespective of country, has shown higher rates of alcoholism among relatives of alcoholics than in the general population (Goodwin, 1971)?

It had been widely assumed that this was due to imitation rather than inheritance. However, in 1973 Goodwin and his colleagues reported that the sons of alcoholics separated from their alcoholic parents in early life and raised by foster parents were nearly four times more likely to become alcoholics than were adoptees without alcoholic biological parents. Another study (Goodwin et al, 1974) comparing adopted-away sons of alcoholics with their brothers raised by the alcoholic parent revealed rates of alcoholism of 25 per cent and 17 per cent, respectively. These controversial findings have been supported by two other adoptive studies. Cadoret and Gath (1978) investigated 84 American adoptees separated from their parents at birth and found alcoholism more frequently in those with a heavy-drinking biological relative. Bohman (1978) used the Swedish criminal and alcoholic registers to examine the biological and adoptive parents of 2000 adoptees. Once again there was a significant correlation between alcoholism in biological parents and in their adopted-away sons.

Kaij (1960) located 174 twin pairs where one member had appeared on the Swedish register of alcohol abusers. When one twin was a heavy abuser so was the other in 70 per cent of MZ but only 32 per cent of DZ twins. Subsequently, Partanen et al (1966) interviewed 902 Finnish male twins. Although there was no difference between MZ and DZ twins in regard to consequences of drinking, the frequency of drinking and the amount drunk at a session showed moderate heritability.

Despite deficiencies in both the twin and adoptive studies, it seems likely that genetic factors do contribute to liability to alcoholism. Is what is inherited an underlying personality of psychiatric abnormality, or is there some biochemical predisposition? There is little evidence in favour of a primary personality defect, and there has been a similar paucity of support for the suggestion of Winokur et al (1971) that alcoholism and depression are genetically linked.

It is known, however, that there is considerable genetic control over alcohol metabolism in both animals and humans (Kopun and Propping, 1977). Inbred strains of rats and mice differ in their preference for, or avoidance of, alcohol and some reports have suggested that the drinker strains tend to have higher alcohol dehydrogenase activity. The existence of an atypically active human form of alcohol dehydrogenase has also attracted a great deal of notice, and this enzyme variant's supposed ability to produce higher acetaldehyde levels has been blamed by some for the unpleasant flushing reaction which makes alcohol less rewarding for many Asians. Paradoxically, Schuckit and Rayses (1979) have reported that the relatives of alcoholics develop higher acetaldehyde levels in response to alcohol than controls. This confusing situation, in which a propensity to develop high acetaldehyde levels has been said to predispose both towards and against alcoholism, is probably a consequence of the technical difficulties involved in estimating acetaldehyde levels.

Murray and Gurling (1980) have proposed a polygenic model in which the pertinent genetic factors are conceptualized as operating at three related levels:

1. For pharmacogenetic reasons some individuals experience an unusually large excess of positive over negative effect of alcohol; such individuals are more likely to proceed to heavy drinking
2. Liability to dependence on alcohol includes a genetic component which can be manifest only after exposure to chronic heavy drinking but may be transmitted independently of heavy drinking
3. Individuals differ in their genetic predisposition to alcohol-related disorders, but again this difference can only become manifest following chronic heavy drinking. In this manner the possession of a particular HLA type may predispose the excessive drinker towards cirrhosis of the liver.

Conclusion

Early research tended to focus on the presence or absence of a genetic effect in various neuroses. More recent work has assumed that genes and environment interact to cause individual variations in personality and psychopathology in the same way that they do for other quantitative human characteristics such as height and skin colour.

For any given set of twin or family data the genetic component (or heritability) can be calculated, but specific heritabilities depend on the instrument used, the size of the population, and the sampling methods.

Although individual results cannot always be generalized, heritability values have tended to be lower for the neuroses than for the functional psychoses. This may, of course, be because the phenotype being assessed is further from the genotype. One of the aims of current research is to identify biological correlates of psychological traits and to identify precisely their inheritance. In this way we may advance our understanding of part of the complex interactive system that determines human behaviour.

References

Arkonac, O, Guze, SB (1963) *New England Journal of Medicine*, **268**, 239
Beard, GM (1869) *Boston Medical and Surgical Journal*, **3**, 217
Black, A (1974) *in* Obsessional States (edited by Beech, HR). Methuen, London. p.19
Bohman, M (1978) *Archives of General Psychiatry*, **35**, 269
Brown, FW (1942) *Proceedings of the Royal Society of Medicine*, **35**, 785
Cadoret, RJ. Gath, A (1978) *British Journal of Psychiatry*, **132**, 252
Carey, G (1978) PhD Thesis, University of Minnesota
Christiansen, K O (1974) *in* Determinants and Origins of Aggressive Behaviour (edited by de Wit. J. Hartnup, W W). Mouton. The Hague p. 233
Cloninger, C R, Reich, T, Guze, S B (1975) *British Journal of Psychiatry*, **127**, 23
Cohen, M E, Badel, D W, Kilpatrick, A. Reed, E W, White, P D (1951) *American Journal of Human Genetics*, **3**, 126
Cooper, J, McNeill, J (1968) *Journal of Child Psychology and Psychiatry*, **9**, 173
Cowie, V (1961) *Acta psychiatrica Scandinavica*, **37**, 37
Crowe, R R (1974) *Archives of General Psychiatry*, **31**, 785
Ey, H, Henric, G (1959) *Évolution psychiatrique*, **24**, 287
Goodwin, D W (1971) *Archives of General Psychiatry*, **25**, 545
—, Schulsinger, F. Hermansen, L, Guze, S B, Winokur, G (1973) ibid. **28**, 238
—, —, Moller, N, Hermansen. L, Winokur, G, Guze, SB (1974) ibid. **31**, 164
Gottesman, J I (1963) *in* Heredity and Achievement (1970) (edited by Robinson, D N). Oxford University Press, New York. p. 171
Hare, E H, Price, J S, Slater, E T O (1972) *British Journal of Psychiatry*, **121**, 197
Helgason, T (1978) *Acta psychiatrica Scandinavica*, **58**, 256
Hutchings, B, Mednick, S A (1974) *in* Genetics, Environment and Psychopathology (edited by Mednick, S A, Schulsinger, F A, Higgins, J, Bell, B). North-Holland/American Elsevier, New York. p.215
Juel-Nielsen, N(1980) Individual and Environment: Monozygotic Twins Reared Apart. International Universities Press, New York
Kaij, L (1960) Alcoholism in Twins. Alonquist and Wiksell, Stockholm
Kopun, M, Propping, P(1977) *European Journal of Clinical Pharmacology*, **11**, 337
Kraulis, W (1931) *Zeitschrift für die gesamte Neurologie und Psychiatrie*, **136**, 174
Lange, J (1929) Verbrechen als Schicksal, Studien an Kriminellen Zwillingen. Thieme Leipzig
Lewis, A J (1936) *Proceedings of the Royal Society of Medicine*, **29**, 325
Lewis, A (1975) *Psychological Medicine*, **5**, 9
Ljungberg, L (1957) *Acta psychiatrica Scandinavica*, Suppl. 112
Loehlin, J C, Nichols, R C (1976) Heredity, Environment and Personality. University of Texas Press, Austin and London

McInnes, R G (1937) *Proceedings of the Royal Society of Medicine*, **30**, 895

Murray, R M, Clifford, C, Fulker, D W, Smith. A (1980) *in* Genetic Tissues in Epidemiology (edited by Tsuang, M), Washington University Press, Washington

—, Gurling, H M D (1980) *in* Psychopharmacology of Alcohol (edited by Sandler, M). Raven Press, New York. p.89

Newman, H H, Freeman, F N, Holzinger, K J (1937) Twins: A Study of Heredity and Environment. University of Chicago Press, Chicago

Nielsen, J, Nyborg, H, Dahl, G (1977) *Acta Jutlandica*, **45**, Medicine series 21

Noyes, R J, Clancy, J, Crowe, R, Hoenk, R P, Slymen, D J (1978) *Archives of General Psychiatry*, **35**, 1057

Oppenheimer, B S, Rothschild, M A (1918) *Journal of the American Medical Association*, **70**, 1919

Partanen, J. Bruun, K, Markkanen, T (1966) Inheritance of Drinking Behaviour. Finnish Foundation for Alcohol Studies, Helsinki

Pitcher, D R (1975) *in* Contemporary Psychiatry (edited by Silverstone, T, Barraclough, B) *British Journal of Psychiatry* Special Publication No. 9. Headley Brothers, Kent. p. 316

Reveley, A, Murray, R (1980) *British Journal of Hospital Medicine*, **24**, 166

Robins, E, Guze, S B (1972) *in* Recent Advances in Psychobiology of the Depressive Illnesses (edited by Williams, T A, Katz, M M, Shields, J A). Government Printing Office, Washington. p. 283

Rosenberg, C M (1967) *British Journal of Psychiatry*, **113**, 405

Rüdin, E (1953) *Archiv fur Psychiatrie und Nervenkrankheiten*, **191**, 14

Rutter, M L (1966) Children of Sick Parents: An Environmental and Psychiatric Study. Maudsley Monograph No. 16. Oxford University Press, London

Schuckit, M A, Rayses, V (1979) *Science*, **203**, 54

Schulsinger, F (1972) *International Journal of Mental Health*, **1**, 190

Shapiro, R W (1970) *Acta Jutlandica*, **42**, No. 2

Shields, J (1962) Monozygotic Twins Brought Up Apart and Brought Up Together. Oxford University Press, London

— (1981) *in* Hysteria (edited by Roy, A). John Wiley, Chichester

Slater, E (1961) *Journal of Mental Science*, **107**, 359

—, Glithero, E (1965) *Journal of Psychosomatic Research*, **9**, 9

—, Shields, J (1969) *in* Studies of Anxiety (edited by Lader, MH) Headley Brothers, Ashford. p. 62

Snowden, J A (1975) MPhil Thesis, University of London

Stenstedt, A (1966) *Acta psychiatrica Scandinavica*, **42**, 392

Theilgaard, A, Nielsen, J, Sørensen, A, Frøland, A, Johnsen, S G (1971) A Psychological-Psychiatric Study of Patients with Klinefelter's Syndrome 47 XXY. Munksgaard, Copenhagen

Torgersen, (1980) personal communication

Vandenberg, S G (1967) *in* Recent Advances in Biological Psychiatry 9 (edited by Wortis, J). Plenum, New York. p. 65

Winokur, G, Rimmer, J, Reich, T (1971) *British Journal of Psychiatry*, **118**, 525

Wood, P (1941) *British Medical Journal*, i, 845

Chapter 2

The genetic contribution to the functional psychoses

Adrianne Reveley/Robin M Murray, Institute of Psychiatry, London

Psychiatric genetics emerged in the first quarter of this century from the attempt to apply simple Mendelian laws of heredity to the supposedly distinct conditions into which Kraepelin had split the functional psychoses. Indeed, when Rüdin carried out the first family risk study of schizophrenia in 1916 he used patients who had in some cases actually been diagnosed by Kraepelin. Subsequently his Munich school became pre-eminent and many of the giants of psychiatric genetics such as Kallman, Essen-Möller, and Slater studied there. Family studies soon confirmed the increased risks of illness in the relatives of psychotic patients but the different psychiatric syndromes stubbornly refused to fit the classic dominant or recessive mode of inheritance.

Twin studies were developed as another way of assessing the possible contribution of heredity to psychiatric disorders. This method, pioneered by Galton in 1883 in total ignorance of Mendel's laws, depends on the fact that identical (monozygotic [MZ]) twins share their family upbringing and all of their genes whereas familial (dizygotic [DZ]) twins share their upbringing but only 50 per cent of their genes. Luxenburger's study in 1928 was the first in the series of classic twin studies that culminated in 1953 with Slater's *Psychotic and Neurotic Illnesses in Twins*. All these early twin studies found much higher concordance rates for psychosis in MZ twins than in DZ twins, thus suggesting a substantial genetic contribution.

But the picture began to change as psychoanalysis, social psychiatry, and behavioural psychology grew in influence and all emphasized the role of environment in shaping behaviour. As a result the nature or nurture conflict came to dominate the 1950s and early 1960s and psychiatrists who still believed in a genetic contribution to abnormal behaviour were criticized as being nihilistic. Evidence in favour of an aetiological role for heredity was often totally dismissed. For instance, Jackson (1960) discounted the contribution of twin studies to the understanding of schizophrenia by stating that since schizophrenia was caused by a confusion of identity MZ twins were uniquely vulnerable.

Nevertheless, many of the criticisms of the early genetic literature were well founded. For example, since no psychiatric syndrome had been shown to follow a Mendelian pattern of inheritance, untestable assumptions such as reduced penetrance or a combination of genes had been invoked. In a series of papers from 1959–62 Rosenthal pointed to the bias introduced by studying nonconsecutive samples of resident inpatient twins: concordant pairs and the more severely ill were likely to be over-represented. He also drew attention to deficiencies in determining zygosity and differing diagnostic standards for the index twin and the co-twin. His assertion that the concordance rates in schizophrenia were too high was borne out by the second wave of twin studies which all reported much lower concordance rates.

Many of the methodological and environmentalist criticisms were assimilated by geneticists into important refinements of the twin and family studies including the examination of reared-apart twins. In addition, the adoptive strategy was introduced to tease apart genes and environment by studying individuals who received their genes from one set of parents but their upbringing from another. The 1960s also saw the development of statistical methods of describing the genetics of common physical and mental disorders (Carter, 1969). The assumption of these models is that liability to such disorders is normally distributed throughout the population in much the same way as height or weight and that environmental variables as well as two or more genes play an aetiological role. Falconer (1965) postulated that the disorders would become manifest when a certain threshold was reached.

Schizophrenia

The role of heredity in schizophrenia has attracted a great deal of controversy over the years. Indeed, many of the old arguments were aired again in response to a critical review by Gottesman and Shields (1976). Fortunately, the highly charged debate that ensued demonstrated that the simplistic nature or nurture argument is redundant. The emphasis now is on the extent of the genetic contribution, its mode of transmission, and the manner of its interaction with environmental variables.

Concordance rates from twin studies might be expected to provide the best estimate of the genetic contribution but determining these rates is complex. The pairwise rate, the proportion of the sample in which both twins are affected, appears straightforward but unfortunately it is an underestimate of the true concordance rate. If one tries to set up a 2 × 2 table with twin data it becomes obvious that the information collected is incomplete since pairs with an unaffected index twin are either not counted or are added to the discordant pairs with an affected index case. The probandwise method ascertains concordance from each index case which appears in the sample whether already a co-twin or not. Although the number of double probands or pairs counted twice varies from study to study, in practice it gives a fairly consistent and reliable estimate of heritability which accords well with the value from family studies.

TABLE 2.1. Twin studies of schizophrenia

		Kringlen (1967)	Pollin et al (1969)	Tienari (1971)	Fischer (1973)	Gottesman and Shields (1972)
MZ twins	no. of pairs	55	95	16	21	22
	*probandwise concordance (%)	45	43	35	56	58
DZ twins	no. of pairs	90	125	21	41	33
	*probandwise concordance (%)	15	9	13	26	12

*Probandwise concordancies recalculated by Gottesman and Shields (1976)

Table 2.1 summarizes the results of the recent twin studies. The three Scandina-vian studies (Tienari, 1963; Kringlen, 1967; Fischer, 1973) identified their twins from national registers and in the cases of Kringlen and Fischer cross-matched them with psychiatric registers. This is theoretically ideal but in practice a number of twins was lost and Fischer's sample had a high proportion of deceased twins. This made clinical and zygosity determination more difficult and may have contributed to the relatively high concordance rate she found in DZ twins. Tienari examined all male twins in a geographically limited area where both were alive and could be traced. He initially reported an MZ concordance rate of zero per cent but this was raised subsequently to 35 per cent (see Gottesman and Shields, 1976).

Pollin et al (1969) surveyed 15 000 pairs of white male twins who served in the US army. Their population was thus selected for health and despite broad diagnostic categories they found a low morbidity risk for schizophrenia. Gottesman and Shields (1972) used the traditional method of examining an unselected series of twins, ascertained after they presented to a psychiatric hospital. Their study is remarkable for a careful diagnostic review by an international panel.

In spite of the differences in diagnostic criteria and in sample collection the range of probandwise concordance rates is relatively small (*Table 2.1*). Pooling the figures produces a concordance rate of 47 per cent for 261 MZ co-twins and 14 per cent for 329 DZ co-twins. This gives a heritability of 0.87 which means that about 87 per cent of the difference in concordance between MZ and DZ twins can be accounted for genetically. Such a heritability estimate is comparable to those found for anencephaly and congenital dislocation of the hip.

MZ twins reared apart (some 27 pairs) are concordant for schizophrenia to about the same extent as those reared together (Gottesman and Shields, 1976) thus confirming the role of heredity. But twin studies also emphasize the importance of the environment since only about half of MZ pairs are concordant for schizophre-nia in spite of sharing the same genes.

Adoption studies

In the first of the adoption studies Heston and Denney (1968) followed-up 47 adopted-away children of chronically hospitalized schizophrenic mothers and a well-matched control group. Five of the experimental group but none of the controls had become schizophrenic.

A series of papers then came from a large Danish-American adoption study which utilized careful design and exemplary methodology. Rosenthal et al (1971) studied in a blind fashion the adopted-away offspring of known shizophrenics. Of these, 18.8 per cent received a diagnosis of definite or uncertain schizophrenia compared with 10.1 per cent of control adoptees and 4.8 per cent of children of normal people crossfostered to schizophrenics. Furthermore, 31.6 per cent of the index adoptees and only 17.8 per cent of controls were considered to have a schizophrenia spectrum disorder; this is a broad concept that includes not only borderline schizophrenia but also schizophrenic personality disorders.

As part of the same fruitful collaboration Kety et al (1978a) blindly rated extensive psychiatric assessments of the biological and adoptive relatives of 33 known schizophrenic adoptees. Twenty one per cent of the biological relatives fell into the schizophrenia spectrum compared with only 5 per cent of the adoptive relatives. One of their further strategies was to compare the rates of schizophrenia in paternal versus maternal half-siblings as a way of controlling for intrauterine and very early rearing factors. The paternal half-siblings had the higher rate suggesting that these factors were not relevant.

No attempt was initially made to examine the second parent. Such a strategy is rather like Mendel crossing a known plant with an unknown one and then attempting to relate the characteristics of the second generation only to the familiar plant. To remedy this Rosenthal (1974) examined 54 spouses of the schizophrenic parents of adopted children. They reported that assortive mating had taken place at an appreciable rate and that the prevalence of a schizophrenia spectrum disorder in the offspring was more than three times as frequent when the coparent also had a spectrum disorder.

Mode of inheritance

All the evidence suggests that what is inherited is not the certainty of developing schizophrenia but rather a vulnerability to it. The twin studies in particular show that environmental factors must be necessary for the expression of this vulnerability in at least half the cases. What can be said about the mode of transmission of this vulnerability?

Current models fall into four categories: single gene, two interacting genes, polygenic, and heterogeneous. Slater (1958) put forward a monogenic theory and later Heston (1970) suggested that such a dominant gene might express itself either as classic schizophrenia or in a partial form as schizoid disease. Pollin (1972) tested this theory by studying 15 MZ pairs discordant for schizophrenia and showed that the nonschizophrenic co-twins were not particularly schizoid. Two-locus models have often been suggested over the years, initially by Rudin (1916) and most recently by Böök et al (1978) who propose a dominant gene affecting monoamine oxidase activity and a recessive gene affecting dopamine beta hydroxylase.

Polygenic models (Gottesman and Shields, 1972) assume that the genetic contribution to schizophrenia is the result of the combined effect of at least three genes, no one of which is essential. The genetic predisposition in the population would therefore be graded but once the combination of genetic and environmental factors results in the crossing of a threshold (Falconer, 1965) schizophrenia would occur.

Theories of genetic heterogeneity consider that schizophrenia can be subdivided into different conditions in some of which environmental factors may be crucial while in others genetic factors predominate. For instance, Bocklage (1977) drew attention to the unusual distribution of handedness in Gottesman and Shields' (1972) sample of twins. Fourteen of the 22 pairs contained at least one left-handed member. In these pairs the concordance rate was lower and the illness less severe than in the eight both-right-handed pairs, seven of whom were concordant for chronic schizophrenia. This raises the possibility that the hazards of being born a twin might increase the risk of altered cerebral dominance and later schizophrenia; such a twin's schizophrenia would be nongenetic and so the pair would be discordant. However, although twins are more often left-handed than singletons there is no consistent evidence that schizophrenia is more common in twins.

Recent reviews (Kidd and Matthysse, 1978; Rieder and Gershon, 1978) recommend strategies designed to take into account clinical and biochemical heterogeneity. Homogeneous subgroups of schizophrenia might be found either by isolating those, for example, with low monoamine oxidase levels or by limiting studies to single families in which the process leading to schizophrenia might be the same.

Environmental factors might also define a homogeneous subgroup. Schizophrenics are known to be born more often than expected in the early months of the year (Dalen, 1975). Kinney and Jacobsen (1978) suggest that the genetic loading may be less in these winter-born schizophrenics.

Linkage studies might also be used to define a subgroup, perhaps through linkage with the histocompatibility (HLA) complex. The principle involves knowledge of the location of a particular marker gene, in this case the HLA gene on chromosome 6. If it is linked to schizophrenia then a specific combination of HLA subtype and the presence of schizophrenia should always appear together in members of any given family (McGuffin, 1979).

Affective disorder

Estimates of the prevalence of affective disorder in the general population and in the relatives of those with affective disorder have varied widely, largely because of the difficulty in defining the illness. Nonetheless, almost all studies have agreed that the first-degree relatives of those with affective disorder have a morbidity risk of about 10–15 per cent (Price, 1968), well above that of the general population. The risk appears to be greater in female than in male relatives and in the relatives of those who fall ill at a younger age. For instance, Gershon et al (1976) estimated that the morbidity risk for relatives of probands with an early onset (<40 years old) was 19.4 per cent and that for relatives of probands with a later onset ($\geqslant$40 years old) was 10.4 per cent.

Unipolar and bipolar illness

Without doubt the major contribution of genetics to psychiatric nosology in the last 20 years has been the validation of the division of affective disorder into unipolar (UP) and bipolar (BP) illnesses: the former is characterized by one or more episodes of depression and the latter by both depressive and manic episodes. This distinction was, of course, first made by Leonhard. Then in 1966 Perris published a monograph on 277 probands and 2396 relatives in which the differences between BP and UP illnesses were documented. By a strange coincidence Angst (1966) published a similar study independently.

The results of these and more recent studies are summarized in *Table 2.2*. It can be seen that the overall risks are generally higher for the relatives of BP as opposed to UP probands. The relatives of patients with a BP disorder are at risk of both BP and UP disorders while the relatives of UP probands generally have an increased risk of UP but not BP illness. Perris (1966) found very few relatives with a UP disorder of BP probands and very few relatives with a BP illness of UP probands, thus suggesting quite distinct inheritances for the two disorders. However, the dichotomy is less complete in the other studies.

TABLE 2.2. Risk of affective disorder in first-degree relatives

		Angst (1966)	Perris (1966)	Reich et al (1969)	Helzer and Winokur (1974)	Gershon et al (1975)
Morbidity risk (%) in relatives of BP probands	BP	4.3	10.2	10.2	4.6	3.8
	UP	13.0	0.5	20.4	10.6	6.8
Morbidity risk (%) in relatives of UP probands	BP	0.3	0.3	—	—	2.1
	UP	5.1	6.4	—	—	11.5

Winokur (1979) and Schlesser et al (1979) attempted to subdivide UP depression into sporadic depression and two supposedly genetic conditions, pure depressive disease and depressive spectrum disorder. Family pure depressive disease, Winokur (1979) states, is characterized by nonsuppression with dexamethasone, whereas depressive spectrum disorder is commoner in women and is genetically linked to alcoholism and antisocial personality. There are, however, obvious environmental reasons why the relatives of alcoholic or personality-disordered individuals should have an increased likelihood of depression. Consequently, the concept of depressive spectrum disorder has not been widely accepted.

Twin studies

The results of twin research are less easy to evaluate in affective disorder than in schizophrenia. Gershon et al (1976) reviewed the six reports with the fewest methodological flaws. The overall concordance rate for 91 MZ twin pairs was 69.2 per cent and that for 226 DZ pairs was 13.3 per cent. If one assumes that the intrapair environmental influences are the same for MZ and DZ twins, then this difference indicates a considerable genetic contribution. Price (1968) provided some support for this assumption through his literature survey of affective disorder in 12 MZ twin pairs reared apart. Their concordance rate at 67 per cent was very similar to that of MZ pairs reared together.

The above rates refer to all affective disorders and naturally interest has now turned to the comparative heritabilities of BP and UP illnesses. In a reanalysis of all reported twin studies Allen (1976) showed that in comparing rates for BP and UP illnesses there was a significant difference in concordance rates for MZ twins (72 per cent and 40 per cent, respectively) but not for DZ twins (14 per cent and 11 per cent). Subsequently, Bertelsen et al (1977) specifically addressed this question. For BP disorder they reported pairwise concordance rates of 74 per cent in MZ and 17 per cent in DZ twins; for UP disorder the rates were 43 per cent and 19 per cent, respectively. Thus, it appears that genetic factors are more important in BP than in UP illness.

Mode of transmission

Although the data reviewed above strongly suggest a genetic transmission of affective disorder the exact mode of inheritance remains unclear. A single dominant gene effect can only fit the pedigree data if one assumes variable penetrance (Johnson and Leeman, 1977). However, one possible explanation for the greater frequency of the disorder in women would be X-linkage, that is the location of the relevant gene on the X chromosome. A sex-linked dominant transmission would imply that generally an affected male would not have an ill father or son but could have an ill mother or daughter. Winokur (1970) examined this question in the families of 89 manic probands and reported striking findings. There were no ill-father/ill-son pairs although there were 13 or more for each of the other combinations. Helzer and Winokur (1974) and Reich et al (1969) also found data suggesting X-linkage for BP illness but Perris (1966) reported 13 father–son pairs and others have also reported that such pairs are not infrequent (Johnson and Leeman, 1977).

Winokur and Tanna (1969) then examined marker genes on the X chromosome for linkage with BP illness and reported significant evidence of linkage with colour blindness and suggestive evidence of linkage with the Xg blood group. Unfortunately this is confusing since these marker genes are at opposite ends of the chromosome so linkage with both would be impossible. Some but not all subsequent studies have confirmed their findings for colour blindness and the argument for and against X-linkage continues. Kidd and Weissman (1978) sum up the situation by saying that some BP illnesses may be determined by an allele or alleles at an X-linked locus but the evidence is not compelling that this is involved in more than a small fraction of BP illnesses.

Schizoaffective disorder

Nosologists have repeatedly puzzled over those cases of psychosis that appear to have both schizophrenic and affective features. Are these atypical cases to be regarded as a mixture of the two main functional psychoses or as variants of one or the other, or do they constitute a separate third psychosis? Dual mating studies provide no support for the notion that such cases result merely from inheriting a predisposition to both schizophrenia and affective disorder. Among the children of 19 clearly schizophrenic and clearly manic-depressive matings, Elsässer (see Slater and Cowie, 1971) found six schizophrenics and six manic-depressives but only one with atypical psychosis. Furthermore, the children of 17 atypical × atypical psychotic marriages included 10 with atypical psychosis, five with manic-depressive illness, and five with schizophrenia.

Fischer and Gottesman (1980) similarly found that schizophrenic × manic-depressive matings produced 17 per cent schizophrenic and 17 per cent manic-depressive offspring, but only one case of schizoaffective psychosis. Kringlen (1978) reported that six schizophrenic × manic-depressive marriages produced no children with what he termed reactive psychosis.

Tsuang (1979) used the elegant method of comparing the diagnosis in pairs of siblings where both had a functional psychosis. He found a dearth of pairs where both were schizoaffective and suggests that schizoaffective disorder is heterogeneous, comprising variants of both affective disorder and schizophrenia. In other work he found that 7.6 per cent of the first-degree relatives of schizoaffectives were suffering from affective disorder but only 1.3 per cent from schizophrenia (Tsuang et al, 1976).

A number of studies have compared good and poor prognosis schizophrenia and noted a similar increase in affective disorder among the relatives of those with a good prognosis (Clayton et al, 1968). Evidence from the Danish adoption study is consistent with this—schizophrenia spectrum disorder is found more frequently among the biological relatives of adoptees with chronic schizophrenia than those with acute schizophrenia (Kety et al, 1978b). Thus, within what we currently call acute schizophrenia and schizoaffective disorder there may exist a subgroup with a closer genetic relationship to affective disorder than to chronic process schizophrenia.

However, this does not exclude the possibility that there exists an independent third psychosis. Such a notion receives some support from Elsässer's demonstration (quoted by Slater and Cowie, 1971) that dual matings of atypical psychotics often breed true, and from the finding by Cohen at al (1972) of a higher concordance rate in MZ twins for schizoaffective disorder than for schizophrenia or affective disorder. Both Mitsuda (1967) and Perris (1974) noted a significant loading of atypical or cycloid psychosis in the families of probands with these hypothetical conditions. Perris (1974) found no evidence for combined schizophrenic/manic-depressive heredity in the families and now believes he can reliably distinguish cycloid psychosis from the other two functional psychoses on clinical grounds. It remains to be seen whether this is a transferable skill.

References

Allen, M G (1976) *Archives of General Psychiatry*, **33**, 1476
Angst, J (1966) *Monographien aus dem Gesamtgebiete der Neurologie und Psychiatrie*, **112**
Bertelsen, A, Harvald, B, Hauge, M (1977) *British Journal of Psychiatry*, **130**, 330
Bocklage, C E (1977) *Biological Psychiatry*, **12**, 19
Böök, J A, Wetterberg, L, Modrzewska, K (1978) *Clinical Genetics*, **14**, 373
Carter, C O (1969) *British Medical Bulletin*, **25**, 52
Clayton, P J, Rodin, L, Winokur, G (1968) *Comprehensive Psychiatry*, **9**, 31
Cohen, S M, Allen, M G, Pollin, W, Hrubec, Z (1972) *Archives of General Psychiatry*, **26**, 539
Dalen, P (1975) Season of Birth: A Study of Schizophrenia and Other Mental Disorders. North-Holland, Amsterdam
Falconer, D S (1965) *Annals of Human Genetics*, **29**, 51
Fischer, M (1973) Genetics and Environmental Factors in Schizophrenia. Munksgaard, Copenhagen
—, Gottesman, II (1980) *in* The Social Effects of Psychiatric Disorder (edited by Robins, L, Wing, J K). Brunner-Mazel, New York
Gershon, E S, Mark, A, Cohen, N, Belizon, N, Baron, M, Knobe, K E (1975) *Journal of Psychiatric Research*, **12**, 283
—, Bunney, W E, Leckman, J F, Van Eerdewegh, M, De Bauche, B A (1976) *Behaviour Genetics*, **6**, 227
Gottesman, II, Shields, J (1972) Schizophrenia and Genetics: A Twin Study Vantage Point. Academic Press, New York
—, —, (1976) *Schizophrenia Bulletin*, **2**, 360
Helzer, J E, Winokur, G (1974) *Archives of General Psychiatry*, **31**, 73
Heston, L L (1970) *Science*, **167**, 249
—, Denney, D (1968) *in* The Transmission of Schizophrenia (edited by Rosenthal, D, Kety, S S). Pergamon Press, Oxford. p.383
Jackson, D D (1960) The Etiology of Schizophrenia. Basic Books, New York
Johnson, G F S, Leeman, M M (1977) *Archives of General Psychiatry*, **34**, 1074
Kety, S S, Rosenthal, D, Wender, P H, Schulsinger, F, Jacobsen. B (1978a) *in* The Nature of Schizophrenia: New Approaches to Research and Treatment (edited by Wynne, L C, Cromwell, R L, Matthysse, S). John Wiley, New York. p.25
—, —, — (1978b) *in* Critical Issues in Psychiatric Diagnosis (edited by Spitzer, R, Klein, D). Raven Press, New York. p.213
Kidd, K K, Matthysse, S (1978) *Archives of General Psychiatry*, **35**, 925
—, Weissman, M M (1978) *in* Depression: Biology, Psychodynamics, and Treatment (edited by Cole, J, Schatzberg, A F, Frazier, S H). Plenum Press, New York, p.107
Kinney, D K, Jacobsen, B (1978) *in* The Nature of Schizophrenia: New Approaches to Research and Treatment (edited by Wynne, L C, Cromwell, R L, Matthysse, S). John Wiley, New York. p.38
Kringlen, E (1967) Heredity and Environment in the Functional Psychosis. Heinemann, London
— (1978) *in* The Nature of Schizophrenia: New Approaches to Research and Treatment (edited by Wynne, L C, Cromwell, R L, Matthysse, S). John Wiley, New York. p.9
Luxenburger, H (1928) *Zeitschrift für die gesamte Neurologie und Psychiatrie*, **116**, 297
McGuffin, P (1979) *Psychological Medicine*, **9**, 721
Mitsuda, H (1967) Clinical Genetics in Psychiatry. Igaku Shoin, Tokyo
Perris, C (1966) *Acta psychiatrica Scandinavica*, Suppl. 194
— (1974) *ibid.* Suppl. 253
Pollin, W (1972) *Archives of General Psychiatry*, **27**, 29
—, Allen, M G, Hoffer, A, Stabenau, J, Hrubec, Z (1969) *American Journal of Psychiatry*, **126**, 597
Price, J (1968) *in* Recent Developments in Affective Disorders (edited by Coppen, A, Walk, A). British Journal of Psychiatry, Special Publication No. 2. Headley Bros, Ashford, Kent. p.37
Reich, T, Clayton, P J, Winokur, G (1969) *American Journal of Psychiatry*, **125**, 1358
Rieder, R O, Gershon, E S (1978) *Archives of General Psychiatry*, **35**, 866

Rosenthal, D (1974) *in* Genetics Environment and Psychopathology (edited by Mednick, S A, Schulsinger, F, Higgins, J, Bell, B). North-Holland, Amsterdam. p.167
—, Wender, P H, Kety, S S, Welner, J, Schulsinger, F (1971) *American Journal of Psychiatry*, **128**, 307
Rüdin, E (1916) Zur Vererbung und Neuentstehung der Dementia Praecox. Springer Verlag, Berlin and New York
Schlesser, M A, Winokur, G. Sherman, B M (1979) *Lancet*, i, 739
Slater, E (1953) Psychotic and Neurotic Illnesses in Twins. MRC Report Series No. 278. HMSO, London
— (1958) *Acta Genetica et Statistica Medica (Basel)*, 7, 20
—, Cowie, V (1971) The Genetics of Mental Disorders. Oxford Unversity Press, London
Tienari, P (1963) *Acta psychiatrica Scandinavica*, Suppl. 171
— (1971) *in* Psychiatria Fennica 1971 (edited by Achté, K A). Helsinki. p.97
Tsuang, M T (1979) *Archives of General Psychiatry*, **36**, 633
—, Dempsey, G M, Rauscher, F (1976) *ibid.* **33**, 1157
Winokur, G (1970) *British Journal of Psychiatry*, **117**, 267
— (1979) *Archives of General Psychiatry*, **36**, 47
—, Tanna, V (1969) *Diseases of the Nervous System*, **30**, 89

Chapter 3

Violent behaviour by psychiatric patients

Eamonn Fottrell, Tooting Bec Hospital, London

Violence is a generic word and covers a multitude of phenomena. It exists on psychological, social and physical planes and ranges from blackmail, through self-defence and warfare, to suicide and homicide. The type that causes greatest concern is, of course, personal physical violence to self or others.

Throughout history there has been a tendency to ascribe violence as a characteristic of places, groups or classes of individuals. Insane persons were widely believed not only to possess superhuman strength but also to be characterized by outbreaks of uncontrollable physical violence. According to Nunnally (1961) many still viewed the psychiatrically ill as dangerous and unpredictable. How valid is this view now?

Violent behaviour and the mentally ill

Most of the studies in this field have examined the arrest records of patients not only for violence and assault but also for rape and robbery. The earlier studies like those of Pollock (1938), Cohen and Freeman (1945), and Brennan (1964) found either no difference or lower arrest rates among mental patients compared with the general population. Later studies tempered this picture somewhat. Rappeport and Lassen (1965, 1966) found higher rates of arrest for robbery and rape among male expatients and for aggravated assault among female expatients than in the general population. Giovanni and Gurel (1967) and Zitrin et al (1976) obtained results supporting the findings of Rappeport and Lassen. The tendency to discover a positive relation between the mentally ill and criminality (including violence) has continued with the most recent findings of Gruneberg et al (1977), Lagos et al (1977) and Sosowsky (1978).

Researchers in this field are very aware of the difficulties in drawing valid conclusions from their findings and of the dangers in generalizations. For example, the incidence of violent behaviour by psychiatric patients may vary from one catchment area to another because of the differing admission policies of hospitals. Patients may be subject to considerable harassment and exploitation by landlords and employers resulting in frustration and violence. A study of the innate violent tendencies of an individual (or group) is only meaningful when it is closely related to the social setting in which he is functioning and the particular stresses under which he is labouring at the time. Although the threshold of tolerance varies, everyone is potentially violent, and psychiatric patients will exhibit violence either because of, independently of, or in spite of their illness should their frustrations, real or imagined, become intolerable. Such patients would also be more likely to draw attention to themselves and less likely to evade detection than the general population. This fact may be offset by an opposite tendency for few of them to be prosecuted. However, most crime, assaultive or otherwise, goes undetected.

Although the pendulum of more recent research findings, based generally on arrest records, has swung a little towards the view that psychiatric patients may be more violent than the general population, this must also be seen against the general level of prevailing violence in homes and public houses and on the roads. Steadman et al (1978) observed that the arrest rates of patients in their sample were considerably higher than the general population rates primarily because of the large percentage of their patients who had previously been arrested. Such individuals are more apt to be re-arrested than those without prior arrest are to be arrested.

In the USA, where most studies in this field have been carried out, many patients previously caught in a revolving cell door now find themselves in a revolving hospital door or bouncing back and forth between hospital and jail. It must also be taken into consideration that although the rates of most major psychiatric illnesses have in general remained the same over the last 100 years, the rates for violent crimes have shown a steady increase. The comment of Tennent (1971) that "the mentally ill contribute proportionally very little to the general problem of dangerous behaviour" is probably valid. There is no substantial body of evidence that proves that the mentally ill as a group are either less violent or more inherently violent than the general population. The observation of Mark Twain, made in the pre-Watergate era, that "It could probably be shown by facts and figures that there is no distinctly native American criminal class except Congress", is astute in the context of this review.

Personality and violent behaviour

The underlying personality of a patient may be the determining factor in deciding whether the end result of an aggressive thought or fantasy is a violent act. Authors have commented on the role played by personality in various psychiatric syndromes. Blackburn (1968) concluded that in schizophrenia the premorbid personality of the patient was more important in determining hostile behaviour than his illness, and Hill (1964) stated that there were strong counterforces within the personality of the schizophrenic that prevented the expression of aggressive drives and this led to withdrawal and preoccupation with delusional ideas. Nicol et al (1973) in a study of the relation of alcoholism to violent behaviour commented on the personality disorders of the alcoholics. Similarly Lewis (1968) and Ellinwood (1971) concluded that while the use of particular drugs in drug-dependent individuals may be associated with violent crime it is likely that a particular type of personality is necessary to produce violence.

The group par excellence within the psychiatric field in which personality structure is the most closely related to thoughtless, irresponsible, and violent behaviour is the psychopathic or sociopathic group. Unfortunately there is no universally accepted concept or definition of this group. Henderson and Gillespie (1969) described such subjects as "individualistic, rebellious, emotionally immature, lacking foresight and behaving like dangerous children, they fail to learn from their mistakes and the stupidity of their actions is appalling". The principal features of the group may be exhibited in the form of physical assault, suicide, and abuse of alcohol and drugs. This behaviour cannot be explained on the basis of madness or badness in isolation and the existence of the syndrome as a "disease" is disputed. However, Robins (1966) demonstrated the persistence of the disorder from childhood to adulthood; he showed that it ran in families and carried a poor prognosis with death commonly resulting from self-neglect, suicide, fighting, careless accidents, and the effects of too much alcohol or other drugs.

The life history of a psychopath was described by Lloyd and Williamson (1968). Harry, a psychopath, was the offspring of a brutal sadistic father and a vagrant teenage girl. His mother reared him in the most calamitous circumstances and throughout his life he found all relationships difficult; this was especially so with women, whom he assaulted frequently. He spent his life in and out of jail and died at the age of 39 by swallowing open safety pins.

There is a diversity of views on the cause of the condition and psychopathic behaviour has been described as predominately aggressive, inadequate or creative. Craft (1969) stated that improvement may be noted with time, but Whiteley (1970) advised that the so-called burning out of psychopathy in middle age should be viewed with caution. Psychopaths form the most socially irresponsible and physically aggressive category in psychiatry. The view of Brill and Malzberg (1954) that "an attack of mental illness with hospitalization does not tend to leave an inclination towards criminal activity greater than that which existed prior to the illness" is valid today and emphasizes the role of personality in behaviour.

Certain psychiatric states and violent behaviour

Although the premorbid personality of the individual is important in determining violence, certain psychiatric conditions appear to be associated with this behavioural characteristic. For example, people who abuse or are dependent on alcohol or other drugs and those with morbid jealousy and sadistic tendencies commonly exhibit assaultive behaviour. There are well known stereotypes of substance abuse in the public mind, for instance the belligerent drunk, the mugger desperate for heroin, and the frenzied speed freak striking out at all.

Substance-induced violent behaviour

Alcohol   Alcohol has been responsible for more aggression and violence than any other drug. Its use dates at least from the Babylonion period and has been found in the majority of cultures. Physically assaultive behaviour is commonly encountered in public houses or in the adjoining neighbourhoods after closing hours. The association between alcohol abuse and the time of a violent incident has been commented on by McClintock (1963) and Gibbens and Silberman (1970).

Powers and Kutash (1978) concluded that aggression or violence is most likely to occur during alcohol use if:

1. The premorbid personality is characterized by aggressive and sociopathic tendencies
2. Dosages are at medium levels (blood alcohol content of 0.10–0.35 per cent)

3. Stereotypes of alcohol-induced behaviour serve as cues for aggression or are used to excuse the individual from responsibility for his aggression
4. Drinking occurs during close interpersonal interactions particularly in social and/or competitive situations.

A high percentage of murderers and their victims are intoxicated at the time of the crime. In a study of 116 cases of criminal homicide, Virkkunen (1974a) found that in 92 cases (79 per cent) alcohol was detected in either the murderer or the victim. Alcoholics kill themselves at a much greater rate than the general population. Kessel and Grossman (1961) followed-up two series of alcoholics in London and found that the males had 75–85 times the expected rate of suicide for men of their age. Of course abuse of or dependence upon alcohol could appear as only one aspect of an antisocial personality, and also individuals of previously normal personality may turn to crime and violence at a late stage of their dependence to subsidize their drinking.

Drugs   Drug dependence or abuse is commonly associated in the public mind with assaultive behaviour. Although drug misuse is relatively new to Western culture (when compared with alcohol abuse) it is not difficult to envisage how violence might result from the direct effects of drugs or their withdrawal on vulnerable personalities or from the hustling that takes place to ensure supplies.

When drugs are taken, several factors determine the nature and extent of aggression expressed. The most important of these are the drug type and dosage, the individual's expectations from it, the premorbid personality, and the setting in which the drug is taken.

The field of substance-induced aggression has been very well reviewed by Powers and Kutash (1978), and it is evident that most drugs used by drug-dependent individuals of differing personality types can result in aggressive and violent behaviour if the dosage and the setting are appropriate. Gordon (1971) suggested that heroin addicts are slightly more likely than other kinds of addicts to have criminal convictions for violence. Amphetamine abuse has also been associated with violent crime (Ervin and Lion, 1969; Ellinwood, 1971). Aggression and violence may be observed in amphetamine users if the dosage levels are high and the individual is unaware of the negative psychoactive experiences such as paranoid feelings that may occur. The evaluation of the effects of individual drugs on violent behaviour is complicated by the fact that most individuals who abuse drugs are found to abuse more than one substance.

Morbid jealousy and violent behaviour

Morbid jealousy, a symptom of psychiatric illness, has been of special interest to psychiatrists since it may culminate in serious assault or homicide. It may be a symptom of alcoholism, schizophrenia, depression or personality disorder. Shepherd (1961) reviewed the topic and studied 80 cases. He found that the symptom usually appeared in one partner of a marriage who came to believe that his or her spouse had been unfaithful. Paroxysms of rage frequently end in serious assault, homicide or suicide. The best known English study of the syndrome was done by Mowat (1966) who found that it accounted for 12 per cent of insane male murderers and 3 per cent of insane female murderers. Complete separation of the married pair may be indicated. This may not be sufficient to prevent violence as a second partner may well be a potential victim.

Sadistic impulses and violent behaviour

Individuals with sadistic impulses are found in psychiatric practice and attempts have been made by Brittain (1968, 1970) to define the sadistic murderer. Such individuals are invariably male and have been described as quiet and introverted with bizarre sexual sadistic fantasies and an interest in Neo-Nazism, guns, torture and black magic. There may also be a masochistic component in their make-up, involving forms of bondage. Little is known about the prevalence of these features in the psychiatric population but it is thought that in the light of present knowledge such individuals may be very violent.

Suicide and homicide

Homicide is phenomenologically related to suicide and the two frequently occur together (West, 1965). All suicides do not of course involve physical violence to the self in the general meaning of the term, yet statistically suicide is a much more common form of violent death than homicide. Blom-Cooper (1965) observed that "between 1900 and 1950 there were some 7500 murders known to the police but the suicide rate was running at something like 5000 per year". Stengel (1964) found a positive correlation between suicide and alcohol consumption, mental illness, the single state and the divorced state. Suicide is not specific to any particular type of mental disorder although there is an association with psychotic depression.

Fire raising and the mentally ill

Three out of every eight fires that cause more that £10 000 worth of damage are started deliberately (Scott, 1978). Fire raising is a serious and increasing problem and may be associated with loss of life, intentional or otherwise; little research has been done on it. It may be carried out for political or financial gain or may be motiveless and it is much more indulged in by men, especially by those in the 16–25-year age-group. Schizophrenic patients may set fire to their house or their ward in response to auditory hallucinatory voices, and manic-depressive patients may set fire to their property either when manic or when depressed. Alcohol, by lowering the level of inhibition, may lead to a spree of fire setting. In a study of arsonists in a special hospital, McKerracher and Dacre (1966) found that as a group they had a higher psychotic morbidity level and a more marked history of attempted suicide than the other patients in the hospital. Nurcombe (1964) stated that children who raise fire come from disturbed home environments, have been emotionally deprived, or have been regularly moved from home to home. Schools may be particularly vulnerable to child fire raisers. It is unknown how many child fire raisers become adult fire raisers.

The firebug has been described by Scott (1978) as very frequently having a background of personality disorder and experiencing periods of mounting tension that are relieved by fire setting. The number of fires necessary to relieve tension varies from individual to individual. The fires are usually well planned and lit in concourses or places where the public have access, such as stairs or passages, in contrast to an arsonist working for financial gain who lights his fire in the heart of a building ensuring that considerable damage occurs before it is detected.

There is a small group described as fire fetishists who gain overt sexual satisfaction from their indulgence. These are usually withdrawn solitary individuals, some being vagrants or subnormal. They generally get sexual satisfaction by masturbating while watching conflagrations.

Sexual offenders and violent behaviour

Sexual crimes are sometimes accompanied by violence. According to the report of HMSO (1970) sexual offenders numbered less than 0.5 per cent of all offenders in England and Wales in 1969. Most sexual offences go undetected and it is difficult to provide accurate statistics. Males commit the vast majority of sexual offences; soliciting is the main female offence.

Most sexual offenders are, of course, within the "normal" range mentally. Randzinowicz and Turner (1957) did a study on 2000 who had been detected and found that most of them could be categorized as aggressive, irresponsible, and deviant but would not be regarded as mentally ill. Gunn (1976) in a review of 90 long-term prisoners found that overt sexual activity played a significant role in the offence of 20 of them and commented that some seriously dangerous and violent men may also have considerable sexual problems that are sometimes related to their dangerousness. Sexual jealousy should be noted as a special danger. The relation between subnormal intelligence and sexual offences is probably more direct than that between general psychiatric illness and sexual offences. As a group sexual offenders have slightly lower intelligence levels than other offenders (Woodward, 1955). Walker (1965) compared the indictable offences of all male offenders aged 17 or more who appeared in English courts in 1961 with those committed by subnormals of similar age and found that the percentage of sexual offences among the latter was six times as high as that among the former. He drew attention to their difficulty in competing with normal men in getting heterosexual experience.

Psychotic illness and violent behaviour

In surveys on populations of psychiatric patients, schizophrenic or personality-disordered subjects are often prominent among the assaultive groups. Henderson and Gillespie (1969) stated that the largest clinical group involved in aggressive and violent behaviour were the aggressive psychopaths and these were followed by the schizophrenics. Fottrell (1980) in his study of violence found that schizophrenic patients were the most prominent, and Mowat (1966) noted that 6 per cent of the male and 2 per cent of the female admissions to Broadmoor for homicidal offences were schizophrenic. The study of Böker and Häfner (1973) on homicidal or lethal attacks by severely mentally ill offenders in the Federal Republic of Germany suggested that there is a very much higher potential for violence in schizophrenics than in psychotic depressives or subnormals and that 84 per cent of homicidal schizophrenics have been ill for over one year and 55 per cent for more than 5 years before they commit the act. They also concluded that suicide is a far greater risk in schizophrenia than homicide (6–10 per cent of schizophrenics commit suicide).

While the contribution of schizophrenics to patient violence would appear to be quite considerable it must also be borne in mind that schizophrenia is a common illness (one per cent of the general population), that many mental hospitals contain large numbers of such patients at risk of exhibiting violence over many years, and that there may be a small group within the schizophrenic population who account for most of the assaultive behaviour by exhibiting frequent violence. Young male patients with prominent paranoid symptomatology may be the most likely among the schizophrenic group to exhibit serious violence. Reichard and Tillman (1950) stressed that schizophrenics can only commit violence against themselves or others under the influence of delusions or hallucinations, and Planansky and Johnston (1977) stated that homicidal aggression is most probable during the active phase of the illness. However, Virkkunen (1974b) found that only 37 per cent of acts of schizophrenic violence took place during the psychotic episode.

The depressive homicide is one of the classic forensic psychiatric problems but the relation of psychotic depression to violent behaviour, apart from violence to the self, has not been established. West (1965) stated that in the UK the incidence of murder associated with depression is high and indicative of this is the high proportion of murders that are connected with the suicide of the offender—about one in three English murderers kill themselves. It has not been established, however, that they kill themselves because of depression.

Fottrell (1980) found in a study in three psychiatric hospitals that depressed patients did not present with a problem of violence to others. The psychoanalytical view that depression is a turning inwards of aggressive impulses has been studied by Kendell (1970) and there appears to be considerable support for it. An inverse relation between homicide and suicide rates has been found by Henry and Short (1954) in certain cultures. The theory on the inwardly aggressive basis of depression would help to explain the behaviour of the Hutterites (an Anabaptist sect with about 9000 members). They religiously inhibit all aggressive responses and have a very low level of murder but a very high level of depression. The vast majority of depressed patients met in practice present with problems of violence to the self rather than to others.

Violent behaviour in psychiatric hospitals

The belief that psychiatric hospitals are particularly violent places has been fostered not only by the widespread publicity given to serious violent acts committed by patients but also to the far more regrettable violence occasionally emanating from staff to patients. It would appear that although physical assault by patients in psychiatric hospitals is not uncommon, serious physical assault is relatively rare especially in the UK. This was the finding of Folkard (1957) in a study confined to disturbed wards of a psychiatric hospital and of Fottrell et al (1978). In a study in three psychiatric hospitals in the UK, Fottrell (1980) found that the vast majority of incidents were of a petty nature; psychotic women with a history of violence and under the age of 50 were the most frequent offenders. Most of the incidents were perpetrated by a small percentage of patients who repeatedly exhibited violence (3–4 per cent of patients accounted for 60–70 per cent of incidents). They took place in the wards, especially acute or special treatment wards, and nursing staff were by far the commonest victims.

The most common diagnoses among the offending patients were schizophrenia, drug dependence and personality disorders. Ekblom (1970) found that only 17 out of 300 patients labelled as dangerous had been placed in that category for acts of violence committed while in hospital. Marten et al (1970) observed that there was no difference in the incidence of belligerent behaviour (behaviour ranging from aggressive thoughts to violent acts) in a group of 314 patients in an emergency ward between black and white patients; however, males were more belligerent than females and younger patients more belligerent than older ones. Fottrell (1980) noted that females were more often violent than males in hospital—it may be that frequent petty violence is more characteristic of the hospitalized female patient and serious violence more characteristic of the male. In the UK, however, the most seriously violent patients are likely to be excluded from psychiatric hospitals and to be found either in the special hospitals or in prison.

Ekblom (1969) found a favourable comparison between psychiatric hospital staff and staff in other work settings as regards risk of injury. Group violence by patients in hospital appears to be rare. Some authors have described a "body buffer-zone" in relation to violence by patients in hospital: this is defined as an area around an individual which if encroached on to excess by another instils anxiety and provokes a violent response (Kinzel, 1970). Schizophrenics are particularly sensitive to this. It would help to explain the common observation that overcrowding, especially in a ward with a poor therapeutic atmosphere and a locked door, may be conducive to aggressive behaviour. Overall the modern psychiatric hospital is not a particularly violent place.

Prediction of violent behaviour

Few psychiatrists believe they can predict when or where an individual patient will exhibit violence. Accurate prediction is very desirable because it would alleviate the anxiety of psychiatrists caring for potentially dangerous individuals. In the USA approximately 50 000 mentally ill persons per year are predicted to be dangerous and preventively detained for society's and their own protection (Rubin, 1972). A major problem is the high rate of error associated with efforts to predict infrequent events and even with a dangerous individual violence may be infrequently exhibited. There is of course a tendency to overpredict violence because the error to be avoided is the one that would incur undesirable publicity, for example if a released psychiatric patient predicted to be nonviolent exhibited violence in the community. Cocozza and Steadman (1974) suggested that a history of violence and an age under 50 were the only factors of help in distinguishing those who were from those who were not arrested for dangerous behaviour after release from hospital.

If statistical accuracy is to be achieved then with present methods it appears that the best procedure is to predict that no patient would behave violently. But the fact remains that some patients are dangerous and such a strategy would not be acceptable. Scott (1977), in an article on assessing dangerousness in criminals, concluded that as regards accurate prediction "no such magical process will be possible" and that any attempt at prediction entails involvement with the individual on a long-term basis.

Some authors have criticized the practice of predicting and labelling patients as dangerous. Rubin (1972) commented that society has a way "of labelling some mentally ill as criminals, overpredicting violence and then acting on that prediction to exact retributive costs". He continued, "The poor, the mentally incompetent, the drifter and the black are very likely to be labelled in this way for social reasons unrelated to any violent behaviour but rather to society's need to find objects who represent projections of its own violence". Scheff (1963) wrote persuasively about the labelling of patients and indicated that this process of categorizing was the single most important cause of "a career of individual deviance". Further research is needed to establish the effects of labelling.

Prediction of violence for short-term emergency commitment of persons considered imminently violent may be more accurate than prediction over the long term (Monahan, 1978). Overprediction of violence with the resultant detention of many nonviolent individuals so that a few will not be violent is the price society is prepared to pay at present for protection. More accurate methods of prediction would reduce this overkill.

Victims of patient violence

Often the victim of patient violence is a friend, a relative, or else someone known to the patient and with whom he has frequent personal interaction. In acts of impulsive violence the victim may well be the person in closest proximity. Planansky and Johnston (1977) in a study of homicidal aggression in schizophrenic men found that the closely related families were the prime targets, especially wives, and if the patient was in the forces fellow servicemen came under attack. Nursing staff are the commonest victims of attack in hospital; the report of the Confederation of Health Service Employees (1977) stated that 311 assaults were made on nursing staff in England and Wales in a 3½-year period.

Quite frequently it is found that depressive patients kill their children and the crimes have the characteristics of altruistic murders. The patient may well believe, during the course of his depressive illness, that the future is particularly bleak and dreadful and that the children are better out of the world, so he proceeds to kill them. An infant may be at risk from a mother suffering from depression in the puerperium and a spouse may fall victim to a patient with morbid jealousy. Victims of alcoholic and alcohol-intoxicated individuals are commonly found to have partaken of alcohol and of course victims of drug-dependent individuals are frequently found to be drug-dependent themselves or involved in the trade.

Victims of patient violence may also play a considerable role consciously or subconsciously in provoking an attack. Virkkunen (1974a) in a study of criminal homicide and alcohol found that the aggressive behaviours and altercations that preceded the crimes had been initiated by the victims as frequently as by the offenders. Levy and Hortocollis (1976) discussed the ways in which nursing staff may unconsciously provoke violence in patients, and Brailsford and Stevenson (1973) stressed the need for instruction in violence prevention and control for nursing trainees.

The response of the victim to the assault also often determines the nature and seriousness of the act and this is probably particularly true in sexual assaults. Gunn (1976) described the differing responses of three women to a rapist with a knife and the nature of each crime was coloured by the response of the woman. Sexual crimes involving children are particularly abhorrent yet many children participate and cooperate in assaults. Gibbens and Prince (1963) estimated that two thirds of child victims participate in sexual offences and only one third of assaults are by complete strangers (friends and relatives are the usual offenders). Personal violence is an interaction between two or more people and the role of the victim may be considerable in initiating the act and in determining its final nature. "Victimology" (Mendelsohn, 1963) has been proposed as a special field of study of its own.

Summary

There is no substantial body of evidence to prove that psychiatric patients as a group are more violent than the general population. In determining whether violence is exhibited, the underlying personality of the individual is far more important than the psychiatric illness from which he suffers. Individuals with psychopathic personalities, those who abuse or are dependent on alcohol or drugs, and those with pronounced paranoid or sadistic traits may be characterized by aggressive and violent behaviour. There is at present no reliable method of predicting if or when an individual patient will exhibit assaultive behaviour. Psychiatric hospitals, especially in the UK, are characterized more by frequent petty violence than by serious violence. Victims of assaults by patients are often related or known to them and interact with them on a personal level; they may also play a considerable role consciously or otherwise in instigating the assault.

My thanks to Dr Thomas Bewley (Tooting Bec Hospital, London), Professor John Gunn (Institute of Psychiatry, London), Dr Michael Pritchard (St Thomas' Hospital, London), and Dr Zahid Mahmood (Duke Street Hospital, Glasgow) for advice; and also to Mrs Florence Bunwell for secretarial help.

References

Blackburn, R (1968) *British Journal of Psychiatry*, **114**, 1301
Blom-Cooper, L (1965) *Howard Journal*, **11**, 297
Böker, W, Häfner, H (1973) Crimes of Violence by Mentally Disordered Offenders in Germany—a Study in Psychiatric Epidemiology. Springer-Verlag, Berlin. p.292
Brailsford, D S, Stevenson, J (1973) *Nursing Times*, January 18, p.9
Brennan, J J (1964) *American Journal of Psychiatry*, **120**, 1181
Brill, H, Malzberg, B (1954) Statistical Report on the Arrest Record of Male Expatients, age 16 and over, Released from New York State Mental Hospitals during the period 1946–48. New York State Department of Mental Hygiene, Albany
Brittain, R P (1968) Grodwohl's Legal Medicine (edited by Camps, F E). John Wright, Bristol
— (1970) *Medicine, Science and the Law*, **10**, 198
Cocozza, J J, Steadman, H J (1974) *American Journal of Psychiatry*, **131**, 1012
Cohen, L H, Freeman, H (1945) *Connecticut State Medical Journal*, **9**, 697
Confederation of Health Service Employees (1977) The Management of Violent or Potentially Violent Patients. Confederation of Health Service Employees, Banstead
Craft, M (1969) *British Journal of Psychiatry*, **115**, 39
Ekblom, B (1969) *Svenska Läkartidningen*, **66**, 2106
— (1970) Acts of Violence by Patients in Mental Hospitals. Almquist and Wiksells Boktycheri A B, Uppsala
Ellinwood, E H (1971) *American Journal of Psychiatry*, **127**, 1170
Ervin, F R, Lion, J R (1969) *in* Staff Report to the National Commission on the Causes and Prevention of Violence, Vol. 13, Appendix 24. Government Printing Office, Washington, p.1163
Folkard, M S (1957) A Sociological Contribution to the Understanding of Aggression and its Treatment. Netherne Monographs, 1. Netherne Hospital, Coulsdon
Fottrell, E (1980) *British Journal of Psychiatry*, **136**, 216
—, Bewley, T, Squizzoni, M (1978) *Medicine, Science and the Law*, **18**, 66
Gibbens, T C N, Prince, J (1963) Child Victims of Sex Offenders. Institute for the Study and Treatment of Delinquency, London
—, Silberman, M (1970) *in* The Drunkenness Offence (edited by Cook, T. Gath, D. Heusmann, C). Pergamon Press, Oxford. p.35
Giovanni, J T, Gurel, L (1967) *Archives of General Psychiatry*, **17**, 146
Gordon, A M (1971) Patterns of Delinquency in Drug Addiction. Unpublished MPhil Thesis, University of London
Gruneberg, F, Klinger, B, Grumet, B (1977) *American Journal of Psychiatry*, **134**, 685
Gunn, J (1976) *British Journal of Hospital Medicine*, **15**, 57

Henderson, D K, Gillespie, R D (1969) Textbook of Psychiatry. Oxford University Press, Oxford. p.528
Henry, A F, Short, JF (1954) Suicide and Homicide. Glencoe Publishers, Illinois
Hill, D (1964) *in* The Natural History of Aggression (edited by Corth, J D, Ebbing, F J). Academic Press, New York
HMSO (1970) Criminal Statistics for England and Wales 1969. Command paper no. 4398. HMSO, London
Kendell, R E (1970) *Archives of General Psychiatry*, **22**, 308
Kessel, N, Grossman, G (1961) *British Medical Journal*, ii, 1671
Kinzel, A F (1970) *American Journal of Psychiatry*, **127**, 59
Lagos, J M, Perlmutter, K, Saexinger, M D (1977) *American Journal of Psychiatry*, **134**, 1134
Levy, P, Hortocollis, P (1976) *American Journal of Psychiatry*, **133**, 429
Lewis, A J (1968) Cannabis—A Review of the International Clinical Literature. Home Office Advisory Committee on Drug Dependence. HMSO, London. p.40
Lloyd, R, Williamson, S (1968) Born to Trouble:Portrait of a Psychopath. Faber, London
McClintock, F H (1963) Crimes of Violence. Macmillan, London
McKerracher, D W, Dacre, A J (1966) *British Journal of Psychiatry*, **112** 1151
Marten, S, Minog, R A, Gentry, K A, Robins, E (1970) Belligerence, its Frequency and Correlates in a Psychiatric Emergency Room Population. Paper read at the 1970 meeting of the American Psychiatric Association, San Francisco. American Psychiatric Association, San Francisco.
Mendelsohn, B (1963) The Origin of the Doctrine of Victimology. *Excerpta Criminologica*, **3**, 239
Monahan, J (1978) *American Journal of Psychiatry*, **135**, 198
Mowat, R R (1966) Morbid Jealousy and Murder. Tavistock Publications, London
Nicol, A R, Gunn, J, Gristwood, J, Foggit, R H, Watson, J P (1973) *British Journal of Psychiatry*, **123**, 47
Nunnally, J C (1961) Popular Conceptions of Mental Health. Holt, Rinehart and Winston, New York
Nurcombe, B (1964) *Medical Journal of Australia*, **1**, 579
Planansky, K, Johnston, R (1977) *Acta psychiatrica Scandinavica*, **55**, 65
Pollock, H M (1938) *Psychiatric Quarterly*, **12**, 236
Powers, R J, Kutash, I L (1978) *in* Violence. Perspectives on Murder and Aggression (edited by Kutash, I L, Kutash, S B, and Schlesinger, L B). Jossey-Bass, San Francisco. p.317
Radzinowicz, L, Turner, J W C (1957) Sexual Offences. Macmillan, London
Rappeport, J R, Lassen, G (1965) *American Journal of Psychiatry*, **121**, 776
—, — (1966) *American Journal of Psychiatry*, **123**, 413
Reichard, S; Tillman, C (1950) *Journal of Clinical Psychopathology*, **11**, 149
Robins, I. (1966) Deviant Children Grow Up. Livingstone, London
Rubin, B (1972) *Archives of General Psychiatry*, **27**, 397
Scheff, T J (1963) *Behavioral Science*, **8**, 97
Scott, D (1978) *British Journal of Hospital Medicine*, **19**, 259
Scott, P D (1977) *British Journal of Psychiatry*, **131**, 127
Shepherd, M (1961) *Journal of Mental Science*, **107**, 687
Sosowsky, L (1978) *American Journal of Psychiatry*, **135**, 33
Steadman, H J, Cocozza, J J, Melick, M E (1978) *American Journal of Psychiatry*, **135**, 816
Stengel, E (1964) Suicide and Attempted Suicide. Penguin, Harmondsworth
Tennent, T G (1971) *British Journal of Hospital Medicine*, **6**, 269
Virkkunen, M (1974a) *British Journal of Addiction*, **69**, 149
— (1974b) *Acta psychiatrica Scandinavica*, **50**, 145
Walker, N (1965) Crime and Punishment in Britain. Edinburgh Press, Edinburgh
West, D J (1965) Murder Followed by Suicide. Heinemann, London
Whiteley, J S (1970) *British Journal of Hospital Medicine*, **3**, 263
Woodward, M (1955) Low Intelligence and Delinquency. Institute for the Study and Treatment of Delinquency, London
Zitrin, A, Hardesty, A S, Burdock, E I, Drossman, A K (1976) *American Journal of Psychiatry*, **133**, 142

Chapter 4

The problems of malicious fire raising

Donald Scott, The London Hospital

Open a newspaper almost any day and there is a story about a fire leading to destruction of property and sometimes to loss of life. The surprising point is not the frequent occurrence of fires but the fact that of those that cause more than £10 000 worth of damage, three out of every eight are started deliberately. Malicious fire raising, according to the Fire Protection Association which is concerned with prevention and control of fires, is currently the leading cause of serious conflagrations. Targets include warehouses, schools, shops, industrial premises, engineering works and farms. Of particular note is the fact that the losses incurred in these fires have risen from £1.4 million in 1964 to £224.1 million in 1973. The latter figure is of significance, even allowing for inflation, because there has been more than a threefold increase in the number of incidents. Yet fire raising has received little attention in this or other countries. An official report (Fisher et al, 1976) on arson concludes that "it is the most neglected crime in the USA and probably elsewhere".

Since fire raising is not only a serious but an increasing problem it is perhaps surprising that this subject has been neglected in textbooks and that reports of research in the journals are sparse. The only major contribution to the field is the study on pathological fire setting by Lewis and Yarnall which was published as long ago as 1951, at which time malicious fire setting was less of a problem than it is today. Because of the lack of interest and the dearth of readily available information, the subject of the motivation of incendiarists was recently comprehensively reviewed (Scott, 1974).

For the purpose of this article fire raising is taken to include all kinds of malicious incendiarism. At first sight, as with other types of abnormal behaviour, arsonists seem to form a heterogeneous group with an age range from infancy to senility. However, men always predominate and are responsible for more than 85 per cent of fire-raising incidents (Lewis and Yarnall, 1951). Although fire setting is clearly an irrational act, sometimes a definite motive is expressed by the perpetrator. In other instances the arsonist can give no explanation. Between these two extremes stretches a continuum in which the motives given become more and more blurred until to the outside observer they are nonexistent. However, in the first instance it is useful to put forward a simple classification dividing the incendiarists into those with clear-cut motives and those with none. In this paper the various types of fire setter are described and some of the problems of assessment and management discussed.

The motivated fire setter

The most obvious of the motivated arsonists are the ones who work for profit. This is an important subject as it is certain, at least in the USA, that arson for profit is probably the most rapidly increasing form of fire setting (Levin, 1976). The profit-seekers can be divided into those who set light to their own premises to collect the insurance and those who hire arsonists for the same reason. The former group includes the affluent housewife who sets a smoky fire so that she can collect the insurance money and have the room redecorated and, at the other end of the scale, the welfare recipient who starts a blaze in his apartment to collect relocation expenses. Arson for profit may involve many people and therefore the risk of detection is high but, as the case of Leopold Harris in the 1920s and 30s showed, financial success is possible and the activity can go undetected for years.

Fire setting for financial gain still happens, as a recent court case indicated: a mill in Norfolk was burned down and thousands of pounds were illegally collected. However, retribution did come later. A variation on this theme was the famous Rouse case. He set light to his own car with the body of a vagrant inside intending that it should be thought that he had committed suicide, presumably so that insurance could be collected by his family. However, Rouse was discovered and brought to justice.

There is little in the literature about the psychology of those who set fires for profit. It is debatable whether the behaviour would be regarded as "normal" even though the motive is clear cut. This is certainly the case where fire is used to destroy evidence, for example a murder victim, or other evidence that could be used to establish guilt for a certain crime. This can result in a calamitous conflagration as in 1974 at Port Chester, New York, when a fire in a discotheque led to 24 deaths (Levin, 1976). Arson may also be part of a complex criminal gang activity. Recently, again in the USA, stores that failed to buy supplies of a particular detergent promoted by a certain criminal organization were burned to the ground (Scott, 1974).

Political fire setting

Historically, fire and bombs have figured in events as widely separated in time as the Gunpowder Plot and the burning of the Reichstag. Recently we have been reminded by the troubles in Northern Ireland that fire is still a weapon of the political activist. Not only has property been destroyed but families have been burnt to death in their homes. The impact on life in general and on the economic viability of the province as a whole has been severe. Somewhat surprisingly it has been shown (Lyons, 1972) that during spells of violence there is a decline in the number of suicides, although there is obviously a notable rise in the number of murders as well as an increase in the incidences of arson, bomb explosions and rioting. This is of interest because it gives us insight into depressive illness. When the individual is able to externalize his aggressive feelings then internalized destructive tendencies leading to suicide are diminished.

Political fire setting, although it may be carried out by a single individual, is not normally a solitary pursuit like most other types of arson. Indeed, it may be the work of a group. These fire setters have not been studied in depth but it is quite clear that the presence of others encourages their behaviour, whereas most other types of arsonists would feel inhibited. Vandals also usually work in groups but often carry out the act for excitement rather than to cause destruction (Moll, 1974).

Sometimes a pair of boys sets fires together but one is usually in a dominant role and the other submissive, a relationship similar to that found in homosexual pairs (Shaw, 1966).

Another type of group fire setting occurs in the context of racial tension and social unrest. As in fire raising for political ends, it appears that criminal elements infiltrate the mob and spur on the others to commit acts of arson, loot property and attack the police and the fire brigade when they arrive.

Suicide by fire

In the 1960s political activists in desperate situations turned to the unusual and terrifying act of self-immolation and set themselves on fire. This was carried out in public places as a protest against the authorities, for example, in Vietnam Buddhist monks set light to their petrol-soaked clothing. Similar acts have occurred in various parts of the world. Perhaps the best known instance is that of Jan Palach, the young Czechoslovakian student who set fire to himself in Wenceslas Square in Prague in 1969 after the Russian invasion.

The motives for such behaviour probably have something in common with those of the Christian martyrs since their deaths often resulted from acts of provocation towards the authorities as in the case of Joan of Arc. The underlying psychology of all these acts is unknown but in some instances it is related to mental disturbance. Fortunately this form of suicide is relatively uncommon but, for example, seven instances were reported in the national press during the year 1971 (Scott, 1974). It appears that such suicides generally occur in the context of a severe depressive or schizophrenic illness.

The "motiveless" fire setter

The remaining types of arsonist are more complex. The term motiveless has been used since to the observer the motive is either trivial, totally misguided, or virtually absent. These fire raisers work alone and as a result detection may be difficult. It follows that our view of them is mainly based on those who are caught, but an attempt to find out how arsonists reveal their behaviour to medical practitioners is also in progress (Scott, 1977). Nevertheless, the psychiatric background of this group of fire setters is probably better understood than that of those who work for profit. These motiveless fire raisers can be divided into three main groups, as follows.

Patients with overt psychiatric disorder or organic brain disease

In this first group it can be appreciated that in a period of confusion the individual may start a fire partly accidentally and partly intentionally. Those with a schizophrenic illness may in an acute phase be directed by auditory hallucinatory voices to set fire to their house or hospital ward. Similarly patients with a manic-depressive psychosis may also destroy their property or other possessions by fire, either when severely depressed or when manic. One such patient, for example, set fire to the curtains in a hospital ward and then attempted to put out the blaze remarking jovially "Wasn't it lucky I was here when this all started?".

Alcoholism is related to fire-raising activities since it lowers the level of inhibition and may thus lead to the occurrence of a particular fire-setting spree. On the other hand, in phases of the alcohol withdrawal syndrome, hallucinosis (Scott, 1967) may occur and the patient may barricade himself in his house and set light to it in order to escape from the imagined besieging forces.

Patients with no overt psychiatric disorder or organic brain disease

In the second group the arsonist when challenged puts forward a reason for his act of incendiarism which is quite out of proportion to the effect. He may say that it is for revenge or to spite a particular individual. These fires can obviously cause tremendous damage and the perpetrator does not seem to realize the effects or in any case to care. For example a serious fire may be caused in a hospital by an employee sacked from a catering department, and a student may set light to a college library because he has failed an examination.

Also in this category are some teenagers who give such reasons for fire setting as boredom, desire for excitement, or merely to impress equally outrageous hooligan colleagues. These individuals can cause serious damage but often such acts are a single event or perhaps repeated only once or twice. Thus they pose less of a threat to the community than the final group who do not have any tangible motive.

Patients with no motive

This third group of fire setters have no reason for their actions other than creating and watching the fire itself, and the pleasure derived is sufficient to lead to repeated episodes. In a detailed study of pathological fire setting in the USA, Lewis and Yarnall (1951) found that of 1145 men in their series 688 were of this type, that is about half the men started blazes deliberately for no real reason. In addition, these men set fires again and again. Some, for example the fire bugs (see below), gave as explanations a wish to see the firemen, to be heroes, or to enjoy the destruction of property, but most merely said that they had an irresistible inner desire. It is probably to this group that the term "pyromania" is best applied, but its use has been avoided since it has been rather loosely employed for all who enjoy the spectacle of fire even if they do not participate actively.

There are also the fire fetishists who gain overt sexual satisfaction from their pursuits. These people form a relatively small group; some are vagrants and some are mentally subnormal, but all are solitary and withdrawn from society. They have ecstatic dreams of fires and these become their only means of achieving gratification. The pleasure is initially derived from seeing images of flames while masturbating and later from experimenting with harmless blazes. However, the impulse grows and grows and there is a desire for larger and larger conflagrations.

Age and sex incidence

Lewis and Yarnall (1951) found that there were only 201 women, just under 15 per cent, in their total group of fire setters. It seems, therefore, that women less commonly turn to fire for a solution to their problems. The age incidence in the two sexes is different: women appear in small numbers steadily from childhood to old age whereas men show the highest incidence in the 16–25 age-group. The former distribution is different from that which might have been expected, namely a peak incidence in women at the menarche.

Women can be equally dangerous and dramatic in their fire-setting activities but their motives are somewhat different from those of their male counterparts. They often desire to attract attention, create excitement, or (perhaps most important and understandable) wreak revenge against their husbands or lovers. Fires, therefore, tend to be concentrated on their own home or their husband's property, for example a farmer's wife set fire to stacks and buildings because her husband spent all his spare time away from home drinking and playing cards.

Detailed information is available on women arsonists in the study by Tennent et al (1971) from the special hospitals such as Broadmoor, where psychiatric help is available to arsonists and others with serious antisocial personality disorders. On the whole the arsonists were no different from other delinquent women. The former too suffered from problems of immaturity and mixed feelings in relation to their sexual role as well as from poor rapport with their parents. Fire for these women had on the one hand a sadistic aggressive form representing their ability to destroy their mates and on the other a self-destructive element, a feature that is rarely observed in male fire setters. Indeed a proportion of women commit suicide by fire, although the intense excitement that surrounds the physical strength and energy of the fire engines and the firemen and which appeals to many male fire raisers is generally of little interest to them.

Children and adolescents merit study as they present an increasing problem, particularly in relation to school fires. Bender (1953) carried out a detailed investigation of 60 children who had a history of fire raising and were admitted to the children's ward in a hospital in New York. They can be conveniently divided into two groups—those younger than 10 years and those older. The former were characterized by minor brain dysfunction syndromes with clumsiness, poor hand and eye coordination, and learning difficulties. Some were of below average intelligence and a proportion were bed-wetters.

A more recent survey by Nurcombe (1964) reached similar conclusions. He studied 21 cases, the age of onset of symptoms ranging from 2 to 11 years with a maximum frequency at 6 years. Thirteen of the children set fires solely at home, seven at home and elsewhere, and only one always away from the place of residence. There was no unequivocal mental retardation in the series, but nine of the children were of low or borderline intelligence. In none of these patients was fire setting the solitary symptom: in 10 it was combined with stealing and in nine with sadistic behaviour to young siblings and a variety of other disorders. Over half had nocturnal enuresis at the time they were studied. Severe family disorganization was characteristic with absent parents, parental rejection, and institutionalization. The majority were solitary and markedly retarded in scholastic achievements.

The polymorphic nature of the behaviour disorder in the younger children is also present in the second group, that is older than 10 years. Fire setting occurred against a background of theft and truancy. They had a nonchalant attitude to their fire-raising activities and expressed neither anxiety nor regrets. Indeed, Macht and Mack (1968) observed that they had an unemotional matter-of-fact attitude and that fire raising was in no way regarded as alien to their way of life. Unlike the younger children they planned the blazes and carried them out away from the family home. They gained enjoyment from the noise and excitement as the fire engines arrived, for example in a recent case a boy set fire to a school sports pavilion and sat in a nearby tree to enjoy his handiwork. The headmaster spotted him and confronted him with the act.

There has recently been a marked increase in the number of school fires—from 37 in 1969 to 90 in 1975. The latter fires caused £8 million worth of damage and were the subject of an investigation by the Fire Protection Association. It was found that the majority occurred outside school hours and thus caused considerable damage prior to discovery. Two thirds were definitely started maliciously and in some of the remainder this could also have been the case. These fires almost certainly represent the most serious aspect of vandalism in schools and are a subject of great concern since it appears that the perpetrators are neither all boys nor necessarily have reached their teens.

Information on another related matter emerges from the Report of Her Majesty's Chief Inspector of Fire Services for 1975 (1976). This is the incidence of false fire alarms of which there were 59 000 during that year. Unhappily, some of these false alarms can end in disaster when the fire brigade is involved in an accident or called away just before a genuine fire alarm is received. Although there is relatively little information about who is responsible, many false alarms are probably the work of children or adolescents who enjoy the sight and sound of the fire brigade and it is conceivable that they choose this in preference to setting a blaze.

The fire bug

All those who are involved in malicious incendiarism have a background of personality disorder. This is most obvious with the fire bug. He suffers from periods of mounting tension, becoming increasingly restless and edgy, and then suddenly his actions are out of control having been triggered off, for example, by a quarrel at home or dismissal from work.

The fire bug has learnt that starting a blaze releases tension and so may begin a fire-setting spree. Some fire bugs may find only one blaze sufficient to discharge tension while others start many fires within a short period. The fires are usually unplanned and lit in hallways, staircases and passages where the general public has access. This is in contrast to the arsonist who works for profit and makes sure that his conflagration starts in the heart of a building where it will continue undetected for a considerable period. The fire bug is more likely to thrust a match into a brimming dustbin and rush away to start others elsewhere in the neighbourhood, creating chaos and confusion. After such acts he may return home feeling calm, a sensation akin to that which follows sexual excitement and satisfaction.

Fire bugs appear unable to obtain sexual gratification in the usual way. Lewis and Yarnall (1951) observed that only about a third were married compared with two thirds of the population in the same age range, and that these relationships were usually unsatisfactory ending in separation or divorce. Other characteristics include poor physical qualities, facial disfiguration and low intelligence, as well as poor adjustment to general life with unstable personal and work relationships. Over-indulgence in alcoholic beverages is also an important feature. These factors may, against a background of mounting tension, render the fire bug more susceptible to loss of control and thus act as a trigger to a fire-setting spree.

Assessment

As with other antisocial persons, fire raisers present problems in assessment and the answer to the crucial question "Will it happen again?" can be difficult. The points to be taken into consideration in their assessment are set out in *Table 4.1*, and the single most important factor is whether there have been previous episodes. Of course, initially this may not be honestly answered; the truth may only emerge after further probing. Evidence of personality disorder, not only the admission to other types of antisocial behaviour but also to poor overall social adjustment, has to be taken into account. Furthermore, evidence of a depressive mood swing before a fire-setting episode is sometimes found and there may be trigger factors such as problems at work or at home.

TABLE 4.1. Points in assessment of fire raisers

Is there overt psychiatric disorder, for example depressive illness or schizophrenia?
Is there organic disease, for example confusional states, dementia, or alcoholism?
Is there evidence of psychopathy, for example other antisocial acts?
Is social adjustment satisfactory?
Have there been previous episodes?
What reasons are given?
Are there trigger factors?
Was the act carried out alone or with others?

Another question that arises is why the individual chose fire as a weapon. This almost certainly dates back to childhood as the fascination for fire starts at an early age, young children having an almost universal interest in playing with matches. Most outgrow this and learn the dangerous nature of fire fairly soon since it is part of the basic instruction given by parents. Not surprisingly therefore, as noted by Nurcombe (1964), unsatisfactory family relationships are one of the features of child arsonists. They have learnt that fire is the most destructive element and quite different from water. Certainly flooding a building can cause serious damage but water does not have the living, growing quality of fire. Furthermore, setting a fire requires little effort and the striking of a match is utterly trivial in comparison with the destructive power unleashed. The fire raiser lets the flames take over and then slips into an entirely passive role.

Nurcombe (1964), in his study of child arsonists, made a detailed attempt to obtain evidence about their fantasies. He found that they saw fire as a means of venting aggression on adults and siblings, and that there was a mingling of rage and desperation in their acts. The reason why a particular child or individual chooses fire is more difficult to determine. In one instance accidental burning in childhood is cited and in another the observation of a forest fire at a very early age. One of the children studied by Bender (1953) was kicked by a fireman at the age of 8 years and always said he wanted to revenge this act. Information on this matter is difficult to obtain, especially with adult arsonists, and generally the reason for the choice of fire by an individual is speculative.

Management

The management of fire raisers, as of those responsible for other types of antisocial behaviour, is difficult. A balance has to be struck between consideration of the individual patient and of the community at large. In recent years there has been a change of attitude and more attention is increasingly being paid to treatment and rehabilitation rather than to punishment. Nevertheless, accurate assessment of the patient is a prerequisite for management. If an overt psychiatric disorder is present then a treatment order in a mental hospital may be appropriate. However, for the repeated fire setter with a severe personality disorder such a course of action would be unsuitable and a prison sentence during which psychiatric help can be given seems to be the best course of action. This is possible at special hospitals and allows detailed research on which rational treatment can be based (see Tennent et al, 1971).

One of the many questions that remains unanswered is the extent to which child fire setters become adult fire setters. If there is such a tendency then treatment in childhood, if possible, would be an important preventive measure. This has been attempted on a limited scale using behaviour therapy techniques. Welsh (1971) reported two separate cases of 7-year-old boys of average intelligence who, apart from other behavioural problems at home, had been involved in fire setting. The approach was to use stimulus satiation to eliminate interest in fires. Each child was given the opportunity to strike matches one by one for an hour a day until he no longer wanted to do so. In both instances after several sessions the child asked to stop the "game" and fire-setting incidents at home ceased. The follow-up period was, however, somewhat limited.

A different approach was used by Holland (1969). He did not deal directly with the child but with the father. The child was rewarded with money for bringing to his father any matches that he found about the house. He was also given an opportunity to strike 20 matches and offered a penny for each match that he chose not to strike. The outcome in this case was also satisfactory. Whether behaviour therapy could be employed for adult fire raisers is uncertain, although a great variety of other disorders have been treated successfully by this method.

Conclusion

Arson is an important subject for us, both as members of the community and as doctors, particularly in view of the recent increase in the number of incidents and the consequent damage to property and in some cases loss of life. Unfortunately, the subject has been neglected and little detailed research has been done. This is essential, since only then can there be a rational approach to the assessment and management of fire raisers and the prevention of fire setting.

References

Bender, L (1953) Editor. Aggression Hostility and Anxiety in Children. Thomas, Springfield, Illinois. p.116

Fisher, P.E., Hillenbrand, L J, Suchy, J T (1976) Arson, America's Malignant Crime. US Department of Commerce, Washington, DC

Holland, C J (1969) *Behaviour Research and Therapy*, 7, 135

Levin, B (1976) *Fire Journal*, **70**, 36

Lewis, N D C, Yarnall, H (1951) Pathological Firesetting. Nervous and Mental Diseases Monograph, No. 83. Coolidge Foundations, New York

Lyons, H (1972) *British Medical Journal*, i, 342

Macht, L B Mack, J E (1968) *Psychiatry*, **31**, 277

Moll, K D (1974) Arson, Vandalism, and Violence. United States Department of Justice, Washington, DC

Nurcombe, B.(1964) *Medical Journal of Australia*, **1**, 579

Report of Her Majesty's Chief Inspector of Fire Services for 1975 (1976) HMSO, London

Scott, D F (1967) *British Journal of Addiction*, **62**, 113
— (1974) Fire and Fire-Raisers. Duckworth, London
— (1977) *Practitioner*, **218**, 812
Shaw, C R (1966) The Psychiatric Disorders of Childhood Prentice Hall, Englewood Cliffs, New Jersey
Tennent, T G, McQuaid, A, Loughnane, T, Hands, A J (1971) *British Journal of Psychiatry*, **119**, 497
Welsh, R S (1971) *in* Behaviour Therapy with Children (edited by Graziano, A M) Aldine Publishing, Chicago, Illinois. p.283

Chapter 5

Self-mutilation

Michael A Simpson, Temple University, Philadelphia

Self-mutilation occurs for diverse reasons: to frighten an enemy or make oneself a more attractive suitor, as an initiation rite or a religious sacrifice, and to seek magical cures, malinger, or simulate a disease. Some varieties are culturally accepted and we bite our nails, cut hair and nails, and pierce earlobes without attracting much attention.

But one variety of self-mutilation, when an emotionally disturbed person cuts himself, is commonly seen in many different medical settings. It usually attracts an inordinate amount of concern, disturbing others to a degree far out of proportion to the gravity of the act. Such patients are almost always badly managed by the doctors and nurses they encounter, which arouses strong feelings of frustration and hostility. The typical example of the self-cutting syndrome is the wrist-slasher. However, two other less common, distinctive, and more lethal variations must be distinguished: the psychotic individual who mutilates himself (often bizarrely) in response to his disordered thoughts, and the person (usually male and older than the others) who makes one deep and dangerous cut in a highly lethal suicide attempt. The larger group of self-mutilators presents a characteristic clinical problem and they share many attributes.

Incidence

Self-mutilation is quite common but there have been no adequate studies to quantify this. Phillips and Muzaffer (1961) reported an incidence of 4.3 per cent among psychiatric patients (women outnumbering men by 3:1) and Ballinger (1971) found that 14.9 per cent of a population of subnormal patients and 3.4 per cent of general psychiatric patients had injured themselves in the course of a month. Many cases fail to be reported or noted at all, especially if the wounds are minor and are cared for by the patient herself. Also, in casualty departments the wounds may be recorded as simple lacerations or classified inappropriately as a suicide attempt.

Whitehead et al (1972, 1973), in an unusually thorough survey, estimated the incidence of all forms of self-injury (including suicide and overdoses) as 730 per 100 000 population per annum, a figure far higher than previous estimates which varied between 40 and 220 per 100 000 per annum. Johnson et al (1973) found that of previous self-injuries the patients' doctors were aware of only 20 per cent of such incidents (and unsure of a further 28 per cent) and only 46 of the patients had themselves initially reported these previous episodes.

Much higher incidences have been found among subnormal and schizophrenic children (Green, 1968; Shodell and Reiter, 1968) and among prisoners (Panton, 1962; Fully et al, 1965; Beto and Claghorn, 1968; Reiger, 1971; Wilmotte and Plat-Mendlewicz, 1973). In prisons self-cutting and hanging are the favoured means of suicide (Cooper, 1971; Danto, 1971; Beigel and Russell, 1972). Most clinical studies have been of hospitalized patients and in these women have markedly outnumbered men (Graff and Mallin, 1967; Pao, 1969; Nelson and Grunebaum, 1971; Novotny, 1972; Rosenthal et al, 1972). Clendenin and Murphy (1971) studied suicide attempters reported to the police. They found that 11.5 per cent of all attempts were by self-cutting and that the cutters were more often male than non-cutters (40 per cent compared with 28 per cent) although women still outnumbered men by 1.5:1.

Suicidal lethality

Although the wrist-cutter may be highly perturbed, such acts are usually of low lethality (Goldwyn et al, 1967; Grunebaum and Klerman, 1967; Rinzler and Shapiro, 1968; Asch, 1971; Siomopoulos, 1974; Simpson, 1975).

Symptomatology

The principal symptoms wrist-cutters complain of are tension and chronic feelings of emptiness, and less commonly depression (Rosenthal et al, 1972; Simpson, 1975). Rapidly fluctuating mood swings (not usually prolonged into classic depression) were reported by Grunebaum and Klerman (1967) and Simpson (1975), and these, like the tension, respond poorly or briefly to phenothiazine or other tranquillizers or to antidepressant medication.

Clinical diagnosis

These puzzling patients are allotted many diagnoses, most of which are unhelpful. Psychopathy, schizophrenia, borderline personality disorder, depression, and hysteria are the most popular although they are usually more informative about the doctor than the patient. Asch (1971) considered the condition a primitive form of depression called anhedonia, and Siomopoulos (1974) classified it as an impulse neurosis like kleptomania and pyromania. Clanon (1962) proposed the term "psychoschizopathic" which gets us nowhere. Pao (1969) said that cutters typically go "in and out of psychosis in a split second", and that while psychotic they may show "perceptual distortion, hallucinations, tenuously formulated delusional systems, and other primary process experiences". However, other authors stress the infrequency of hallucinations or delusions and I have found them quite rare in practice. Borderline personality disorder would seem the most comprehensive diagnosis for most of the patients.

The typical cutter

A clear composite picture of the typical wrist-cutter emerges from the classic papers. She is likely to be a young (usually 16–24 years of age) attractive woman. She may have worked in nursing or a related paramedical field, or have strong medical interests or connections (five of 13 in McEvedy's [1963] series and 10 of 24 in Simpson's [1975] study). Waldenberg (1972) found that significantly more cutters than controls had a history of trauma at school and of trouble with the police. They have low self-esteem and may express dislike of their own bodies. They tend to behave so as to involve others in their pathology, such as by absconding from hospital.

Dysorexia

Recently it has been recognized that major dysorectic symptoms are common in self-mutilators. In the 1972 series of Rosenthal et al, 15 of 24 patients described either compulsive overeating or severe anorexia, or periods of both, and seven had frequent nausea. In Simpson's (1975) series 75 per cent reported dysorectic symptoms, and McEvedy (1963), Asch (1971), Novotny (1972), Waldenberg (1972), and Siomopoulos (1974) have noted the association. Cutting may be temporally associated with binge-eating or its associated vomiting. Malcove (1933) proposed a relation between bodily mutilation and learning to eat. The cases of binge-eating described by Nogami (1974) in the Japanese literature show similarities to the typical self-mutilator and some 28 per cent cut themselves. He has suggested a similar origin (in self-directed aggression) for self-mutilation and hyperorexia, while Shinosaka (1974) has pointed out the incidence of mutilation in frank anorexia nervosa, and there may be homologous underlying disturbances in the experience of the body image.

Drug and alcohol abuse

Nearly 50 per cent of the cutters reported by Novotny (1972) and Rosenthal et al (1972) and in the two major controlled studies by Waldenberg (1972) and Simpson (1975) used drugs and alcohol in excess. The hallucinogens, by their tendency further to dissolve distinctions between self and object (already a somewhat tenuous distinction in these patients) can be highly anxiety-provoking for cutters, while amphetamines are popular with them because they can amplify sensation and sharpen bodily awareness. Alcohol remains the most commonly abused drug.

Sexual problems

Confusion of sexual identity seems common and was manifested by 66 per cent in Simpson's (1975) study and 59 per cent in Gardner and Gardner's (1975) series. Several authors have been struck by the degree of promiscuity shown by some cutters while others seem to have had no experience at all: sexual behaviour often appears to be an all-or-nothing affair. Few seem to have enjoyed their sexual encounters.

Menstruation

A high proportion of cutters describe a negative reaction to menarche or irregular menstrual periods with quite frequent amenorrhoea. Indeed, Rosenthal et al (1972) have suggested that the more frequent cutters have more irregular menses and described an increase in cutting at the time of menstruation as did Crabtree (1967).

Neither McEvedy (1963) nor Waldenberg (1972), however, found any relation between cutting and the phase of the menstrual cycle.

Childhood

Compared with controls, cutters more commonly come from homes broken by divorce or death (Waldenberg, 1972; Simpson, 1975). Lester (1972) stresses parental deprivation through emotional distancing and inconsistent maternal warmth. Varieties of family pathology have been described (Vereecken, 1965; Graff and Mallin, 1967; Grunebaum and Klerman, 1967; Friedman et al, 1972). Bach-y-Rita (1974) who studied violent prisoners who cut themselves reported similar findings. There seems to be a high incidence of surgery and hospitalization before the age of 5 years and often before 18 months. Mason and Sponholz (1963) have shown a correlation in experimental monkeys between isolation in childhood and self-mutilation. Experiences of abandonment and of very limited physical handling may also be relevant.

Verbalization

Graff and Mallin (1967) and Grunebaum and Klerman (1967) have emphasized the difficulties these patients seem to have in expressing their emotions and needs, and this limits their accessibility to conventional psychotherapy. In Simpson's (1975) series 66 per cent showed significant difficulties in verbalization, and an improved facility in verbal expression was associated with clinical improvement and cessation of cutting. Shodell and Reiter (1968) found that among schizophrenic children the more verbally fluent were significantly less likely to mutilate themselves.

The pattern of cuts

A single cut is rare. Typically the wrist-slasher tends to make multiple relatively superficial incisions, some of which are so delicate as to heal without scarring although a spidery network of up to several hundred fine scars may be seen. The forearms are the commonest sites to be used although almost any accessible part of the body may be cut. Bach-y-Rita (1974) found an average of 93 scars per patient (range 3–150). Rosenthal et al (1972) found that half of their patients had cut on more than five occasions, three patients alone totalling more than 200 cutting episodes. The cuts vary in depth from very superficial scratches to full-thickness lacerations although they usually draw blood. Other techniques of self-mutilation may be seen in the same patient including burning with cigarettes, dermatitis artefacta, and tattooing (Taylor, 1968). Favoured instruments are razor blades and broken glass, with a preference for materials obtained by breaking or bending hospital rules or property.

Precipitants

The commonest precipitants are experiences of loss or abandonment (or the threat of these), separation, rejection, the loss of a meaningful person, or an impasse in personal relationships. Rosenthal et al (1972) described a peak incidence of cutting on the ward when the residents were away, during active planning for discharge, or when the doctor went on holiday. Two other factors I have noticed with some consistency are frustration at experiencing strong emotions that the patient cannot express in words, and the turning of passive into active (transforming the experience of being hurt by malevolent others into the active harming of oneself).

Epidemics

The technique of self-cutting can be learned and propagated in hospitals and institutions, and there may even develop a sense of competition between patients as they cut to demonstrate who is the most unhappy. Matthews (1968) and Simpson (1975) have described epidemics of self-cutting in inpatient units.

The act of cutting

The sequence of events when cutting is almost stereotyped and the descriptions of most authors already cited are in general agreement as are those of Burnham and Giovacchini (1969), Kafka (1969) and Yap (1970). The precipitants described above lead to feelings of anger, self-hatred, and/or depression but tension soon becomes the dominant effect and rises steadily. During the mounting tension the patient may realize that she is going to cut and can experience some mild relief as she plans this. She will usually seek solitude at this stage, if she is not already alone. As the tension becomes unbearable a transition into a state of depersonalization often occurs and may be described as "numb" or "empty". She becomes self-engrossed, withdrawn, and dissociated. Suddenly she cuts, often expressing lack of direct awareness of cutting: "I find that I have cut myself". Some describe cutting repeatedly until they have had "enough blood". Suicidal ideation is quite uncommon and far from an act of suicide the self-mutilator is committing what amounts to antisuicide, using the cutting as a means to gain reintegration, repersonalization, and a return to reality and life from her state of numb unreality.

Blood

Blood has a special significance for the self-mutilator, functioning partly as a transitional object (Simpson, 1976a,b) and partly as a potential security blanket carried within oneself and capable of giving warm and comforting envelopment. It seems to be a necessary component of the process by which the cutter recathects her depersonalized body image and, thus re-establishes a functioning sense of the boundaries between inside and outside, self and non-self. The patients often spontaneously comment very positively on their reactions to the sight and feel of their blood, especially its colour and warmth. One of my patients described: "The pleasure of it coming, crawling and dribbling over your flesh—you know that it's really you coming out. Deep rich red, the colour ... like liquid rubies or a vintage claret ... the velvety warmness." Some patients explicitly liken the experience to intercourse or masturbation, the rising tension leading to the orgasmic quality of the relief and pleasure as the blood flows, followed by relaxation and calm so that they may even fall asleep.

Pain

A complete absence of pain during the actual cutting is typical and most interesting. Gross lacerations may be inflicted without any apparent suffering, severing tendons (Grunebaum and Klerman, 1967) and lacerating vagina and cervix (Gerstle et al, 1957; Goldfield and Glick, 1970; Simpson, 1973; Simpson and Anstee, 1974). Even a bilateral orchidectomy (Lowy and Kolivakis, 1971) or hysterectomy of a prolapsed uterus (Vedrinne et al, 1969) may be performed without pain. One may be able to suture the wounds without needing further anaesthetic. Pain may return at any time from a few hours to a couple of days later.

Management

All those who have written any account of this condition agree that it is very difficult to treat and can provide exquisitely awkward management problems. Few studies have offered much useful advice but some general principles can be identified.

Many problems arise from the effects wrist-slashing has on the staff. Pao (1969) has suggested that it evokes castration anxiety in them. They may feel menaced by the rapidity with which the patient can regress to the intensely self-engrossed object-unrelated state which is out of their reach. The primitive aggression of the cutting may also be threatening. Staff attitudes are usually highly aroused after a slashing and fluctuate between feelings of rage, guilt, sympathy, resentment, and the bitter sensation of being quite unable to cope with a clinical situation.

The unpredictability of the mood swings and of the cutting is also upsetting to staff who rely on their abilities to understand patients and to predict their behaviour. The anxiety and conflict among the staff contribute to the patient's instability and may help to precipitate further cutting. If cutting continues the patient becomes a centre of staff discussion. There can be intense disagreement about her proper diagnosis and management, particularly about the amount of supervision needed and the restrictions to be applied. Retaliatory strictness may be sought. Most members of the therapeutic team feel sure they could handle the patient better than her therapist, usually accusing him of being too permissive and seeking more exacting limit-setting.

The patient is often rejected by the staff who rationalize medically by pejorative labelling, for example "manipulative" or "attention-seeking", as if such labels automatically absolve us of the responsibility to understand the patient. The therapist can be forced into an adversary position, taking the patient's part in all confrontations. The patient may add to this by seeking out a junior staff member or another patient in whom she confides specially, asking them to promise not to reveal what she says, and thus forming what Grunebaum and Klerman (1967) called a co-conspiratorial dyad. Faced with such conflict between professional and personal obligations I have even known nurses to cut themselves.

It is useful, therefore, to establish and maintain a clear and coherent policy, leaving one therapist in complete charge of all significant decisions but ensuring that every other staff member knows what decisions have been made. So far as is possible an attitude of acceptance of the patient herself, despite a dislike of her actions, should be maintained and communicated to her. Excessive restrictions are not helpful—they seldom if ever inhibit cutting and the eventual and unavoidable lifting of each restriction can provide precipitants for further cuts.

Setting of limits should be done with firmness and consistency, distinguishing between appropriate restrictions and retaliation. Psychotherapy is difficult but challenging and feasible, although highly traditional approaches may be unhelpful. Increasing the self-esteem, nurturing the positive aspects and strengths of the personality, improving the ability to talk about her emotions (without using such self-destructive, if graphic, body language), and using alternative techniques for reduction of tension are all to be sought.

The pursuit of insight into the genesis of the cutting is not useful and analytical interpretations are of no help. One may need to respond to the patient's regressive features by reactions appropriate to the degree of regression. Despite our general inhibitions about touching patients there is both theoretical and practical evidence to suggest that comforting physical contact, like putting an arm around the patient's shoulders, may be helpful. The patient should be helped to become more aware of the emotional effect she has on others (they often seem genuinely unaware of this) and encouraged to explore more satisfactory ways of relating to others.

Where needed, medical treatment of the injuries, such as suturing, should be done with minimal interpersonal reinforcement (for the patient may become so isolated as to receive staff attention only when she has cut). When practical, the patient can be given gauze and tape to apply by herself as required, and she should not be excused from social and other responsibilities after a cut.

Other techniques of impulse-control should be explored and I encourage the patient to come to a designated staff member whenever the familiar state of rising tension begins, to talk it over, and to receive help and encouragement to control the impulse. In my experience, the use of autogenous relaxation training combined with relaxation-based deconditioning of specific precipitants can be successful. Sedation by drugs seems seldom to be of value. Benzodiazepines seem unhelpful and the possibility of inducing paradoxical aggression should not be overlooked. If a sedative must be used, the phenothiazine pericyazine may be more effective than its alternatives.

When the patient's discharge nears she may act in such a way as to force one to keep her in hospital. Further slashing, drunkenness and similar challenges should not lead to automatic reimposition of special attention and restrictions. Emphasize the patient's continuing responsibility for her own actions and carry on planning for discharge and beyond. It may be important to stress that discharge will not lead to abandonment but that further support will be available.

Outcome

Disappointingly, but not surprisingly in view of the elusiveness of some of these patients, there have been no adequate follow-up studies. Grunebaum and Klerman (1967) refer to the frequency with which such patients may be transferred to custodial institutions with less intense staff involvement. Watson's case (1970), on becoming more disturbed was transferred to a long-stay mental hospital where the self-mutilation ceased. Others are simply discharged abruptly when the hospital will no longer tolerate their behaviour, but despite this some appear to recover reasonably well. Only Nelson and Grunebaum (1971) have managed to follow 19 self-cutters for 5–6 years after their initial hospital contacts. Ten were regarded as well or improved (by criteria of social adjustment and decrease of psychiatric symptoms); four showed no significant change and continued wrist-slashing, thus requiring frequent hospital admissions; and three who had been regarded as intermittently psychotic (one with psychotic depression and two with strong self-destructive impulses and delusions of guilt, possibly not representative of the group we are discussing) had committed suicide.

Theories, mechanisms and explanations

Theories on self-mutilation have been multiple and highly varied without either very much evidence for the theories or many practical applications of them. A classic attempt to conceptualize the subject was presented in Menninger's (1938) book *Man Against Himself*, and he advanced the idea of focal suicide which concentrates the aggression on a part of the self as a substitute for the whole. More fanciful psychodynamic theories have been offered, for example those by Dabrowski (1937), Deutsch (1944), Hoffer (1950), Declich (1956), Bettelheim (1962), Graff and Mallin (1967), and Friedman et al (1972).

There are traces of the beginnings of a biological approach to explaining the syndrome. An animal model may emerge. In addition to Mason and Sponholz's (1963) work with infant monkeys, Tinkelpaugh (1928) has described self-mutilation in an adult male rhesus separated from his mate and the author has reported mutilation in a bereaved chimpanzee. Genovese et al (1969) induced self-mutilation in rodents by injecting pemoline, and Peters (1967) produced similar effects with caffeine. Another intriguing, although possibly misleading model, exists in the Lesch–Nyhan syndrome (Nyhan, 1968) where a defect in hypoxanthine-guanine phosphoribosyltransferase leads to hyperuricaemia, mental retardation, and persistent and grossly disfiguring self-mutilation.

Mizuno and Yugari (1974) reported cessation of mutilation on administering L-5-hydroxytryptophan but further studies in other centres, unpublished as yet, have not tended to confirm or extend this finding. Cooper and Fowlie (1973) have described the cessation and long-term control of gross self-mutilation in a severely subnormal girl by the use of lithium carbonate, a finding that deserves further study. The possible implication of temporal lobe phenomena also merits investigation, perhaps by the use of telemetric leads and prolonged EEC monitoring, for some of the patients' descriptions of their experiences resemble such epileptic symptoms. Similarly, the trial of anticonvulsant therapy might be of interest.

Conclusion

As may be seen there exists a clearly identifiable and relatively common variety of self-mutilation, often involving wrist-cutting, which exhibits much of the stability of a syndrome. Much more is known about these puzzling and often infuriating patients than is generally recognized and a detailed survey of the literature is available (Simpson, 1976a). A more rational approach to the management of such patients can be attempted with the hope of a more satisfactory outcome.

References

Asch, S S (1971) *Psychoanalytic Quarterly*, **40**, 603
Bach-y-Rita, G (1974) *American Journal of Psychiatry*, **131**, 1018
Ballinger, B R (1971) *British Journal of Psychiatry*, **118**, 535
Beigel, A, Russell, H E (1972) *Hospital and Community Psychiatry*, **23**, 361
Beto, D R, Claghorn, J L (1968) *American Journal of Correction*, **30**, 25

Bettelheim, B (1962) Symbolic Wounds. Collier Books, London
Burnham, R C, Giovacchini, P L (1969) *British Journal of Medical Psychology*, **42**, 223
Clanon, T L (1962) *Corrective Psychiatry and Journal of Social Therapy*, **11**, 96
Clendenin, W W, Murphy, G E (1971) *Archives of General Psychiatry*, **25**, 465
Cooper, A F, Fowlie, H C (1973) *British Journal of Psychiatry*, **122**, 370
Cooper, H H A (1971) *International Journal of Offender Therapy*, **3**, 180
Crabtree, L H (1967) *Psychiatry*, **30**, 91
Dabrowski, C (1937) *Genetic Psychology Monographs*, **19**, 1
Danto, B L (1971) *Police Chief*, **8**, 64
Declich, M (1956) *Rassegna di studi psichiatrici*, **45**, 603
Deutsch, H (1944) Psychology of Women, Vol 1. Grune and Stratton, New York. p. 168
Friedman, M, Glasser, M, Laufer, E, Laufer, M, Wohl, M (1972) *International Journal of Psycho-Analysis*, **53**, 179
Fully, G, Hivert, P E, Schaub, S (1965) *Annales de médecine légale, criminologie, police scientifique et toxicologie*, **45**, 108
Gardner, A R, Gardner, A J (1975) *British Journal of Psychiatry*, **127**, 127
Genovese, E, Napoli, P A, Bolego o-Zonta, N (1969) *Life Sciences*, **8**, 513
Gerstle, M L, Guttmacher, A F, Brown, F (1957) *Journal of the Mount Sinai Hospital*, **24**, 641
Goldfield, M D, Glick, I D (1970) *Diseases of the Nervous System*, **31**, 843
Goldwyn, R M, Cahill, J L, Grunebaum, H U (1967) *Plastic and Reconstructive Surgery*, **39**, 583
Graff, H., Mallin, R (1967) *American Journal of Psychiatry*, **124**, 36
Green, A H (1968) *Archives of General Psychiatry*, **19**, 171
Grunebaum, R, Klerman, G L (1967) *American Journal of Psychiatry*, **124**, 527
Hoffer, W (1950) *International Journal of Psycho-Analysis*, **31**, 156
Johnson, G G, Ferrence, R G, Whitehead, P C (1973) *Canadian Psychiatric Association Journal*, **18**, 101
Kafka, J S (1969) *British Journal of Medical Psychology*, **42**, 207
Lester, D (1972) *Psychological Bulletin*, **78**, 119
Lowy, F H, Kolivakis, T L (1971) *Canadian Psychiatric Association Journal*, **16**, 399
McEvedy, C (1963) Self-Inflicted Injuries. DPM dissertation, University of London
Malcove, L (1933) *Psychoanalytic Quarterly*, **2**, 557
Mason, W A, Sponholz, R R (1963) *Journal of Psychiatric Research*, **1**, 299
Matthews, P C (1968) *International Journal of Social Psychiatry*, **14**, 125
Menninger, K (1938) Man Against Himself. Harcourt, Brace and World, New York
Mizuno, T-I, Yugari, Y (1974) *Lancet*, i, 761
Nelson, S H, Grunebaum, R (1971) *American Journal of Psychiatry*, **127**, 1345
Nogami, Y (1974) personal communication
Novotny, P (1972) *Bulletin of the Menninger Clinic*, **36**, 505
Nyhan, W L (1968) *Federation Proceedings*, **27**, 1027
Panton, J H (1962) *Journal of Clinical Psychology*, **18**, 63
Pao Ping-Nie (1969) *British Journal of Medical Psychology*, **42**, 195
Peters, J M (1967) *Archives internationales de pharmacodynamie et de thérapie*, **169**, 139
Phillips, R H, Muzaffer, A (1961) *Psychiatric Quarterly*, **35**, 421
Reiger, W (1971) *Archives of General Psychiatry*, **24**, 532
Rinzler, C, Shapiro, D A (1968) *Journal of the Mount Sinai Hospital*, **35**, 485
Rosenthal, R J, Rinzler, C, Wallsh, R, Klausner, E (1972) *American Journal of Psychiatry*, **128**, 1363
Shinosaka, N (1974) personal communication
Shodell, M J, Reiter, H H (1968) *Archives of General Psychiatry*, **19**, 453
Simpson, M A (1973) *ibid*. **29**, 508
—(1975) *Canadian Psychiatric Association Journal*, **20**, 429
— (1976a) *in* Suicidology: Contemporary Developments (edited by Shneidman, E.S.). Grune and Stratton, New York
— (1976b) *in* Das Borderline-Syndrom in Theorie und Praxis. Pinel, Berlin
—, Anstee, B H (1974) *Postgraduate Medical Journal*, **50**, 308
Siomopoulos, V (1974) *American Journal of Psychotherapy*, **28**, 85
Taylor, A J W (1968) *British Journal of Criminology*, **8**, 170
Tinkelpaugh, O L (1928) *Journal of Mammology*, **9**, 293
Vedrinne, J et al (1969) *Médecine légale et réparation du dommage corporel*, **2**, 156
Vereecken, J L (1965) *Nederlandsch tijdschrift voor geneeskunde*, **109**, 2280
Waldenberg, S S A (1972) MPhil dissertation, London University
Watson, J P (1970) *Psychotherapy and Psychosomatics*, **18**, 67
Whitehead, P C, Ferrence, R G, Johnson, F G (1972) Life-Threatening Behaviour, **3**, 137

—, Johnson, F G, Ferrence, R (1973) *American Journal of Orthopsychiatry*, **43**, 142
Wilmotte, J N, Plat-Mendlewicz, J (1973) *in* Jail House Blues (edited by Danto, B L). Epic Publications, Michigan. p.55
Yap, K B (1970) Automutilatie van Loghum Slatems. Deventer, Holland

Addendum

Since this article was originally published, several areas of this field of study have shown significant developments. Our clarification of the concept of indirect self-destructive behaviour (Farberow, 1979) has added a major dimension to the understanding of the psychopathology of everyday life, risk-taking, noncompliance, and self-endangering. Within that body of work Simpson (1979) has given a very detailed account of the phenomenology and psychodynamics of this behaviour and its meanings. The functions and significance of the diagnosis of the borderline syndrome in many such cases (Mack, 1975; Simpson, 1977, 1979) have become clearer, and this raises important questions about the relevance of very early life experiences, especially during the separation–individuation phase of ego development, in the aetiology of self-aggression later in life. Roy (1978) and Green (1978) have found relations between excessive physical punishment and abuse in childhood and later self-destructive behaviour. Carroll et al (1980), comparing self-mutilators with a control group, found that the mutilators recalled more major separations before the age of 10 years (including loss of a parent), more family violence, more physical abuse, and prohibition of the expression of anger.

Two other areas of clear aetiological significance that continue to produce intriguing results and to need further study are the role of biochemical factors (Chamove and Harlow, 1970; Razzak et al, 1975) and the relevance of animal models (Levison, 1970; Lewis and McKinney, 1975; Allyn et al, 1976; Jones and Barraclough, 1978; Jones et al, 1979). Much of the psychological literature remains unhelpful (for example Carr, 1977) by failing to distinguish between the many varieties of self-mutilation and assuming that a unitary (usually behavioural) explanation will apply to them all.

The one significant account of therapeutic intervention is that reported in the recent monograph by Ross and McKay (1979). Working in an institution for delinquent girls, they began with a descriptive and phenomenological study and followed with an elegantly designed evaluation of varying treatment methods based on orthodox behavioural strategies. Although the incidence of self-cutting dwindled to zero while they were simply studying it, the behavioural regimens had little or no benefit, leading in some cases to a substantial increase in cutting. They recognized the function of cutting within such an institution as a means by which the girls could very predictably control staff behaviour. With rare insight they re-examined their results and capitalized on their accidental success. They adopted a very different approach which sought to "co-opt" the cutting, depathologizing and deromanticizing it. While not yet fully developed or conceptualized, this approach, along with those of Masterson (1972) and others in managing the borderline syndrome, constitutes the most promising management strategies for such patients.

References

Allyn, G, Demye, A, Begue, I (1976) *Primates*, **17**, 1
Carr, E G (1977) *Psychological Bulletin*, **84**, 800

Carroll, J, Schaffer, C, Spensley, J et al (1980) *American Journal of Psychiatry*, **137**, 852

Chamove, A S, Harlow, H F (1970) *Journal of Abnormal Psychology*, **75**, 207

Farberow, N L (1979) Editor. The Many Faces of Suicide: Indirect Self-Destructive Behaviour. McGraw-Hill, New York

Green, A H (1978) *American Journal of Psychiatry*, **135**, 579

Jones, I H, Barraclough, B M (1978) *Acta psychiatrica Scandinavica*, **58**, 40

—, Congiu, L, Stevenson, J et al (1979) *Journal of Nervous and Mental Disease*, **167**, 74

Levison, C A (1970) *American Journal of Mental Deficiency*, **75**, 323

Lewis, J L, McKinney, W T (1975) *Archives of General Psychiatry*, **33**, 699

Mack, J E (1975) Editor. Borderline States in Psychiatry. Grune and Stratton, New York

Masterson, J F (1972) Treatment of the Borderline Adolescent: A Developmental Approach. John Wiley, New York

Razzak A, Fujiwara M, Ueki, S (1975) *European Journal of Pharmacology*, **30**, 356

Ross, R R, McKay, H B (1979) Self-Mutilation. Lexington Books, Lexington, Massachusetts

Roy, A (1978) *British Journal of Medical Psychology*, **51**, 201

Simpson, M A (1977) *Dynamische Psychiatrie*, **42**, 42

— (1979) *in* The Many Faces of Suicide (edited by Farberow, N L). McGraw-Hill, New York. pp. 257–283

Chapter 6

Psychiatric management of attempted suicide patients

Keith Hawton/Jose Catalan, Warneford Hospital, Oxford

The dramatic increase in the incidence of deliberate self-poisoning and self-injury during the 1960s and early 1970s (Wexler et al, 1978) appears to be levelling off (Holding et al, 1977; Gibbons et al, 1978a). However, attempted suicide patients continue to make considerable demands on general medical and psychiatric services. In this article we review the psychiatric assessment and treatment of such patients in order to provide guidelines for general hospital physicians, psychiatrists, and others involved in their care. The characteristics and problems of this population are summarized first so as to supply a background to the assessment and treatment procedures.

Characteristics of patients who deliberately poison or injure themselves

Female suicide attempters outnumber males by 1.5:1–2:1. The majority are young, at least two thirds being under the age of 35, and attempts by persons under the age of 16 are by no means uncommon. The highest rates are found among females aged 15–30 of whom as many as one in 100 make attempts in any one year (Bancroft et al, 1975; Holding et al, 1977).

Approximately 90 per cent of suicide attempts involve deliberate self-poisoning, the rest being self-injuries or a combination of both. Many overdoses involve prescribed drugs, particularly tranquillizers (Jones, 1977; Proudfoot and Park, 1978), although nonopiate analgesics (for example salicylates) are used in approximately a quarter of cases and in considerably more of the attempts of young persons (Morgan et al, 1975). There has been a recent increase in overdoses of paracetamol (Gazzard et al, 1976) and paracetamol and dextropropoxyphene combinations (Young and Lawson, 1980).

Although psychiatric symptoms are commonly detected in attempted suicide patients (Newson-Smith and Hirsch, 1979a), formal psychiatric disorders requiring psychiatric treatment are found in a minority (Urwin and Gibbons, 1979). The most common disorder is depression.

The majority of suicide attempters have recently experienced threatening or undesirable life events (Paykel et al, 1975) and these usually reflect interpersonal problems. Attempts often follow a major row in the setting of a chronic relationship difficulty with a spouse, boyfriend or girlfriend (Bancroft et al, 1977). Approximately half of male attempters have serious employment problems.

Recently an association has been demonstrated between child abuse and attempted suicide (Roberts and Hawton, 1980). High rates of attempted suicide are found in many patients with epilepsy (Mackay, 1979; Hawton et al, 1980). There is also a marked association between attempted suicide rates and both lower social class (Bancroft et al, 1975; Holding et al, 1977) and living in an area of relative social deprivation (Skrimshire, 1976; Gibbons et al, 1978a).

Two thirds of patients consult their GPs in the month prior to making a suicide attempt. As a result of their visits, many are prescribed psychotropic drugs which are subsequently used in overdoses (Hawton and Blackstock, 1976).

Association with suicide

Although different types of people are usually involved in attempted suicide and completed suicide, there is considerable overlap between the two groups (Ovenstone, 1973). One to 2 per cent of suicide attempters kill themselves in the year following attempts (Kreitman, 1977) and between a third and a half of those who complete suicide have a history of previous attempts (Barraclough et al, 1974; Kreitman, 1977). In addition to previous attempts, the risk of completed suicide is increased by the presence of psychiatric illness especially depression and alcoholism (Barraclough et al, 1974), male sex, older age, living alone, and being recently bereaved (Sainsbury, 1978).

Repetition of attempted suicide

Repetition of attempts is common, with 16–25 per cent making further attempts within one year (Morgan et al, 1976; Bancroft and Marsack, 1977; Kreitman, 1977). Repeats are most frequent during the 3 months after an attempt (Bancroft and Marsack, 1977). There is a small subgroup of chronic repeaters which makes particularly heavy demands on health services.

Assessment

The assessment of patients following deliberate self-poisoning or self-injury should not be a cursory procedure but should be carried out with care, attention being paid particularly to the following:

1. Evaluation of risk of suicide
2. Evaluation of risk of repetition
3. Identification of psychiatric disorder
4. Clarification of current problems faced by the patient
5. Obtaining information from other sources, including the GP, relatives, and friends
6. Making arrangements for appropriate help after discharge from hospital

Method

During the assessment the patient should be interviewed in surroundings conducive to discussion of personal matters. The open ward or a cubicle in the casualty department should be avoided, and a side room or office where the patient can be interviewed without interruptions should be used. Sufficient time must be allowed to carry out an unhurried interview.

The patient should be assessed as soon as he is fit, that is as soon as the pharmacological effects of an overdose have worn off. A drowsy or confused patient is unlikely to give reliable information. The pharmacological effects of an overdose may persist after a patient appears to have become alert. Equally, early assessment allows a clearer understanding of the circumstances and motives associated with the act. Subsequently they may be rationalized or made socially acceptable.

The approach developed in Oxford consists of a semistructured interview schedule (Hawton and Catalan, 1982) which includes evaluation of the various factors that help to determine the degree of risk of subsequent suicide, the presence of psychological disorder, and the nature of the patient's current problems. The assessment interview proceeds in stages which are summarized in *Table 6.1.*

TABLE 6.1. Stages in the assessment interview

Establishing rapport	Introduction by name and explanation of the purpose of the interview
Understanding the attempt	Detailed account of events in the 48 hours preceding the attempt Circumstances surrounding the act—degree of planning, isolation, suicide note, motives, actions after attempt, and whether alcohol was taken Previous attempts
Clarification of current difficulties	Nature of problems and their duration, and recent changes Areas to be covered—psychological and physical problems, relationship with partner and other family members, children, work, friends, and consumption of alcohol
Background	Relevant family and personal history Usual personality
Coping	Current coping resources—personal resources and external resources (such as friends, social agencies, and GP) Previous ways of coping with difficulties
Assessment of mental state at interview	Especially mood and cognitive state
List of current problems	Formulated together with patient
Establishing what further help is required	What the patient wants and is prepared to accept Who else should be involved (for example the partner or other relatives)
Contract	Terms of further involvement of the assessor or other agencies are made explicit and agreed

Particular emphasis is placed on understanding the reasons for the suicide attempt and the intended outcome by obtaining a detailed account of the events leading up to and following the attempt. Not only is the degree of suicidal intent assessed but also other reasons for the act are investigated (Bancroft et al, 1979).

Another feature of this model is the use of a problem-orientated approach in preference to a purely diagnostic one. The patient takes an active role in defining his problems together with the assessor and this is often helpful in assisting the patient to understand his current difficulties and to plan the steps that have to be taken to deal with them. Typical problems faced by such patients are disturbed marital relations (especially infidelity and poor communication), employment and accommodation difficulties, financial problems, and inability to cope with care of children.

In assessing possible psychiatric disorders, particular attention should be paid to symptoms suggestive of depression (for example severe mood disturbance, suicidal preoccupation, impaired appetite and weight loss, sleep disturbance, forgetfulness, impaired concentration, feelings of hopelessness and guilt, loss of interest, and impaired libido) and alcoholism.

After interviewing the patient, the assessor should always try to interview the partner, other relatives, or friends in order to check the accuracy of the information obtained from the patient and to assess their contribution to the difficulties and their potential role in providing help. The GP should always be contacted before definite arrangements are made. Not only is he likely to provide valuable information about the patient but he may also wish to take an active part in the follow-up.

In assessing the risk of suicide, attention should be paid to the factors mentioned earlier. The degree of suicidal intent of the attempt must be evaluated and the Beck suicide intent scale (Beck et al, 1974) can be a useful aid. It consists of two sections, the first covering the circumstances of the attempt (for example precautions taken to avoid or ensure discovery and a suicide note) and the second the patient's thoughts and feelings at the time of the attempt (such as the wish to die and the degree of premeditation). A simple scale is available to predict the risk of a further attempt (Buglass and Horton, 1974). It contains six items: problems in the use of alcohol, diagnosis sociopathy, previous inpatient psychiatric treatment, previous outpatient psychiatric treatment, a previous attempt leading to hospital admission, and not living with relatives.

Who should assess suicide attempters?

The official policy in this country (Hill Report, 1968) is that all suicide attempters should be seen by a psychiatrist before they are discharged from the general hospital. However, the policy has often been disregarded and some patients have either not been referred or, if referred, left hospital before being seen by the psychiatrist. In addition, the increased numbers of attempters have put consider-able strain on psychiatric services As a result, alternative approaches involving nonpsychiatric personnel have been developed in some hospitals. It has been demonstrated that social workers (Newson-Smith and Hirsch, 1979b) and nurses (Catalan et al, 1980) can safely and reliably assess suicide attempters, and that attempters assessed by general medical teams do not have a higher suicide or repetition rate than those seen by psychiatrists (Gardner et al, 1977). However, the latter approach requires further examination in view of the heavy demands already being made on house physicians and the negative attitudes shown by some to suicide attempters (Patel, 1975; Ramon et al, 1975).

Our experience has been that a multidisciplinary team including nursing, social work, and psychiatric personnel, who have all been specially trained, is very satisfactory for the assessment and management of suicide attempters, particularly because of the combination of skills available to meet the diverse needs of these patients. The enthusiasm and experience developed by counsellors in the team is reflected in the high percentage of patients who keep their follow-up appointments (Hawton et al, 1979). A similar model could be implemented in hospitals with fewer resources by training a nurse and a social worker who would then carry out the assessments in collaboration with a psychiatrist. Such an approach would make use of the skills and experience of the nurse and the social worker while reducing the demands on the psychiatrist's time, and it could lead to a reduction in medical bed occupancy by suicide attempters.

Patients presenting special problems

Patients who refuse to be interviewed   Sometimes patients feel very threatened by the prospect of a psychiatric interview because of the implication of being mentally ill and the fear of possible psychiatric hospital admission. Explanation of the assessor's role and his willingness to offer further help if appropriate is usually sufficient to reassure most patients. For a patient who still refuses to speak it is essential to interview other informants and obtain the GP's opinion. Sometimes reticence is due to guilt or regret concerning a failed serious attempt.

The very young   The assessor may be regarded as an authority figure by young patients, resulting in distorted information. They may also be terrified at finding themselves in hospital. Special care is necessary in interviewing such patients and a young assessor may be preferable.

Patients at risk of late complications   Some substances (for example paracetamol and paraquat) can cause delayed complications occasionally resulting in death. Tragically, the patient is usually unaware of the potential effects and did not intend to die. The assessor may have to concentrate on helping the patient deal with the uncertainty of his recovery, and on supporting the relatives.

Treatment

Although a thorough assessment may itself have therapeutic value, most patients are offered further help after discharge from hospital. Such treatment varies according to the nature of each patient's problems and particularly the risk of suicide and the presence of psychiatric disorder. The disposal of 2512 patients referred to the general hospital in Oxford for attempted suicide during 1976–78 was as follows (Hawton et al, 1979): psychiatric hospital inpatient care, 9 per cent; psychiatric hospital outpatient care (most were already in treatment), 12 per cent; outpatient or domiciliary care by general hospital emergency psychiatric service, 47 per cent; returned to care of GP, 23 per cent; other forms of care, 5 per cent; and made their own discharge from hospital, 4 per cent. We shall now consider the indications for the different forms of management and the nature of treatment that may be provided.

Psychiatric hospital inpatient care

Admission to a psychiatric hospital is required for patients with serious psychiatric illness and those at risk of suicide. Careful observation in the general hospital is necessary for some of these patients to prevent suicide occurring there (Farberow et al, 1971). When psychiatric hospital admission is essential to protect the patient but he refuses this, compulsory admission will be necessary. Brief admission may be desirable for some patients who are in need of sanctuary or whose coping resources are temporarily exhausted.

In hospital, traditional methods of treatment of psychiatric disorders can be instigated. However, an initial period of observation is recommended while further assessment of the patient's problems is carried out. Sometimes the crisis preceding an attempt rapidly resolves and early discharge is possible. Unfortunately further attempts or successful suicide can occur in hospital (Hawton, 1978). A set of policy rules is used in some hospitals to maintain appropriate surveillance of patients according to their risk of suicidal behaviour (Morgan, 1979).

Outpatient care

Although the majority of attempted suicide patients are not in need of psychiatric inpatient care, many are contending with considerable difficulties and welcome help with these. A brief treatment approach has been developed in Oxford which seems well suited to the needs of such patients (Hawton and Catalan, 1982). The therapist tries to help the patient overcome his problems as rapidly as possible in a way that ideally leads to resolution of the crisis that precipitated the overdose, a general improvement in social adjustment, and a greater ability to cope with similar situations in future. The emphasis is on encouraging the patient to overcome his own problems, with the therapist helping set goals and suggesting means of obtaining them.

If a patient's problems centre around a relationship with a partner or family member(s) and if the relationship is to continue, it is important to include this person in the setting of goals and in the treatment sessions. The timing of sessions should be flexible according to each patient's needs. It is usually appropriate to organize appointments one to three times per week at first. Subsequent sessions can be more spaced out. Few patients require help for longer than 3 months and many need be seen only two or three times. Sessions of 30–40 minutes' duration are usually adequate.

The principles followed by the therapist and the patient during the brief treatment are as follows:

1. Define the problems clearly
2. Establish suitable and clear goals
3. Clarify the steps necessary to obtain the goals, and their likely consequences
4. Agree what the patient has to do before the next session.

At each session the patient's progress is reviewed in detail and praise and encouragement offered for any improvement made. During the course of treatment the following aspects may need special attention.

Communication   Many attempted suicide patients have difficulty discussing their needs and emotions with their partners or families. In joint sessions the exchange of information and the expression of emotions can be encouraged. Where loss has occurred, either through death or separation, the expression of grief may need to be facilitated.

Attitude change   Obstructive attitudes may prevent progress and these can usually be identified by carefully analysing the patient's attempts to achieve goals and the reasons for failure. In order to help the patient modify his attitudes, confrontation and simple interpretations can be useful.

Drug prescribing   In the management of this group of attempted suicide patients it is seldom necessary to introduce psychotropic drugs; it is often more appropriate to consider stopping psychotropic drugs already prescribed. Medication is unlikely to alter the problems in personal relationships frequently associated with suicide attempts.

Referral to other agencies   During or at the end of treatment the patient may be recommended to seek advice from other helping agencies (for example FPA, Citizen's Advice Bureau, or Campaign for Homosexual Equality) or referred elsewhere for further help (for example Social Services, a long-term group, or a psychosexual problems clinic) in order that his special needs can be met.

   In preparing patients for future crises it may be found useful, towards the end of treatment, to discuss the *meaning* of the attempt with the patient and/or his family. In particular the communication aspects of the behaviour may need to be clarified. Alternative means of coping can then be explored, including rehearsing them in the session and perhaps using role play. Finally, some services operate an "open access" telephone line whereby patients can seek help after discharge if faced with a situation that they find difficult to overcome.

Who should carry out treatment?

The outpatient care of attempted suicide patients has traditionally been the responsibility of psychiatrists. Recently, interest has turned to the use of nonmedical personnel. Gibbons et al (1978b) demonstrated a superior effectiveness of social workers using a structured treatment approach as compared with traditional care (psychiatric outpatient clinics and referral to Social Services and to the care of the GP). In Oxford, treatment is provided by nursing, social work, and psychiatric members of the multidisciplinary team working under the supervision of senior psychiatrists (Hawton et al, 1979). This has the advantage that a patient can be allocated to the team member whose expertise is most suited to his needs. The individual who made the initial assessment usually provides subsequent treatment, thus ensuring continuity of care.

Is treatment effective?

At present the effectiveness of treatment has not been properly evaluated. Retrospective studies have suggested that patients who receive psychiatric attention after their attempts do better than those who do not (Greer and Bagley, 1971; Kennedy, 1972). Prospective studies have been confined to comparisons of special forms of treatment with traditional care. An intensive aftercare service was found to be no more beneficial than traditional care for chronic repeaters in terms of further repetition, but was associated with somewhat superior social adjustment particularly for female patients (Chowdhury et al, 1973). Special treatment by social workers also resulted in better social adjustment than traditional care in the study by Gibbons et al (1978b). Home-based treatment has not proved any more effective than treatment carried out in outpatient clinics although it is more acceptable to patients (Hawton et al, 1981). It may be preferable for patients with family problems when other members of the family cannot get to the hospital.

Clearly, further evaluative research is required. Until then there is no reason to abandon the present policy of offering help with social problems to those who want it.

Return to the care of the GP

Not all patients appear to require special treatment after attempts. The assessment procedure may have helped to resolve the situation. In other cases the behaviour is trivial and out of character. Returning the patient to the GP's care after discussion with him is all that is required. However, this decision can only be made after a thorough assessment, as already described.

Patients posing particular management difficulties

Two groups of suicide attempters pose particularly difficult problems for management.

Chronic repeaters   It is often very difficult to understand why some patients make many repeat attempts. There is a danger that the attempts may come to be dismissed as trivial by hospital staff who become increasingly frustrated by the behaviour. However, such patients appear to be particularly at risk of subsequent suicide. The best approach to this very resistant problem may be to conduct a careful analysis of the patient's behaviour with all those concerned with his care in order to identify the benefits the patient appears to be getting from repeat attempts and to try to meet his needs by a more acceptable means. In some cases, long-term support may be the only method of reducing the frequency of attempts.

Wrist-slashers   Patients who cut their wrists, often repeatedly, appear to be rather different from the bulk of patients who take overdoses (Simpson, 1976). The act of cutting is usually carried out in a state of detachment and appears to alleviate intolerable tension. Apart from tackling the personality and interpersonal difficulties of these patients, methods of tension reduction probably offer the best means of treatment. These include relaxation exercises and alternative means of expressing anger and frustration such as very vigorous exercise. At present such an approach has not been evaluated.

Prevention

It is often suggested that the best means of managing attempted suicide is to prevent it in the first place. However, it is not known how to achieve this. The Samaritans do not appear to play a major role in prevention of attempted suicide (Holding, 1974). Because of the frequent use of psychotropic drugs in self-poisoning it has been suggested that more careful prescribing of these could be one means of prevention. Greater use of counselling by GPs has been put forward as an alternative. Given the high proportion of young attempters, educational approaches have also been proposed (Morgan, 1979). None of these possibilities has been evaluated.

Summary

Although the recent epidemic of deliberate self-poisoning and self-injury may have passed its peak, attempted suicide patients continue to make considerable demands on medical and psychiatric facilities. There is no doubt that careful assessment of such patients is essential and that subsequent help should be provided in many cases. Appropriately trained and supervised nonmedical staff can play a useful role in management. In hospitals where services are being established for attempted suicide patients a small multidisciplinary team supported by senior psychiatrists probably offers the most satisfactory solution.

References

Bancroft, J H J, Marsack, P (1977) *British Journal of Psychiatry*, **131**, 394
—, Skrimshire, A, Reynolds, F, Simkin, S, Smith, J (1975) *British Journal of Preventive and Social Medicine*, **29**, 170
—, —, Casson, J, Harvard-Watts, O, Reynolds, F (1977) *Psychological Medicine*, **7**, 289
—, Hawton, K E, Simkin, S, Kingston, B, Cumming, C, Whitwell, D (1979) *British Journal of Medical Psychology*, **52**, 353
Barraclough, B, Bunch, J, Nelson, B, Sainsbury, P (1974) *British Journal of Psychiatry*, **125**, 355
Beck, A T, Schuyler, D, Herman, I (1974) *in* The Prediction of Suicide (edited by Beck, A T, Resnik, H L P, Lettieri, D J). Charles Press, New York. p.45
Buglass, D, Horton, J (1974) *British Journal of Psychiatry*, **124**, 573
Catalan, J, Marsack, P, Hawton, K E, Whitwell, D, Fagg, J, Bancroft, JHJ (1980) *Psychological Medicine*, **10**, 483
Chowdhury, N, Hicks, R C, Kreitman, N (1973) *Social Psychiatry*, **8**, 67
Farberow, N L, Ganzier, S, Cutter, F, Reynolds, D (1971) *Life Threatening Behaviour*, **1**, 184
Gardner, R, Nanka, R, O'Brien, V C, Page, A J F, Rees, P (1977) *British Medical Journal*, ii, 1567
Gazzard, B G, Davis, M, Spooner, J, Williams, R (1976) *ibid.* i, 212
Gibbons, J S, Elliott, J, Urwin, P, Gibbons, J L (1978a) *Social Psychiatry*, **13**, 159
—, Butler, J, Urwin, P, Gibbons, J L (1978b) *British Journal of Psychiatry*, **133**, 111
Greer, S, Bagley, C (1971) *British Medical Journal*, i, 310
Hawton, K (1978) *British Journal of Medical Psychology*, **51**, 253
—, Blackstock, E (1976) *Psychological Medicine*, **6**, 571
—, Catalan, J (1982) Attempted Suicide: A Practical Guide to its Nature and Management. Oxford University Press
—, Gath, D, Smith, E (1979) *British Medical Journal*, ii, 1040
—, Marsack, P, Fagg, J (1980) *Journal of Neurology, Neurosurgery and Psychiatry*, **43**, 168
—, Bancroft, J, Catalan, J, Kingston, B, Stedeford, A, Welch, N (1981) *Psychological Medicine*, **11**, 169
Hill Report (1968) Hospital Treatment of Acute Poisoning. HMSO, London
Holding, T A (1974) *British Journal of Psychiatry*, **124**, 470
—, Buglass, D, Duffy, J C, Kreitman, N (1977) *ibid.* **130**, 534
Jones, D I R (1977) *British Medical Journal*, i, 28
Kennedy, P (1972) *ibid.* iv, 255
Kreitman, N (1977) Parasuicide. John Wiley, London
Mackay, A (1979) *British Journal of Psychiatry*, **134**, 277
Morgan, H G (1979) Death Wishes? The Understanding and Management of Deliberate Self-Harm. John Wiley, Chichester
—, Burns-Cox, C J, Pocock, H, Pottle, S (1975) *British Journal of Psychiatry*, **127**, 564
—, Barton, J, Pottle, S, Pocock, H, Burns-Cox, C J (1976) *ibid.* **128**, 361
Newson-Smith, J G B, Hirsch, S R (1979a) *Psychological Medicine*, **9**, 493
—, — (1979b) *British Journal of Psychiatry*, **134**, 335
Ovenstone, I M K (1973) *British Journal of Preventive and Social Medicine*, **27**, 27
Patel, A R (1975) *British Medical Journal*, ii, 426
Paykel, E S, Prusoff, B A, Myers, J K (1975) *Archives of General Psychiatry*, **32**, 327
Proudfoot, A T, Park, J (1978) *British Medical Journal*, i, 90
Ramon, S, Bancroft, J H J, Skrimshire, A M (1975) *British Journal of Psychiatry*, **127**, 257

Roberts, J, Hawton, K (1980) *ibid.* **137**, 319
Sainsbury, P (1978) *British Journal of Hospital Medicine*, **19**, 156
Simpson, M A (1976) *ibid.* **16**, 430
Skrimshire, A M (1976) *Journal of Biosocial Science*, **8**, 85
Urwin, P, Gibbons, J L (1979) *Psychological Medicine*, **9**, 501
Wexler, L, Weissman, M M, Kasl, S V (1978) *British Journal of Psychiatry*, **132**, 180
Young, R J, Lawson, A A H (1980) *British Medical Journal*, **280**, 1045

Chapter 7

Hysterical phenomena

H Merskey, University of Western Ontario/London Psychiatric Hospital, Ontario

The peculiar notion that healthy patients can suffer from physical symptoms that involve loss of function in one part of the body and in which they firmly believe requires careful theoretical formulation. By definition such symptoms differ physiologically from states of autonomic discharge such as weeping, laughing and blushing which are mostly involuntary behaviour. In contrast, conversion symptoms are those that produce a change in the body which corresponds to an idea of impairment of function and not to any abnormal discharge or defect in the nerve pathways that serve movement or sensation.

This concept was apparently first made explicit by Reynolds (1869) who described three cases of paralysis resulting from an idea. Interestingly they were all related to railway injuries. The careful work of 19th century neurologists, including Charcot, furthered Reynolds' concept. Neurologists have distinguished symptoms due to an idea by demonstrating that, although the patient thinks he has lost function in a limb, movement is possible if he is appropriately distracted or asked to undertake a particular task (Head, 1922). For example, a "paralysed" leg which is tested by resting the patient on a bed and asking him to raise the other leg may be observed to press down if a hand is placed under the heel. With regard to sensory losses of function the same sort of technique is less readily available but physiological impossibilities may be demonstrated such as the loss of vibration sense on only one side of the sternum. Tests like these have often served to demonstrate ample evidence of power or function which the patient believes to be lost.

The next advance made by Freud (Breuer and Freud, 1955) was to recognize that the idea might be unconscious and might result from conflict. Others had perhaps foreshadowed these notions but Freud was the first to make them explicit and perfectly clear. His elegant and almost incredible concepts remain the basis for the current view of conversion symptoms. This is that the patient is unconscious of the source of the symptom (otherwise he is malingering) which corresponds to his idea of a paralysis or anaesthesia and not to anatomical derangement or physical pathology, except at most indirectly. Freud thought that the ultimate basis for this conflict was always sexual but the Second World War led to general rejection of that idea although it remains true that there is excessive sexual maladjustment in civilian patients with conversion symptoms (Merskey and Trimble, 1979).

The mental mechanism that permits this method of symptom production is called dissociation because feelings and symptoms are split off or separated from each other. When Freud first described it he pictured the feeling or effect attached to the symptom converted into a bodily change. This was analogous to the way that he saw certain forms of anxiety as a consequence of damming up undischarged emotion; thus coitus interruptus was thought to produce anxiety as a result of a physical change. Hence anxiety neurosis was classed as an actual neurosis, that is one having an organic or chemical basis, while psychoneurosis was supposed to occur solely on psychological grounds.

The mechanism of dissociation a priori need not be restricted to bodily symptoms: any symptom that a fertile mind can imagine may be employed in the same way. Thus pain or nausea, hallucinations of dead relations or fairies at the bottom of the garden, or any sort of psychological event can be the reflection of a hysterical experience; even depression which is now widely socially acceptable as a symptom can be utilized as a complaint that avoids the resolution of a conflict and provides medical attention. The logical outcome of this position was demonstrated by a medical student who sought the status of a patient saying simply "Just help me doctor, I'm sick".

More specific dissociative symptoms that have long been recognized as hysterical, *pari passu* with somatic conversion symptoms, include particularly hysterical disorders of awareness or memory. Thus hysterical amnesia and fugue are regarded as classic dissociative phenomena. In the former the individual loses the ability to recollect significant portions of past experience sometimes including personal identity. The same applies in a fugue state in which there is also a tendency to wander. Hysterical amnesia and fugue may both develop in the special manner called multiple personality and such cases can often be shown to have specific clinical characteristics.

Discrepancies from typical organic memory impairments are often readily demonstrated by skilled psychological testing and may also be shown clinically. For example, patients are not demented if they cannot remember their personal identity or discrete periods of time within their lives but have good general knowledge of the world at large and retain specific skills such as the ability to read and write, play chess, and do arithmetic. If they have suffered a limited period of memory loss evidence of some clear cerebral insult, for example head injury or intoxication, is needed before the disorder can be considered organic in origin. Even if partly associated with organic change the discrepancies of Ganser's syndrome, in which patients may answer that a cow has five legs and so forth, are so gross that they cannot be accepted as directly related to organic disorder when the patient is still able to function in other ways with regard to memory and attention. However, some such patients show confusion (Whitlock, 1967a).

Definition

At this point we can frame a basic definition of conversion or dissociative symptoms as follows:

1. They correspond to an idea in the mind of the patient concerning physical or sensory changes or psychological dysfunction
2. They are definable, if somatic, in terms of positive evidence and, if psychological, by techniques of clinical examination
3. They are related to emotional conflict.

It must be said, however, that there are at least a few cases in which a satisfactory explanation on the basis of adequate current emotional conflict is not found even after exhaustive inquiry. At least five other characteristics are often held to be linked to conversion or dissociative symptoms. These include primary gain, secondary gain, a symbolic choice of symptom, manipulation of the environment and other persons, and a hysterical personality which is characterized by attention-seeking, dramatic, labile, and manipulative behaviour among other traits. However, none of these several features is invariably demonstrated although primary gain can be shown in the vast majority of cases and secondary gain and manipulation are frequent. Hysterical and passive-immature-dependent personality between them appear to characterize about 40 per cent of patients with conversion symptoms (Ljungberg, 1957; Chodoff and Lyons, 1958), a rate much higher than that found in other psychiatric patients (Merskey and Trimble, 1979).

It follows from the discussion so far that on theoretical grounds there is no real need to distinguish between conversion and dissociative symptoms. In the rest of this article the words hysterical symptoms are used to cover both types. Furthermore, although full explanation in terms of conflict is highly desirable for the complete elucidation of a hysterical symptom it is not always a practical possibility.

The occurrence of hysterical symptoms

Hysterical symptoms are seen throughout almost the whole range of psychiatric and medical practice. Nevertheless, classic anaesthesias, paralyses, amnesias, blindnesses, and so forth are now extremely rare except in certain special settings as follows:

1. Imitative group outbreaks for example fainting in a girls' school; see Schuler and Parenton (1943) and Moss and McEvedy (1966)
2. Primitive populations; for example see Armstrong and Patterson (1975) for a vivid and insightful description of the spread of hysterical fits among a North American Indian group of young adults
3. Military medicine and psychiatry
4. Orthopaedic clinics and other centres where compensation problems are common and the symptom is more often pain
5. Children's eye clinics where hysterical amblyopia is not uncommon especially in those approaching examinations
6. Neurological clinics and hospitals, where there is some evidence that patients with hysterical symptoms present not only for differential diagnosis but also because particular cerebral organic diseases may predispose to the development of such symptoms (Slater, 1965; Whitlock, 1967b; Merskey and Buhrich, 1975).

In certain medical clinics pain appears to have replaced other hysterical symptoms. It has long been thought that pain could be hysterical, for example Sydenham (1697) described hysterical clavus (a painful sensation as if a nail is being driven into the head). Some current evidence supports his view in a general way since investigations of psychiatric patients with chronic pain frequently disclose a pattern that is regarded as hysterical (Merskey and Spear, 1967). One of the commonest syndromes of psychological symptoms found with atypical facial pain (Pilling et al, 1967) or low back pain (Sternbach, 1974) is that of the conversion V triad, that is elevation of the hypochondriasis (Hs) and hysteria (Hy) scales on the Minnesota Multiphasic Personality Inventory with a relative lowering of the intervening depression (D) scale. This is important in both theory and practice although the greatest care must be exercised before pain is diagnosed as due to conversion.

There is another group of patients with all sorts of hypochondriacal complaints which tends to be classed as polysymptomatic by physicians. These cases range from extreme to normal. In extreme patients a minimum of 25 symptoms arise before the age of 35 and affect at least nine out of 10 different bodily systems or regions; this has been called Briquet's syndrome by a group of workers at Washington University, St Louis, Missouri. They have shown that it affects about one per cent of the normal population (Woodruff, 1968) and 2 per cent of that of medical clinics (Farley et al, 1968) and that it is durable, consistently diagnosable, and irrecoverable (Guze, 1970). Their work demonstrates a pattern of hysterical symptoms, including pain, that shows unequivocally that pain may function as a psychological symptom of hysterical origin.

Diagnosis

With such a wide range of symptoms that may be called hysterical the question arises whether hysteria can be a valid diagnostic category. Slater (1965) argued that we should accept hysterical symptoms but not hysteria as a disease. Szasz (1961) has sought to deny the status of illness to anyone if their symptoms are hysterical. Still others (for example Chodoff and Lyons, 1958) have questioned the justification of recognizing hysterical personality as a typical associate of hysterical symptoms. Many answers can be offered to these arguments and the most important are discussed below.

First, diagnosis in psychiatry is often said to be multidimensional. We may diagnose from serology (general paralysis of the insane), genetics (Huntington's chorea), symptom pattern (depression), mechanism and site (tension headache), the presence or absence of irrationality (psychosis and neurosis). Such a diagnostic system is manifestly imperfect since the categories employed are not mutually exclusive. However, the same is often true in other fields of medicine: a popular medical textbook (Houston et al, 1975) points out that there is no existing satisfactory classification of nephritis which may be diagnosed on a basis of aetiology, pathogenesis, histology or clinical presentation. What matters is that the system works in practice and allows discussion and comparison of findings between medical practitioners and research investigators. This does seem to happen—often with remarkable consonance in ideas and findings. Every one of us can recognize Briquet's syndrome, there is a host of papers on epidemic hysteria, and for every site in which I have suggested hysterical symptoms might occur there are diverse reports that testify to the facts. Thus hysteria as a mechanism, a concept, a pattern of symptoms, and even a personality style is alive and kicking. As a pattern of symptoms it deserves a place in diagnostic categories. It may therefore be useful to explore subcategories or types of hysteria, for example monosymptomatic hysteria, Briquet's syndrome, hysteria secondary to organic disease, and so on.

Secondly, the argument that hysteria should be divorced from medicine is superficially attractive but unrealistic. Some of the diagnostic groupings already mentioned and various causes of hysteria or background conditions associated with it inevitably lead the patient to doctors and require the continuance of medical care. No other group of professionals, whether psychologists or social workers, is equipped both to diagnose and to treat patients with hysterical symptoms. Moreover unless treatment follows from diagnosis and is sustained at least partly by an authority equal to the diagnosis, it is liable to be unsatisfactory and ineffective. At present, particularly in view of the frequent association between hysterical symptoms and neurological disorders (see below), no approach other than the informed psychiatric one based equally on medicine and medical psychology is likely to be both humane and effective in understanding and management. Even if doctors seek to reject the diagnosed hysteric and hysterical hypochondriac, the patient is very unlikely to go away unless they help him find a better approach to his problems.

Symptoms no longer considered hysterical

Certain symptoms that had formerly been classed as hysterical, partly on insufficient grounds, have now been reclassified as nonhysterical in origin. Globus hystericus is one example. A feeling of a ball, lump, or stick in the throat has traditionally been regarded as hysterical and it may be so. However, difficulty in swallowing is also a psychophysiological symptom of anxiety and more refined investigations have suggested that it has a physical basis in a number of patients.

Malcolmson (1968) showed that in a series of 307 patients only 21 per cent had a completely negative physical and radiological examination. He proposed that globus pharyngis is a better term and emphasized occasional fatal cases. Delahunty and Ardran (1970) gave an acid barium swallow to 25 patients with globus hystericus and showed that 22 of them had reflux oesophagitis resulting in an acid-induced disturbance of oesophageal motility. Hunt et al (1970) showed that elevated resting pressures occurred in the cricopharyngeal sphincters of patients with gastric reflux. Suspicion that there is an organic basis for what was thought to be always a psychological symptom has thus become very strong. Lehtinen and Puhakka (1976) examined 20 such patients both by oesophagoscopy with cinematography and psychiatrically. Two had gastro-oesophageal reflux and eight had abnormalities of the cricopharyngeal folds. No patient was free of psychiatric symptoms but only eight showed any evidence of hysterical personality. These authors took the view that there are two different types of globus hystericus, one in which the aetiological factor is mainly somatic and another in which it is primarily psychological.

Patients with abnormal movements are now recognized as very often having a bizarre symptom due to subtle organic disturbance. Traditionally, such actions were regarded as hysterical phenomena but the proof in terms of neurological examination has never been so convincing as that for paralyses or anaesthesias. The original tendency to classify these symptoms as hysterical was related partly to an older 19th century view that hysteria was in any case an organic disease. Thus hemifacial spasm, facial dyskinesia, spasmodic torticollis, many tics, and even hemichorea (Charcot, 1889) were all classified as hysterical. Certain types of torticollis appear to develop after emotional stress (Tibbetts, 1971) and sometimes remit, and tics are undoubtedly often subject to emotional influences and to remission (Corbett et al, 1969). However, there is also a remarkable lack of evidence of psychological causal factors in torticollis (Cockburn, 1971) while positive evidence exists of supervening organic disorders (Tibbetts, 1971).

The fact that many of the patients are depressed or beseeching, which was taken as evidence that their symptoms were due to hysteria, may only reflect the discomfort and social embarrassment that their symptoms provoke. The fact that these emotions usually fail to respond to persistent and competent treatment for neurosis suggests that they have some other basis. Moreover von Economo (1931) showed that tics and torticollis resembling those thought to be psychological in origin could be produced by encephalitis. Probably the major turn in opinion has come since the introduction of levodopa, an excess of which tends to produce such symptoms, apparently on a chemical basis, in patients with Parkinsonism. Very many abnormal movements like blepharospasm, dystonia and dyskinesia are now therefore regarded as primarily physical in origin although sometimes exacerbated by emotional stress or relieved by relaxation. This is not to deny that some tics are due to anxiety and some to hysteria, but many require an alternative diagnosis.

The significance of brain disease

It has already been mentioned that in settled civilian conditions in developed countries one of the commonest associations of hysteria is with cerebral organic disease. Since hysterical symptoms in psychiatric practice are now rare except in those settings specified, it seems that there may be a special connection between cerebral organic disease and hysterical complaints. I do not suggest that hysterical symptoms are directly due to a lesion that disturbs the ultimate pathways in producing the symptom. However, as Slater (1965) has argued, certain organic lesions may cause a degree of regression or disintegration in the personality which favours the production of hysterical symptoms.

There is a possibility that some parts of the brain may be more specifically implicated than others but at present the only evidence for this is the particular association of hysteria with temporal lobe epilepsy. For example, in patients with epilepsy not only are hysterical fits relatively more common (which could be expected if patients have learned the pattern of attack that may occasion sympathy) but also other symptoms like gross astasias, gross abasias, and paralyses seem to occur more frequently (Merskey and Buhrich, 1975). The production of hysterical symptoms has also been noticed with phenytoin intoxication (Niedermayer et al, 1970). In a survey of 666 patients with temporal lobe epilepsy Currie et al (1971) found 12 with schizophrenia (a number slightly above that anticipated) and 17 with gross hysterical symptoms of the types just mentioned which are now rare.

The contribution of organic disease to hysterical phenomena raises an important question: how can the whole theory of hysterical symptoms be developed to explain their production by mechanisms of both conflict and cerebral damage? No fully satisfactory explanation is yet available but I agree with Whitlock (1976a,b) that an explanation in terms of emotional conflict alone is no longer sufficient.

The clinical significance of hysterical phenomena

This varies considerably and a rough scheme is as follows:

1. Hysteria with one or two symptoms usually motor or dissociative (as in amnesia) and sometimes pain
2. Polysymptomatic hysteria, especially hypochondriasis and Briquet's syndrome
3. Hysterical elaboration of organic complaints
4. Symptoms of self-induced illness or self-damage in abnormal personalities, ranging from anorexia nervosa to hospital addiction

5. Psychotic or pseudopsychotic disorders (such as Ganser's syndrome and hysterical psychosis)
6. Hysterical personality
7. Culturally sanctioned endemic or epidemic hysteria.

Points 4 and 5 have hardly been dealt with at all in this article and are special topics in themselves but the whole seven categories cover the bulk of hysterical manifestations. The aetiology of some cases is often evident from the circumstances in which they are seen, for example battle neuroses, culturally based outbreaks, and compensation settings. Other episodes arise in patients with well-established personality disorders or long histories of psychological illness, the evidence of which assists in reaching a diagnosis.

Apart from the foregoing, it may be helpful to consider the differential diagnosis of monosymptomatic cases seen in Westernized settings. First, they may be explained by a definite conflict situation occurring in young people. Secondly, affective illness occasionally afflicts some patients with classic motor conversion symptoms which precede or accompany the onset of the depression (for example schizophrenia does this, although rarely). Lastly, organic nuerological disease (especially epilepsy but sometimes early brain tumour or dementia) can lead to hysterical manifestations.

Prognosis

The prognosis of hysteria is essentially that of the associated conditions and of the problems that have given rise to it. In general, symptoms of sudden acute onset related to definable conflicts, drug intoxication, or recognizable social changes have a good prognosis and are largely recoverable. Those attached to chronic personality disorders may be correspondingly intractable. Suicide is not frequent among patients with the traditional hysterical symptoms here discussed but perhaps 7–12 per cent of patients may make suicidal attempts and of those followed-up for several years 1–2 per cent may die by suicide. There is probably a small but significant excess of deaths from both natural causes and suicide among patients with hysteria.

In epidemics of hysteria recovery is normally complete in almost all patients with regard to individual symptoms and the same is true for endemic culturally induced conditions. Ljungberg (1957) gives the morbidity risk for schizophrenia as 3.1 ± 1.1 per cent in patients with hysterical symptoms and there are similar small increases over the expected population figures for manic depressive, presenile, and psychogenic psychoses, alcoholism, and drug addiction. There is thus generally accepted evidence that patients diagnosed as hysterics have a modest increase in the rates of physical illness, suicide, and psychoses.

Recovery rates are best initially and Ljungberg showed that after an observation period of one year 43 per cent of men and 35 per cent of women had residual symptoms. With the assistance of Seward, Lewis (1975) traced 98 patients who had been diagnosed as hysterics at the Maudsley Hospital over a 5-year period: 40 were well, working, and free from disability or troublesome symptoms. Ciompi (1969) found 38 patients surviving an average of 34 years after first admission to the University Psychiatric Clinic at Lausanne; he noted two with schizophrenia and two with epilepsy but among the remainder former conversion symptoms had largely disappeared. However, two thirds remained mildly anxious, depressed, or hypochondriacal. Hysterical character patterns showed less amelioration and social adjustment was improved in only 50 per cent. Carter (1949) showed that 70 per cent of 90 patients with acute conversion reactions followed for 4–6 years were well and only seven could not work.

Clearly, the prognosis varies with the selection of patients but these figures should give some guide to the expected outlook. The greater the personality disorder, the more other troubles may be expected in the future. The greater the part played by existing circumstances (either of interpersonal conflict or personal stress), the better the outlook.

References

Armstrong, H, Patterson, P (1975) *Canadian Psychiatric Association Journal*, **20**, 247
Breuer, J, Freud, S (1955) *in* the Complete Physiological Works of Sigmund Freud 1893–1895, Vol. 2 (edited by Strachey, J). Hogarth Press, London. p.1
Carter, A B (1949) *British Medical Journal*, **1**, 1076
Charcot, J M (1889) Clinical Lectures on Diseases of the Nervous System, Vol. 3. New Sydenham Society, London
Chodoff, P, Lyons, H (1958) *American Journal of Psychiatry*, **114**, 734
Ciompi, L (1969) *Journal of Geriatric Psychiatry*, **3**, 90
Cockburn, J J (1971) *Journal of Psychosomatic Research*, **15**, 471
Corbett, J A, Mathews, A M, Connell, P H, Shapiro, D A (1969) *British Journal of Psychiatry*, **115**, 1229
Currie, S, Heathfield, K W G, Henson, R A, Scot, D F (1971) *Brain*, **94**, 173
Delahunty, J E, Ardran, G M (1970) *Journal of Laryngology and Otology*, **84**, 1049
Farley, J, Woodruff, R A, Guze, S B (1968) *British Journal of Psychiatry*, **114**, 1121
Guze, S B (1970) *Seminars in Psychiatry*, **2**, 392
Head, H (1922) *British Medical Journal*, i, 827
Houston, J C, Joiner, C L, Trounce, J R (1975) A Short Textbook of Medicine, 5th edn. English Universities Press, London
Hunt, P S, Connell, A M, Smiley, T B (1970) *Gut*, **11**, 303
Lehtinen, V, Puhakka, H, (1976) *Acta psychiatrica et neurologica Scandinavica*, **53**, 21
Lewis, A J (1975) *Psychological Medicine*, **5**, 9
Ljungberg, L (1957) *Acta psychiatrica et neurologica Scandinavica*, Suppl. 112, p. 1
Malcolmson, K G (1968) *Journal of Laryngology and Otology*, **82**, 219
Merskey, H, Buhrich, N A (1975) *British Journal of Medical Psychology*, **48**, 359
—, Spear, F G (1967) Pain: Psychological and Psychiatric Aspects. Balliere, Tindall and Cassell, London
—, Trimble, M (1979) *American Journal of Psychiatry*, **136**, 179
Moss, P D, McEvedy, C P (1966) *British Medical Journal*, ii, 1295
Niedermeyer, E, Blumer, D, Holscher, E, Walker, B A (1970) *Psychiatria Clinica*, **3**, 71
Pilling, L F, Brannick, T L, Swenson, W M (1967) *Canadian Medical Association Journal*, **97**, 387
Reynolds, J R (1869) *British Medical Journal*, ii, **483**, 378
Schuler, E A, Parenton, V J (1943) *Journal of Social Psychology*, **17**, 221
Slater, E (1965) *British Medical Journal*, i, 1395
Sternbach, R A (1974) Pain Patients: Traits and Treatment. Academic Press, New York
Sydenham, T (1697) Discourse Concerning Hysterical and Hypochondriacal Distempers: "Dr Sydenham's Complete Method of Curing Almost All Diseases, and Description of their Symptoms" to which are now added Five Discourses of the Same Author Concerning the Pleurisy, Gout, Hysterical Passion, Dropsy and Rheumatism, 3rd edn. Newman and Rich Parker, London
Szasz, T S (1961) The Myth of Mental Illness: Foundations of a Theory of Personal Conduct. Harper and Row, New York
Tibbetts, R W (1971) *Journal of Psychosomatic Research*, **15**, 461
von Economo, C (1931) Encephalitis Lethargica: its Sequelae and Treatment. Oxford University Press, London
Whitlock, F A (1967a) *British Journal of Psychiatry*, **113**, 19
— (1967b) *Acta psychiatrica et neurologica Scandinavica*, **43**, 144
Woodruff, R A (1968) *British Journal of Psychiatry*, **114**, 1115

Chapter 8

Morbid jealousy

John Cobb, St George's Hospital, London

"... a swan about Windsor; that finding a strange Cock with his mate did swim I know not how many miles after to kill him and when he had done so, came back and killed his hen" (The Anatomy of Melancholy; Robert Burton, 1621)

Intense possessive feelings towards a sexual mate are widespread in the animal kingdom and deeply rooted in primitive proprietary and competitive instincts. Among humans jealousy is very common, although by no means universal. For instance, in some societies it is considered good manners to share one's wife with an honoured guest (Davis, 1936). On the other hand it has been suggested (Freud, 1922; Pinta, 1978) that the mirror image of jealousy, namely sexual tolerance, can also become pathological.

As with other human emotions such as sadness, joy, and fear the point at which normal jealousy becomes morbid has been much debated. By analogy with these other emotions which may become morbid and be expressed as depression, mania, and phobia there have been attempts in the past to recognize a purely morbid form of jealousy. The lyrical, although inappropriate, eponym Othello syndrome (Schmeideberg, 1953; Todd and Dewhurst, 1955) reflects this tendency. However, a consensus now exists, at least among European psychiatrists, that morbid jealousy is best viewed as a descriptive term and not a diagnosis. It covers a wide range of unacceptable or bizarre overt behaviours in addition to distressing irrational thoughts and emotions, all of which share a unifying dominant theme of preoccupation with the partner's sexual unfaithfulness.

Classification

From the psychiatric point of view jealousy may be classified into three types as shown in *Table 8.1*. Although terminology varies, the agreement between various authorities is remarkably close. This article is mainly concerned with the second and third categories which for the sake of simplicity may be termed neurotic jealousy and psychotic jealousy. As might be predicted the grey area in between these is one of dispute, but this may be more of academic interest than of practical clinical importance.

It is important to appreciate at the outset that it is the form in which the jealousy is expressed that is crucial in determining whether or not it is morbid in the psychiatric sense; the intensity is only of secondary significance. The woman who murders her husband when she surprises him in flagrante delicto is not necessarily morbidly jealous from this point of view, whereas the woman who persistently trails her husband to work and hides to watch his movements during the day is almost certainly pathologically jealous.

TABLE 8.1. Classifications of morbid jealousy showing the apparent spectrum from normality to psychosis

Author	Normal jealousy		Neurotic jealousy		Psychotic jealousy
Mairet (1908)			Hyperaesthetic jealousy	Jealousy monomania	Delusional jealousy
Jaspers (1910)			Unsystematic delusional jealousy		Delusional jealousy
Freud (1922)	Normal jealousy		Projective jealousy		Delusional jealousy
Ey (1950)			Jealousy reactions of abnormal persons		Delusional jealousy
Mooney (1965)		Excessive jealousy	Obsessive jealousy		Delusional jealousy

Othello's jealousy could be viewed as normal or morbid according to one's opinion of the Moor's previous personality and the strength of the incriminating evidence (Mooney, 1965). Emilia suggests that it is morbid when she comments:

But jealous souls will not be answer'd so;
They are not ever jealous for the cause.
But jealous for they are jealous; 'tis a monster
Begot upon itself, born on itself.

Underlying psychopathology

Three large-scale surveys of patients with morbid jealousy as a major symptom give information concerning the underlying psychopathology (*Table 8.2*).

Shepherd (1961) did a retrospective case-note survey of patients encountered in a London postgraduate teaching hospital and a nearby metropolitan observation unit between 1950 and 1960. Langfeldt (1961) studied case notes of patients attending the Oslo University clinic during two 3-year periods (1940–42 and 1946–48) and followed-up these patients for an average of 17 years. In Finland between 1962 and 1965 Vauhkonen (1968) interviewed 55 couples one member of which was morbidly jealous. They were drawn from a variety of sources including the university psychiatric clinic, private practice, and a marriage guidance clinic.

Each author used a different system of diagnostic classification, but in order to provide rough comparability the diagnoses have been simplified in *Table 8.2*. Allowing for this and for the different sources of clinical material, the studies show broad agreement. Between one third and one half of the patients suffered from psychotic disorders. Neuroses and personality disorders also constituted one third to one half. Alcoholism as a primary diagnosis occurred in less than 7 per cent of cases and a miscellaneous group, mostly comprised of patients with organic disorders, accounted for the remainder.

TABLE 8.2. Conditions presenting with morbid jealousy as a major symptom

		Shepherd (1961)	Langfeldt (1961)	Vauhkonen (1968)
All psychoses		(33%)	(48%)	(44%)
	Schizophrenia (including monomania and paranoid psychoses)	14 (17%)	30 (45%)	24 (44%)
	Manic-depressive psychosis	13 (16%)	2 (3%)	
Neuroses and personality disorders		(38%)	(41%)	(57%)
	Neurosis	25 (32%)	6 (9%)	13 (24%)
	Personality disorders (including paranoid personality)	7 (8%)	21 (32%)	18 (32%)
Alcoholism		6 (7%)	3 (5%)	
Others		16 (20%)	4 (6%)	
Totals		81	66	55

Psychotic disorders

Mrs M (age 35 years) had an uncle with paranoid schizophrenia. After 13 years of marriage her relationship with her husband had cooled and the couple slept in separate rooms. Following the discovery of a letter that in a circumstantial way suggested that her husband might be having an affair, she became convinced that another woman was entering the house and having sex with her husband while she was asleep. In order to check on him she insisted on tying a piece of cotton around his penis before going to bed. Her bizarre behaviour persisted and was tolerated by her husband for nearly a year. He only sought medical help when her delusional beliefs extended and she claimed that her husband could not only put thoughts into her head but also exercise remote control over the movements of her body by using electromagnetic waves. She improved considerably on phenothiazines but relapsed when she refused further medication.

A delusional belief in the partner's infidelity can appear as the first sign of a psychotic illness. It may either continue to dominate the clinical picture or be lost in other morbid ideas as the illness progresses. If the delusion remains encapsulated the personality is left otherwise intact, as in other examples of monosymptomatic psychoses. This has led in the past to such diagnostic labels as jealous monomania. Most of the psychotic states fall into the paranoid group and in practice the patient is diagnosed as suffering from paranoid schizophrenia, paraphrenia, paranoid illness, or paranoia.

Usually the psychotic type of morbid jealousy occurs with a rapid onset, at a late stage of life, and in patients without previously jealous personalities (Vauhkonen, 1968).

Depressive illness

Shepherd (1961) draws attention to the fact that morbid jealousy may be a symptom of a depressive illness. In his series 13 patients suffered from affective psychoses and 12 from reactive depressions. Since the jealousy is both distressing and disruptive it may often be difficult to determine whether any associated depression is primary or secondary (Cobb and Marks, 1979).

Neuroses and personality disorders

Mr B (age 27 years) had been plagued by intrusive insistent thoughts concerning his girlfriend's faithfulness when he first went steady at the age of 18. The thoughts disappeared when this relationship ended but recurred during a second long-term relationship and again when he married. They made him anxious, miserable, and irritable and led to extensive checking up and violent confrontation. He would check handbags for addresses and telephone numbers, his partner's body for any marks or love bites, her underclothes for semen stains, and even the carpet for other men's hairs. Although he recognized that his fears were groundless and was convinced that his behaviour was "ridiculous, irrational, and shameful", he nevertheless worked himself up into a fury especially if he had been drinking. Often he attacked his partner and then became deeply ashamed and remorseful.

This patient had an immature dependent personality and was also diagnosed as suffering from obsessive compulsive neurosis. Anxiety neurosis and phobic states, hysterical states, and hypochondriasis may all present as morbid jealousy. So may a variety of personality disorders, especially paranoid personalities, as well as asthenic and sociopathic individuals.

Alcoholism

As early as 1847 Marcel stated that delusions of jealousy were generally met in alcoholics. Kraft-Ebing (1891) claimed that about 80 per cent of male alcoholics who still had sexual relations were afflicted by delusions of jealousy.

Kolle (1932; quoted by Shepherd, 1961) distinguished carefully between three principal subgroups and recognized jealous drunkards, delirious jealousy (exogenous drinkers), and paranoid jealousy in alcoholics (delusional drinkers). Long follow-up of the first group showed that they did not deteriorate nor develop psychotic symptoms, suggesting that they were jealous inadequate men who had become jealous drunkards. The third group, Kolle argued, could be diagnosed as schizophrenic; follow-up confirmed this and revealed a poor prognosis. The second group, the least common, could be diagnosed as alcoholic hallucinoses and their progress was correspondingly bad.

More recent workers (Langfeldt, 1961; Shepherd, 1961) have confirmed Kolle's observations and shown that while alcohol frequently inflames pre-existing symptoms and precipitates violence it is only rarely a primary cause of morbid jealousy (as in Kolle's exogenous drinkers). Alcohol may thus be more of forensic than aetiological importance.

Organic states

Addictions other than alcoholism   Both amphetamine and cocaine addictions (Shepherd, 1961) have been reported to be closely associated with morbid jealousy. Typically the delusional ideas rapidly become intense and frequently lead to violence. They may persist for some time after the drug is withdrawn.

Cerebral disorders   Infections, neoplasms, metabolic and endocrine disorders, and degenerative conditions have all been described in association with morbid jealousy. Examples include general paralysis of the insane, primary and secondary cerebral tumours, lead poisoning, panhypopituitarism, disseminated sclerosis,

Parkinson's disease, and various forms of presenile dementia including Huntington's chorea. Shepherd (1961) described a case of temporal lobe epilepsy in which the jealousy appeared as a postictal phenomenon and Banus (1926) described blindness as a precipitant.

Most of the above refer to single case reports and the importance of organic factors must not be overestimated. Indeed, in a series of 3552 brain-injured exservicemen only 42 developed jealous paranoia (Achté et al, 1967).

Biological factors (ageing and endocrine causes)

Claims have been made that morbid jealousy can occur as an isolated symptom in the elderly. However, it is likely that it is some organic cerebral change rather than age by itself that releases this symptom in old people. The predicament of the elderly man whose waning sexual powers are insufficient to satisfy a younger wife is a favourite theme in literature. Old blind Januarie in Chaucer's *The Merchant's Tale* became jealous of his buxom young wife:

> Which jalousye it was so outrageous
> That neither in halle, n'yn noon oother hous
> Ne in noon oother place, neverthemo
> He nolde suffre hire for to ryde or go.

This literary influence is reflected by Todd and Dewhurst (1955) who emphasized the importance of a large age difference between spouses, especially if the husband is much older than his wife. However, in Vauhkonen's (1968) series of 55 couples only four of the male patients were more than 10 years older than their wives and only one of these mentioned the age difference as a factor leading to conflicts.

Several authors point to the importance of the puerperium and the menopause in producing symptoms. However, it can be argued that the change in self-image associated with these events is just as likely to give rise to jealousy as the change in hormonal balance.

Heritable factors

In none of the relevant studies is it possible to distinguish between inherited and environmental influences. For example, 20 of Vauhkonen's (1968) patients had parents who were reported to have shown jealous behaviour. This could be explained on a genetic basis, but equally the behaviour may have been learned through modelling. In fact when the patients and their spouses were compared in terms of their family backgrounds there was little significant difference, although the patients tended to have experienced more temporary deprivation and come from larger families.

Intrapersonal psychological factors

Evidence concerning psychological factors leading to morbid jealousy comes from two sources: relatively superficial surveys of populations of patients (for example Vauhkonen, 1968), and detailed psychoanalytic studies of individuals (Freud, 1922; Schmeideberg, 1953).

Although in some cases it is impossible to identify any specific personality variables, several authors have described a constellation of characteristics. Sensitive, vulnerable, and suspicious individuals who have poor self-esteem and are unassertive seem over-represented in any group of morbidly jealous patients. Kretschmer (1952) maintained that not only a sensitive personality but also a key catalytic experience was necessary before paranoid delusions, such as morbid jealousy, could develop. In Langfeldt's (1961) series three patients had experienced directly relevant sexual trauma, although in others he found it impossible to isolate specific psychogenic releasing factors. In contrast, morbid jealousy is also found in quick-tempered, egoistic, and aggressive individuals (Langfeldt, 1961).

Psychoanalytic concepts stem from Freud who recognized three types of jealousy: normal or competitive, projected, and delusional (*Table 8.1*). The material produced by the Schreber pathographical study (Freud, 1911), set against a background of Freud's early theories of the bisexual nature of infants and the Oedipus complex, provided the rationale for Freud's suggestions that all jealousy has its roots in early childhood experience and that unconscious homosexual feelings play a part in all jealousy particularly of the delusional type. The mental mechanisms of reaction formation, repression, and denial prevent the subject being aware of his own homosexual feelings. In the milder projected form of jealousy it is the subject's own promiscuous urges that are projected directly onto the partner. Hahn (1933) refers to this as conversion jealousy springing from the subject's own inclination to unfaithfulness. In the more severe delusional form homosexual love is denied using the formula "I do not love him because she loves him."

Vauhkonen (1968) failed to find any particular pattern of early childhood experience and he, Shepherd and Langfeldt all found no evidence that overt homosexuality was in any way associated with morbid jealousy. Doctrinaire psychoanalysts could always argue that they are dealing with unconscious processes and so the findings are irrelevant. However, the importance of Freud's theorizing lies not in the truth or falsity of his ideas but in his concept of the possibility of a dynamic psychological process.

Other nonpsychoanalytic dynamic postulates have been made. Cameron (1943) suggested that the paranoid individual, because of poorly developed interpersonal skills, is unable to test the validity of his thoughts about others. Hyroop (1951) reported the persistence of childhood feelings of omnipotence into adult life, leading to a deep need to control others, particularly close relatives. Hahn (1933) drew attention to tyrannical jealousy arising from a lust for power, and other authors have pointed to jealousy as a means of exercising extreme control over the partner resulting in submissiveness and even subjugation (Vauhkonen, 1968; Morgan, 1975). Hahn (1933) also referred to complex jealousy, that is jealousy arising from past experiences such as realistic infidelity of the partner.

Vauhkonen (1968), who studied the reported fantasies of his patients, suggested that the morbid jealousy may be sexually gratifying. The author has treated a morbidly jealous patient who could only reach orgasm if he fantasized about his wife having intercourse with another man.

Langfeldt (1961) reported that 10 of his 66 patients were mentally handicapped. Lack of insight, immature behaviour, and explosive outbursts in this group may all contribute to the production of morbid jealousy. However, other studies have failed to replicate Langfeld's finding presumably because the patients were drawn from different sources.

All the work described leads one to the conclusion that, as in other psychiatric conditions, there is unlikely to be a single psychological determinant in morbid jealousy.

Gender

The sex ratios in five recent studies are shown in *Table 8.3*. Overall, morbid jealousy appears to be twice as common in men as in women. If alcoholism as a major cause is discounted, it is difficult to explain this sex ratio. Possibly males with this symptom are more likely to cause personal, marital, and social disruption and thus attract more attention.

TABLE 8.3. Sex ratio in the morbidly jealous

Author	Male	Female	Male:female ratio
Shepherd (1961)	64	17	} 3.76:1
Langfeldt (1961)	39	27	1.44:1
Vauhkonen (1968)	37	18	2.05:1
Berner (1965)	69	35	1.97:1
Germano (1960)	51	49	1.04:1
Total	260	146	1.78:1

Sexual dysfunction

Accurate data concerning sexual behaviour and feelings are notoriously difficult to obtain. Subjects are unwilling to give information and interviewers often ask the wrong questions; this may lead on the one hand to extreme overemphasis of sexuality as an aetiological factor and on the other to virtual neglect. Thus on the basis of three cases Docherty and Ellis (1976) suggested that the experience as an adolescent of witnessing the mother engaged in extramarital activity may be an aetiological factor in the production of morbid jealousy in men. However, Langfeldt (1961—despite the title of his paper The Erotic Jealousy Syndrome— scarcely considered sexual dysfunction. Shepherd (1961) found sexual difficulties to be of primary importance in only three out of his 81 cases.

On the other hand Vauhkonen (1968) found that 19 out of 36 male patients described sexual dysfunction (one loss of libido, six erectile difficulties, and 12 premature ejaculation) and 11 of these were subjectively sexually dissatisfied. Among women 13 out of 17 described dysfunction (three total frigidity and 10 orgasmic difficulty), but only seven described subjective sexual dissatisfaction. Clearly it is important to distinguish between objective physiological responses and subjective feelings and, as the author pointed out, take account of what normative data are available. Kinsey et al (1948) stated that erectile weakness occurred in 2 per cent of their sample of adult males under the age of 45 years, while a recent estimate of the prevalence of female orgasmic dysfunction was 60 per cent (Fisher, 1973).

Since morbid jealousy inevitably involves two people, it is important to study sexual function in the partner as well as the patient. Vauhkonen (1968) found that seven out of 16 husbands reported sexual dysfunction (two loss of libido, one erectile difficulty, and four premature ejaculation), while *32 out of 37* wives had problems (15 total frigidity and 17 orgasmic difficulty). This failure in the sexual relationship as a whole appears to be very frequently associated with morbid jealousy, although whether this is primary or secondary it is not possible to say.

It seems probable, as writers have claimed for at least 100 years, that the onset of erectile difficulty is particularly likely to provoke morbid jealousy and that this is closely related to sexual dysfunction in the wife.

Marital and social factors

"We were like two convicts hating each other and chained together, poisoning one another's lives and trying not to see it" (*The Kreutzer Sonata*; Leo Tolstoy, 1889). This book eloquently documents the violent disruption of a relationship ridden with morbid jealousy. In this case Pozdnvshev's "terrible abyss of error" regarding his wife was the cause of the tragedy. Equally, morbid jealousy can be the consequence rather than the cause of estrangement between husband and wife.

Shepherd (1961) identified four cases in which marital problems were a primary cause of morbid jealousy whereas in Vauhkonen's (1968) series drawn partially from a marriage guidance clinic the proportion was much higher. It is of interest that 16 of these male patients (almost half) became pathologically jealous prior to the end of the first year of marriage, while only two of the females developed symptoms in a similar period. This difference was statistically significant. It may be partially explained by the fact that the mean age of males at marriage was 25.7 years and that of females 21.9 years. In addition, it may indicate that a woman's behaviour is more likely to be shaped by the events occurring during a relationship. Both loneliness and neglect were cited by the female patients in Vauhkonen's series as precipitating causes.

The influence of the environmental factor is seen in both the rise in crimes associated with jealousy during the post-war period in the UK and the increased incidence of patients with delusional jealousy following a period of economic depression in the Netherlands (Rumbe, 1959).

It is increasingly accepted that any psychiatric symptom has to be assessed in a social as well as an individual setting. This is particularly relevant in the case of morbid jealousy. Lund (1947) went so far as to view jealousy as "descriptive less of an emotional state than of a social situation", and Blacker (1958) drew attention to the prominent role of jealousy in disrupted marriages.

In Vauhkonen's (1968) series the jealousy only came to light in two cases after the partners had made suicide attempts as a response to persistent unreasonable accusations. A further case was recognized after a homicide attempt on the partner. Vauhkonen also pointed out that the partner frequently does not assess the morbid behaviour realistically: "More often the partner reacts with depression, incredulity, resentment, fear of assault or remorse for previous misconduct". The partner may even become involved in the web of delusional ideas, a sort of delusional paranoia.

Forensic aspects

Two approaches shed light on forensic aspects of morbid jealousy. Either populations of those convicted of violent crimes can be studied to discover what proportion were morbidly jealous or, alternatively, the frequency of violence among patients suffering from morbid jealousy can be measured.

Using the first approach, East (1936) and Brierly (1932) showed that of sane murderers 8–25 per cent killed because of jealousy. Mowat (1966) studied the records of all patients admitted to Broadmoor Hospital (for criminally insane patients) over several years and found that in 12 per cent of the men and 15 per cent of the women morbid jealousy was a significant factor. Christiansen (1956; quoted by Langfeldt, 1961) in a study of 40 jealous murderers found seven to be of normal premorbid personality and 13 to be mentally handicapped. Alcohol was shown to be an important aetiological factor in 25 per cent of both sexes, but 16 (40 per cent) used no alcohol whatsoever.

Looked at from the other approach, three (4 per cent) of Shepherd's (1961) cases and one (2 per cent) of Vauhkonen's (1968) patients manifested homicidal behaviour. The frequency of serious physical injury that fell short of homicide was not recorded but is likely to have been higher than that of murderous attacks. Taking into account the risk of suicide in both the patient and the spouse it is clear that jealousy is a potentially dangerous condition, although the focus on forensic rather than general psychiatric populations has tended to lead to an overestimation of the risk of serious physical harm. This tendency has been encouraged by the use of the dramatic but misleading eponym Othello syndrome (Todd and Dewhurst, 1955; Enoch et al, 1967). Too much consideration of the physical risks diverts attention from the almost invariable psychological damage done to individuals, couples, and families.

Clinical distinction between sane and insane jealousy

East (1936) and Christiansen's (1956; quoted by Langfeldt, 1961) reference to sane jealous murders raises the important practical issue of how to distinguish morbid jealousy from intense and violent but normal jealousy. Clearly the intensity of the jealous reaction is not in itself evidence of psychiatric morbidity. A number of aspects are helpful:

1. The form of the jealous behaviour and thoughts
2. The strength of the evidence on which the jealous ideas are based
3. The recognition of the underlying psychiatric disorder
4. The premorbid personality of the patient
5. The duration of the jealousy and whether or not it occurred in previous relationships
6. The attitude of the partner and the nature of the present relationship.

In assessing the risk of physical violence the same advice can be followed that Scott (1977) advocated in relation to criminals: "Involvement on a long-term basis and good communications are the inescapable bases for assessment of dangerousness".

Management

The management of the morbidly jealous should be based on a careful assessment of the problem. Apart from a conventional clinical history, interviews with the partner both alone and together with the patient should be mandatory. Careful attention should be paid to the factors cueing outbursts of jealousy and to the effect of the spouse's reaction on the patient's thoughts and behaviour. One of the author's patients invariably began a morbidly jealous cross-examination of his wife when he returned home from work. If she tried to argue rationally with him he became more and more angry. However, if she ignored him and walked out of the room his jealousy subsided. This information provided a basis for a treatment plan.

Evidence of violence should always be sought by careful sympathetic questioning to elicit the nature of the violent attacks, whether the patient uses his hands or picks up objects, how quickly he can be controlled, and if he has ever inflicted serious injury.

A detailed sexual history from both partners is important, as is an assessment of the quality of their relationship by direct questioning and observation of the way the couple interact during the conjoint interview.

Examples of delusional paranoid ideas include the belief that the accused is poisoning the patient or providing drugs to impair sexual potency. The partner may be accused of having venereal disease or indulging in sexual intercourse during the patient's sleep. Irrational doubts may be expressed concerning the paternity of any children while certain physical aspects of the sexual act, such as normal secretion, are seen as proof of infidelity.

Strenuous efforts may be made to prove suspicions. Extensive checks of letters and diaries lead to apparent confirmation in innocent phrases. Pieces of cotton are seen as a lover's pubic hairs and any marks on the bedclothes or underwear are viewed as unlawful sexual secretions. Lawyers and private detectives may be hired and the blameless partner may ultimately be goaded into making a false confession.

Paroxyms of rage may alternate with periods of rage, the whole clinical picture meriting the description: "A most violent passion it is where it taketh place, an unspeakable torment, a hellish torture, an infernal plague ... a fury, a continual fever full of suspicion, fear and sorrow, a martyrdom, a mirthmarring monster" (*The Anatomy of Melancholy;* Robert Burton, 1621).

The nature of the underlying psychiatric disorder, the motivation and compliance of the patient, and the risk of violence are the major determinants of a management plan.

If the jealousy is clearly delusional or if there is other evidence of a psychotic disorder, a major tranquillizer should be tried (Mooney, 1965). Chlopromazine in dosages of 50–500 mg/day may produce a remission. Some authorities (Riding and Munro, 1975) recommend that pimozide is particularly likely to be helpful in cases of monosymptomatic delusional states.

Problems can arise when the patient is an unreliable tablet taker, in which case an intramuscular preparation may be preferable. In addition to chemotherapy, supportive psychotherapy is indicated partly to attempt to find ways of minimizing stress and partly to monitor progress. Both partners may benefit from a chance to explore the problem, ventilate their anxieties, and receive practical advice. In cases where outpatient treatment fails, the patient refuses to cooperate and the risk of violence is high, hospital admission may be required. In extreme cases it may be necessary to advise the couple to separate; as a Victorian physician put it, "the best treatment may be geographical".

Where the evidence suggests a neurotic disorder or a personality problem various forms of psychotherapy may be helpful. Short-term symptom-orientated behavioural psychotherapy produced improvement in three cases out of four over an average of 19 hourly sessions and this was maintained at follow-up after 8 months (Cobb and Marks, 1979). Therapeutic strategies that were individually designed for each patient involved exposure in vivo, response prevention, cue modification, and differential reinforcement of appropriate and inappropriate responses. In addition, where suitable, sexual skills training, assertive training, and behaviourally based marital therapy were used.

The importance of planning an individually tailored approach through trial and error is illustrated by the following patterns of interpersonal interaction (Vauhkonen, 1968; Cobb and Marks, 1979)

Couple 1. The patient's husband found that an aggressive response to jealousy-inspired verbal attacks led to a decrease in jealous accusations and his partner calming down.
Couple 2. An aggressive response by the wife led to increasing jealous fury in the husband, while ignoring the jealous accusation by turning away or walking out of the room reduced the frequency of jealous thoughts and quietened the rage.
Couple 3. If the wife tried to evade arguments, the husband became more suspicious and anxious and the jealous thoughts were prolonged.

Other workers (Morgan, 1975; Docherty and Ellis, 1976) have advocated marital therapy based on analytic lines. Finally, there are several case histories of patients treated on an individual basis by psychoanalysis (Seidenberg, 1952).

Morbid jealousy frequently runs a fluctuating course (Todd and Dewhurst, 1955; Vauhkonen, 1968) and is usually dependent on the presence of the partner. It is particularly difficult to evaluate the effects of treatment without a control group and at present no controlled studies are available. Hospitalization may produce an apparent remission through separation from the partner, but the risk of recurrence on discharge is great. Scott (1977) drew attention to the risk of second murders due to pathological jealousy even after years of apparent well-being.

On practical grounds short-term intensive treatment may be preferred, although because of the high risk of relapse it is important to provide long-term follow-up. The importance of seeing the couple together has been emphasized by both behavioural and psychoanalytic therapists (Morgan, 1975; Docherty and Ellis, 1976; Cobb and Marks, 1979).

Prognosis

In general, the prognosis is related to that of the underlying psychiatric situation seen in the light of the nature of the patient's premorbid personality and the quality of the premorbid relationship. The immediate response to treatment is usually better than the long-term results.

Langfeldt (1961) found that 56 per cent of his patients had been rated as improved after treatment. He attempted to follow-up a group of 50 after a 17-year interval. Six had died and 17 could not be traced. Of the remainder only 12 showed full recovery (one of whom was suffering from manic-depressive psychosis), six were periodically better, and nine showed no improvement. Patients with severe personality disorder or psychotic illness had a particularly poor prognosis although because of the nature of his population Langfeldt may have been unnecessarily pessimistic.

Mooney (1965) reported the treatment results of a group of patients from his own private practice supplemented by patients from four other series. The treatment varied, but overall he concluded that "about one third of the patients seemed to be much improved, one third slightly improved, and one third unchanged". Again, he found that those with psychotic disorders did worse.

Although morbid jealousy undoubtedly remains a complex challenge to the psychiatrist, the present state of knowledge suggests that with an eclectic approach involving chemotherapy, behavioural techniques and marital psychotherapy, the outlook need not be as pessimistic as is traditionally believed.

References

Achté, K A, Hillbom, E, Aalberg, V (1967) Reports from the Rehabilitation Institute for Brain Injured Veterans in Finland, Vol. 1

Banus, J S (1926) *Schweizer Archiv fur Neurologie und Psychiatrie*, **18**, 141

Berner, P (1965) Das Paranoische Syndrom. Springer-Verlag, Berlin, Heidelberg and New York

Blacker, C P (1958) *Lancet*, i, 578

Brierly, H C (1932) Homicide in the United States. Chapel Hill, New York

Cameron, N (1943) *Psychological Review*, **50**, 219

Cobb, J P, Marks, I M (1979) *British Journal of Psychiatry,* **134**, 301

Davis, K (1936) *Social Forces*, **14**, 395

Docherty, J P, Ellis, J (1976) *American Journal of Psychiatry*, **133**, 679

East, W N (1936) Medical Aspects of Crime, Churchill, London

Enoch, M D, Trethowan, W H, Barker, J C (1967) Uncommon Psychiatric Syndromes. John Wright, Bristol

Ey, H (1950) Etudes Psychiatriques, Tome 11. de Brouwer et Cie, Paris. p.483

Fisher, S (1973) Understanding the Female Orgasm. Penguin, Harmondsworth

Freud, S (1911) The Standard Edition of the Complete Psychological Works of Sigmund Freud, Vol. XII (translated and edited by Strachey, J, 1958) The Hogarth Press, London. p.9

— (1922) ibid. Vol. XVIII (translated and edited by Strachey, J, 1955). The Hogarth Press. p.221

Germano, G (1960) *Rassegna di studi psichiatrici*, **49**, 1

Hahn, B (1933) *Fortschritte der Medizin*, **51**, 336

Hyroop, M (1951) *American Journal of Psychotherapy*, **5**, 38

Jaspers, K (1910) *Zeitschrift für die gesamte Neurologie und Psychiatrie*, **1**, 567

Kinsey, A C et al (1948) Sexual Behaviour in the Human Male. Saunders, Philadelphia and London

Kraft-Ebing (1891) *Jahrbücher für Psychiatrie und Neurologie*, **10**, 221

Kretschmer, E (1952) Medical Psychology (translated by Strauss, E). The Hogarth Press, London

Langfeldt, G (1961) *Acta psychiatrica et neurologica Scandinavica*, Suppl. 151, p.1

Lund, F H (1947) Emotions. Ronald Press, New York. p.228

Mairet, A (1908) La Jalousie: Etude Psychophysiologique, Clinique-et Médico-Légale. Masson et Cie, Paris

Marcel, C N S (1847) De la folie causée par l'abus des boissons alcooliques. Thesis, Paris. p.461

Mooney. H B (1965) *British Journal of Psychiatry*, **111**, 1023

Morgan, D H (1975) *Psychotherapy and Psychosomatics*, **25**, 43

Mowat, R R (1966) Morbid Jealousy and Murder. Tavistock Publications, London

Pinta, E R (1978) *American Journal of Psychiatry*, **135**, 698

Riding, J, Munro, A (1975) *Acta psychiatrica Scandinavica*, **52**, 23

Rumbe, H (1959) *in* Transcript of Comments and Discussion of the Work Conference on problems in Field Studies in Mental Disorders. American Psychopathological Association (unpublished). p.370

Schmeideberg, M (1953) *Psychoanalytic Review*, **40**, 1

Scott, P D (1977) *British Journal of Psychiatry*, **131**, 127

Seidenberg, R (1952) *Psychoanalytic Review*, **39**, 345

Shepherd, M (1961) *Journal of Mental Science*, **107**, 687

Todd, J, Dewhurst, M (1955) *Journal of Nervous and Mental Disease*, **122**, 367

Vauhkonen, K (1968) *Acta psychiatrica Scandinavica*, Suppl. 202, p.1

Chapter 9

Monosymptomatic hypochondriacal psychosis

Alistair Munro, Camp Hill Hospital, Halifax, Nova Scotia

Monosymptomatic hypochondriacal psychosis (MHP) is an illness characterized by a single hypochondriacal delusion that is sustained over a considerable period, sometimes for many years. The delusion is not secondary to another psychiatric illness and the personality remains otherwise well preserved although the person's way of life is adversely affected, often to an extreme degree, and there is much accompanying agitation and at times paranoid anger (Munro, 1980). The condition may be an illness of itself but at present it is convenient to regard it as a variant of paranoia. Definitions of paranoia such as that of Cameron (1974) also describe MHP fairly well: "...a rare condition in which a delusional system develops logically out of some misinterpretation of an actual event...The condition does not interfere with the rest of the individual's thinking or general personality."

The term monosymptomatic hypochondriacal psychosis is not found in most textbooks, especially English-language ones. It is essentially a German and Scandinavian concept and its background has recently been well reviewed by Skott (1978). There are numerous alternative nomenclatures and Reilly (1977) lists several including monosymptomatic psychosis, chronic tactile hallucinosis, tactile delusional hallucinosis, and hypochondriac paraphrenia. Frequently authors fail to distinguish between MHP, a psychotic illness whose fundamental feature is a hypochondriacal delusion, and superficially similar disorders of a neurotic type such as dysmorphophobia (Hay, 1970) and parasitophobia (Susskind, 1973). This important diagnostic distinction is now being emphasized (Andreasen, 1977; *British Medical Journal*, 1978).

Modes of presentation

MHP is a protean disorder: while the essence of the illness is a hypochondriacal delusion the content of the delusion may vary widely from individual to individual. Nevertheless, it is possible to define a limited number of subgroups as follows:

1. Delusion of skin infestation by an insect (Ekbom, 1938)
2. Delusion of internal parasitosis, often ascribed to a worm (Levy, 1906, quoted by Reilly, 1977)
3. False belief, somewhat similar to the delusion of skin infestation, that there are lumps or small seed-like objects under the skin attributed to organisms or to

inert foreign bodies and often associated with compulsion to pick or excoriate (Reichenberger, 1972; Bjerg Hansen, 1976)
4. Dysmorphic delusion which includes a conviction of personal ugliness or an insistence on misshapenness or overprominence of a bodily part despite all evidence to the contrary (Schachter, 1971)
5. Olfactory delusion in which the individual wrongly insists that he emits a foul smell (Pryse-Phillips, 1971)
6. "Phantom bite" syndrome (Marbach, 1978) where the patient has the persistent delusion that his dental bite is abnormal
7. Delusional body-image disturbance in some cases of anorexia nervosa (Plantey, 1977; Trimble, 1977a)
8. Hypochondriacal delusional quality in some complaints of chronic pain (Trimble, 1977b).

Reilly (1977) suggests that cases of MHP may be divided into two categories. The first category (which would include groups 1–3 above) comprises patients with coenaesthopathia, distinguished by exaggeration or distortion of real proprioceptive, kinaesthetic and haptic sensations of which they are not normally aware. The second category (groups 4–8) involves a distortion of the body image. This is an interesting proposal with some heuristic implications, but in practice it may be somewhat redundant since treatment appears to have similar results in all of the above groups. Incidentally, neither Reilly's (1977) categorization nor the list of eight groups should be regarded as exhaustive because there could well be additional modes of presentation of MHP. For example, some apparent transsexuals who demand mutilating operations have a similar bizarre quality.

Previously, the various forms of MHP were regarded as chronic and largely irremediable, even if they did not usually deteriorate so profoundly as cases of paranoid schizophrenia (Retterstol, 1968). Now that many cases are amenable to simple treatment (see below) it has become eminently worthwhile to diagnose the illness accurately and to distinguish it carefully from other conditions associated with hypochondriasis. Kenyon (1976) proposed that most cases of hypochondriasis are an expression of other underlying psychiatric disorders including affective illness, obsessional neurosis, hysterical or other personality disorders, schizophrenia, and organic brain disease. It is usually not too difficult for a psychiatrist to separate and diagnose these illnesses and some are now readily treatable. The less common conditions in which hypochondriasis is a primary element, for example MHP, have proved much more problematic. Such patients usually attend somatic specialists who may institute inappropriate investigations and treatments. Because relatively few cases come to psychiatric notice they are regarded as uncommon and individual psychiatrists have little opportunity to gather case series or to experiment with treatment. It now behoves us to become much more skilled in diagnosing and helping this chronic and wretched group of patients.

Diagnostic features

Until recently it has been usual to concentrate on the content of the hypochondriacal delusion when making a diagnosis, hence the chaotic situation with regard to nomenclature. To gather such an apparently diverse group of complaints under a single diagnostic rubric demands that there should be notable common features. These do exist and the literature did indicate this, but the incentive to regard MHP as a discrete syndrome has been much stronger since the initial report by Riding and Munro (1975a) that several cases with widely differing symptomatologies all responded well to the psychotropic drug pimozide. Of course, it is perfectly possible that different disorders could improve with the same medication, for example Gilles de la Tourette's disease has also been shown to benefit from the drug (Ross and Moldofsky, 1978). However, increasing clinical experience with cases of MHP has convinced the author that there is a quite characteristic group of features in addition to the hypochondriacal delusion. This impression has been independently confirmed (Reilly and Beard, 1976).

The patient with MHP absolutely insists on a physical aetiology and pathology for his complaint. Skott (1978), quoting Ekbom (1938) on parasitic delusional patients, comments that the subject can tell repeatedly the same stereotyped story about the insects without adding details or speculations but shows great imagination about possible treatments. Some of the patient's views on treatment may be quite bizarre and this contrasts with his sensibleness on other topics. Ekbom also noted another characteristic: the energy and persistence with which the patient seeks out innumerable medical consultations and opinions. Typically, he is very insistent in his demand that the doctor confirm the diagnosis that the patient has already made and expresses anger and disdain if this is not accepted. His demands become increasingly idiosyncratic and irrational and it is common for him to complain in paranoid and very circumstantial fashion about the incompetence of his medical advisers. Any suggestion that the condition is psychiatric is met with vituperation, so physicians often fail to press this point. (Also, it has to be admitted that until now a psychiatric opinion has often been of little practical help to the patient or to the physician.)

When he first sees a patient with MHP, the psychiatrist may well be faced with an irate individual who claims that he has been sent along on a pretext. He may be accompanied by a relative who solemnly corroborates all of his fantastic symptomatology; this can be confusing unless one appreciates that folie à deux is not uncommon (Skott, 1978; also see below). Considerable tact is needed to enlist the patient's grudging cooperation (Gould and Gragg, 1976) and in some cases this is never obtained. Many patients make it clear that the psychiatrist is being given only one chance to help and this paranoid attitude has made it impossible to involve most patients in a structured clinical trial of medication. It is found best not to argue with the patient about his disorder or its aetiology, to play down the fact that one is a psychiatrist, and to talk predominantly of the physical nature of the treatment. It is fascinating that even long after an individual has improved markedly with pimozide he will not usually relinquish the idea that his symptom was due to a physical disorder or a parasite.

The onset of MHP may be insidious but some cases begin quite suddenly with an initiation like that of an autochthonous delusion. Patients who have infestation delusions and report seeing insects or those who claim to be deformed or ugly when this is manifestly not the case, may appear to be visually hallucinated. However, instead they probably have illusional misinterpretations, in the dysmorphic delusional subjects this may be similar to the illusions of body width seen in anorexia nervosa (Slade and Russell, 1973). There is no widespread cognitive or thought disorder but there is a notable absence of normal logic in discussing the delusional complaint. Generalized anxiety symptoms are marked. Although in deference to the diagnosis of paranoia the rest of the personality should be normal, in fact premorbid schizoid and obsessional traits seem common. Skott (1978) found that in her series of patients with infestation delusions a significant number had borderline intellectual handicap, but many of these individuals did not suffer from true MHP.

Frequency of the condition

The frequency of MHP in the population is unknown but the condition is generally regarded as rare. Psychiatrists do not see many cases but dermatologists, venereologists, infectious disease physicians, and plastic surgeons are well aware of them, although each specialty tends to come across one or two variants and to be quite unaware of their relationship to cases observed by other specialists. So far as infestation delusions are concerned, pest control agencies and public health authorities are very conscious of such individuals because of insistent and repeated demands for disinfestation of their premises (Edwards, 1977). Retterstøl (1968) found that only 0.4 per cent of a total psychiatric admission consisted of paranoid psychoses with hypochondriasis as the main content (and it is probable that many of these did not have MHP). In fact the condition is not as rare as this and if a psychiatrist shows a special interest it is not difficult to assemble a case series. The author has collected data on 30 patients with MHP, 28 of them seen personally and two examined by colleagues at the Toronto General Hospital who have kindly provided details (Munro, 1980).

Phenomenology

The following data are largely derived from the above 30 cases.

Age at first presentation

This ranges from 20 to 80 years, but the average age of the males at first contact (39.5 years) is considerably less than that of the females (61.8 years). A sharp rise in frequency occurs after the age of 50, largely due to an excess of older women. In fact there seems a definite possibility that MHP is an illness of younger males and older females, giving rise to speculation that there may actually be two conditions with similar presentations.

Sex distribution

This is virtually equal, with 16 males and 14 females. (This is in contrast to previous reports of a predominance of women [Skott, 1978].)

Nationality

This is very diverse and in this series 10 nationalities are represented—English, Canadian, American, Eskimo, Italian, Danish, Greek, West Indian, Portuguese and Polish.

Socioeconomic status

This appears to be lower than average but is possibly an artifact of the author's psychiatric practice. It may also be that sophisticated paranoid patients who do not wish to see a psychiatrist are better able to resist their physician's suggestion that they do so.

Alcohol and drug abuse

This has been noted in seven male patients, although only three had a serious drinking problem at the time of presentation. Previous drug abuse was admitted by two young males, and in total eight of the 16 males had experienced substance abuse whereas no female reported this. It seems that this may be a factor of some importance.

Duration of illness

At the time of the first interview the duration of MHP is on average just over 2 years, with a range of 2 months to 20 years. In long-standing cases a recent exacerbation has been usual.

Previous psychiatric contact

This is infrequent but many of the patients give evidence of some unstable, eccentric, or asocial premorbid personality traits. There are high frequencies of nonmarriage, separation, and divorce (especially among the men) and in married patients of both sexes the reproduction rate is below average. These findings suggest the presence of habitual problems in initiating and sustaining interpersonal relationships. Folie à ménage is a feature in some individuals; four patients have demonstrated this phenomenon—two with folie à deux and two with folie à trois. The other affected individuals have been close family members and either show a complete belief in the patient's delusion or actually adopt the symptoms themselves. When the index case improves it seems possible for the secondary cases' symptoms to disappear. Skott (1978) found that 25 per cent of her patients were involved in folie à deux.

Treatment and prognosis

Until recently the prognosis has generally been regarded as very poor although follow-up studies are virtually nonexistent. Skott (1978) states that some cases progress to florid schizophrenia, and suicide has been reported (Bebbington, 1976). Connolly and Gipson (1978) have reported on the long-term follow-up of a large number of patients who had rhinoplasties, dividing them into those who had the operation for cosmetic reasons and those who required it following trauma or disease. The cosmetic group, which may be inferred to contain some examples of MHP, had a very much higher psychiatric breakdown rate and included a significant number of schizophrenics.

There was no report of effective treatment for MHP until the use of pimozide was described (*British Medical Journal*, 1978). Nowadays, most patients receive some type of neuroleptic drug at an early stage in their illness and this has been true of most of the patients seen by the author. However, there is no consistent evidence of response to any medication other than pimozide or its parenteral analogue fluspirilene. In the present series three patients refused to accept treatment and one had very suspect compliance. Of the 26 remaining, 19 are regarded as having had an excellent response and seven a fair response. This means that 63 per cent of a group of previously intractable patients with MHP had a more or less complete disappearance of symptoms and a satisfactory return to their social existence while another 23 per cent had a partial remission with reduced anguish and some return to their social life. Good results appear to be dependent on careful diagnosis, and nonpsychotic hypochondriacal disorders do not seem to respond to pimozide—indeed these patients may report that they feel even less well on the drug (Riding and Munro, 1975b).

The treatment regimen is very simple. Pimozide is best administered in a single morning dose; if given later it may cause insomnia in some patients but a few individuals report drowsiness and prefer to take it at night. It often has a stimulating, even mildly euphoriant, effect but occasionally causes lethargy or depression, akathisia, and mild extrapyramidal symptoms. These symptoms are generally easily reversible with reduced dosage and antiparkinsonian medication may be useful. The dose of pimozide usually ranges from 2 to 12 mg daily.

With adequate dosage, improvement generally begins within a week. There is considerable subjective relief of tension, reduction in the intensity of the delusional belief, and much less preoccupation with the delusion. The paranoid anger disappears and many of the patients become almost embarrassingly grateful. Fairly soon most of them feel so much better that they spontaneously stop the medication and the symptoms almost invariably return within a few days. Compliance is usually assured thereafter and improvement is maintained while the drug is continued. In this series, follow-up has ranged from 6 months to 4½ years and until now only three patients have successfully come off their medication, so pimozide appears to be palliative rather than curative in most instances. Other reports of successful treatment of similar cases have begun to appear (Reilly 1975; Reilly and Beard, 1976; Trimble, 1977b; Freeman, 1979).

Discussion

There is no satisfactory explanation, psychological or otherwise, of the aetiology of paranoia and related disorders. Variations on the classic formulation by Freud (1896) continue to be quoted. He held that paranoia is a neuropsychosis of defence. In this view there is a gradual weakening of defences against self-reproaches which have been projected externally but have returned to consciousness in a delusional form and which are ascribed to others rather than the self. There is also a postulated failure to maintain homosexual wishes under repression. It has to be said that such a description, while elegant, is almost totally conjectural and has apparently been of no value in promoting effective therapy in this type of disorder.

If, for the present, MHP can be accepted as a type of paranoia then it would appear to be related to the paranoid states and paranoid schizophrenia. From the data gathered by the author it may be conjectured that MHP is actually two syndromes: one mostly affecting younger men (who often have a previous history of substance abuse) and the other occurring mainly in older women. Clinically, the impression is that the condition seen in younger patients may be more nearly allied to schizophrenia.

It is intriguing that the hypochondriacal symptoms in MHP are so specific and so stable; for example a worm delusion never seems to turn into a delusion of ugliness or of smell. Kenyon (1976) raised the question of whether monosymptomatic delusional states always had to be hypochondriacal and he cited the possible specific example of paranoid jealousy. Interestingly, Dorian (1979) has reported the successful use of pimozide in the treatment of one long-standing case of this disorder. This particular case did not arise in a setting of chronic alcoholism but many examples of paranoid jealousy do, and it would be interesting to see if the postalcoholic type also responded to pimozide.

There is no direct experimental evidence pointing to a specific brain disorder in MHP, but if it is indeed related to schizophrenia then perhaps the hypothetical findings regarding neurotransmitter dysfunction in and around the limbic system in the latter disorder may also apply to the former. Recent studies, including those of Bird et al (1977), Owen et (1978), Bacopoulos et al (1979), and Iversen (1979), all seem to indicate that in schizophrenia there is considerable overactivity of dopamine transmission in those parts of the limbic system concerned with the regulation of emotion or with associative functions for higher mental processes. Dysfunction of the limbic area in schizophreniform illnesses may result in a failure to filter information from the internal or external environment, especially those relating to visceral and sexual percepts.

Connolly (1978) has noted that there seems to be a significant correlation between olfactory hallucination (similar to one form of presentation of MHP) and gender doubt, suggesting some functional interrelationship between these two modalities, probably at, or close to, the limbic structures. If a filtering mechanism breaks down, stimuli can then be passed in a nondiscriminated fashion to higher cerebral centres (Stevens et al, 1979) and Frith (1979) has claimed that such a failure of discrimination may be the basis for delusional thinking since the individual can no longer differentiate accurately between various stimuli or assign origins or priorities to them.

It is well known that dextroamphetamine may cause paranoid disorders, as may levodopa (Carlsson, 1977), and these substances act by inducing dopaminergic hyperfunction especially in mesolimbic areas. On the other hand, Seeman et al (1975) have shown that several neuroleptic drugs can block dopamine transmission to the brain by selective receptor blockade, which is presumably part of their antipsychotic action. Butyrophenones such as haloperidol are especially effective in such blocking but pimozide, a diphenylbutylpiperidine and a highly specific dopamine blocker (Laduron et al, 1978), has been shown by Bianchi et al (1975) to be even more effective in this. In animal studies Bailey and Jackson (1978) have demonstrated that pimozide and haloperidol completely antagonize certain behavioural abnormalities induced by dextroamphetamine.

Patients with MHP suffer from a profound breakdown in their ability to discriminate between normal and abnormal somatic perceptions, and it is being tentatively suggested that their delusion and their hypochondriasis may be mediated by an endogenous dysfunction in the limbic area, which is somewhat similar to the exogenous dysfunction induced by dextroamphetamine. The therapeutic effectiveness of pimozide would indicate that the dysfunction may be the result of pathological overactivity of a dopaminergic system. As well as being deluded many patients with MHP are overalerted, tense, and angry, and those with insect infestation delusions quite often report sleep deprivation since they spend much of the night awake searching for parasites. It is noteworthy that pimozide can attenuate dextroamphetamine-induced sleep changes (again probably mediated through a dopaminergic system) and that it produces a marked improvement in the sleep EEG of psychotic patients (Gillin et al, 1978). In practice patients with MHP often report an improvement in sleep and a sense of relaxation as their delusion diminishes following the administration of pimozide. At this stage their insight usually improves and they seem much more able to distinguish between real and imaginary sensory stimuli.

Conclusion

MHP appears to be a relatively specific clinical syndrome. Speculative evidence points to a dysfunction of a particular brain area, the dysfunction conceivably being due to overactivity of one neurotransmitter—dopamine. There is an unmistakable and clear-cut treatment response to pimozide, a very specific dopamin antagonist. It is suggested that this is one of the most suitable psychiatric disorders for systematic research by psychological, neurochemical and pharmacological means. Evidence is accumulating that MHP is much less rare than previously supposed, so making it very worthwhile to identify and treat it. Although the patients are initially difficult and uncooperative, response to treatment is striking and most gratifying.

The author wishes to thank the following colleagues for their permission to make reference to patients: Drs R W Brooks-Hill, H Wolkoff, and A Seltzer of the Toronto General Hospital, and Dr J D Atcheson of the Clarke Institute of Psychiatry, Toronto.

References

Andreasen, N C (1977) *American Journal of Psychiatry*, **134**, 1313
Bacopoulos, N C, Spokes, E G, Bird, E D, Roth, R H (1979) *Science*, **205**, 1405
Bailey, R C, Jackson, D M (1978) *Psychopharmacology*, **56**, 317
Bebbington, P E (1976) *British Journal of Psychiatry*, **128**, 475
Bianchi, A et al (1975) *Acta psychiatrica Belgica*, **78**, 69
Bird, E D, Barnes, J, Iversen, L, Spokes, E G, MacKay, A V P, Shepherd, M (1977) *Lancet*, ii, 1157
Bjerg Hansen, E (1976) Paranoia Hypochondriaca. Frederiksberg Publishers, Copenhagen
British Medical Journal (1978) ii, 588
Cameron, N A (1974) in American Handbook of Psychiatry. Vol. 3(2nd edn). Basic Books, New York. p.676
Carlsson, A (1977) *Psychological Medicine*, **7**, 583
Connolly, F H (1978) *British Medical Journal*, ii, 963
—, Gipson, M (1978) *British Journal of Psychiatry*, **132**, 568
Dorian, B J (1979) *Canadian Journal of Psychiatry*, **24**, 377
Edwards, R (1977) *British Medical Journal*, i, 1219
Ekbom, K A (1938) *Acta psychiatrica et neurologica Scandinavica*, **13**, 227
Freeman, H (1979) *British Journal of Psychiatry*, **135**, 82
Freud, S (1896) in Standard Edition (1962), Vol. 3. Hogarth Press. London. p.206
Frith, C D (1979) *British Journal of Psychiatry*, **134**, 225
Gillin, J C, van Kammen. D P. Bunney. W E (1978) *Life Sciences*, **22**, 1805
Gould, W M, Gragg, T M (1976) *Archives of Dermatalogy*, **112**, 1745
Hay, G G (1970) *British Journal of Psychiatry*, **116**, 399
Iversen, I (1979) *Scientific American*, **241**, 134
Kenyon, F E (1976) *British Journal of Psychiatry*, **129**, 1
Laduron, P M et al (1978) *Biochemistry and Pharmacology*, **27**, 317
Levy, H (1906) Thesis. Steinheil. Paris
Marbach (1978) *American Journal of Psychiatry*, **135**, 476
Munro. A (1980) *Journal of Psychiatric Treatment and Evaluation*
Owen, F, Crow, T S, Poulter, M, Cross, A S, Longden, A, Riley, G T (1978) *Lancet*, ii, 223
Plantey, F (1977) *ibid*, i, 1105
Pryse-Phillips, W (1971) *Acta psychiatrica Scandinavica*, **47**, 484

Reichenberger, M (1972) *Medizinische Monatsschrift*, **26**, 313
Reilly, T M (1975) *Lancet*, i, 1385
— (1977) *Proceedings of the Royal Society of Medicine*, **70**, Suppl. 10. p.39
—, Beard, A W (1976) *British Journal of Psychiatry*, **129**, 191
Retterstol, N (1968) *Acta psychiatrica Scandinavica*, **44**, 334
Riding, J. Munro, A (1975a) *Lancet*, i, 400
—, — (1975b) *Acta Psychiatrica Scandinavica*, **52**, 23
Ross, M S, Moldofsky, H (1978) *American Journal of Psychiatry*, **135**, 585
Schachter, M (1971) *Annals of Medical Psychology*, **129**, 723
Seeman, P et al (1975) *Proceedings of the National Academy of Sciences of the United States of America*, **72**, 4376
Skott, A (1978) Delusions of Infestation : Reports from the Psychiatric Research Centre, No. 13, St. Jörgen Hospital. Unversity of Göteborg, Sweden.
Slade, P D, Russell, GFM (1973) *Psychological Medicine*, **3**, 188
Stevens, J R et al (1979) *Archives of General Psychiatry*, **36**, 251
Susskind, W (1973) *in* Psychosomatic Medicine (edited by Munro, A). Churchill Livingstone, Edinburgh. p.8
Trimble, M (1977a) *British Medical Journal*, ii, 1541
— (1977b) personal communication

Chapter 10

Management problems in psychogeriatrics

Brice Pitt, The London Hospital

Psychogeriatrics usually deals with psychiatric disorders presenting in those over 65 years of age and thus covers a period of about 30 years. The psychiatry of older people has much in common with that of the young. However, the proportion of those with addiction and personality disorder is less while that of those with organic illness is considerably more, and multiple pathology (physical and mental) is much more frequent.

Morbidity

About 25 per cent of the elderly suffer from psychiatric symptoms of disabilities (Kay et al, 1964). The commonest concern mood, depression and anxiety, but the most troublesome affect cognition, especially dementia which afflicts about 10 per cent of those over 65 and more than 20 per cent of those over 80 (Kay et al, 1970). Fourteen per cent of the population of England and Wales are now over 65 and by the end of the century those over 75 will have increased by a third (DHSS, 1978). So the first management problem for psychogeriatrics is the high morbidity of a large and increasing population at risk.

Who treats them?

The second problem concerns the question of who is going to treat the elderly with psychiatric symptoms. Some geriatricians have done so (Prinsley, 1973; Portsmouth, 1974) but while most of their colleagues are willing to deal with the delirious and those with a significant physical disorder, few wish to tackle the severely depressed and those with paranoid and difficult personalities, let alone the robust demented. It is indeed inappropriate that a training in psychiatry should not be regarded as essential for those dealing with the psychiatry of old age, yet until relatively recently psychiatrists themselves have been slow to offer a comprehensive service to the elderly. While ready enough to treat the more obviously treatable, such as those with depression presenting for the first time in their late 60s, psychiatrists' enthusiasm for the less tractable problems, especially dementia, has been inconspicuous. Consequently the confused elderly and their families and GPs have often fallen victim to buck-passing and demarcation disputes with the Social Services as well as between psychiatry and geriatrics, which may leave them little choice but to confect a medical emergency or engineer a social crisis in order somehow to get a bed somewhere (see below).

Within the last 20 years, however, there has developed a subspecialty of general psychiatry, psychogeriatrics (Jolley, 1976), which is now accorded recognition as a section of the Royal College of Psychiatrists and in about half the Health Districts in the country there is a consultant psychiatrist with a special interest in the elderly to whom he gives the bulk of his time (Wattis et al, 1981). In comparison with general psychiatrists, psychogeriatricians tend to have a larger area to serve, less assistance and worse resources (White, 1979). In comparison with child psychiatrists their training for the task is paltry. There are but a handful of senior registrar posts in geriatric psychiatry and concern has been expressed by the College's assessors (Rawnsley and Kendell, 1979). Meanwhile most consultants learn the job as they go along.

Widespread ageist (Butler, 1975) attitudes of defeatism and disparagement impede training, recruitment, and the practice of good psychiatry and also condone a philosophy of second best as good enough for the elderly. Psychogeriatric beds and clinics are even rarer than geriatric facilities in main teaching hospitals (Pitt, 1980) and too many doctors qualify still believing that psychiatric illness in the elderly signifies dementia which means disposal to somewhere else—a geriatric or mental hospital or a residential home.

Nevertheless the elegant epidemiological, nosological, and prognostic studies of Roth and the Newcastle-upon-Tyne school and of Post at the Bethlem and the Maudsley hospitals have shown to the discerning the fascination of the psychiatry of old age, and the challenge of a neglected area is sufficiently attractive to those with a pioneering spirit for the infant subspecialty of psychogeriatrics to be quite lusty!

The expertise of the psychogeriatrician is as much administrative as clinical (Arie, 1971). He must develop a multidisciplinary team that undertakes responsibility for the problems of old people needing psychiatric help in a defined area. Ready availability, prompt appraisal, swift action where necessary, and deft liaison with the primary health care team, the geriatric and social services, and families and caring neighbours are of the first importance, so a good full-time secretary is particularly essential (White, 1979).

Assessment and diagnosis

Assessment at home is the favoured response to referral. The meagre or inaccurate information so often given over the telephone is particularly inadequate to determine priority where resources are scarce. A domiciliary consultation avoids the expectation that the hospital can provide the answer (perhaps only a quarter may be admitted to a psychiatric bed: Pitt, 1982), and enables the problem to be seen where it presents, family and neighbours to be met, the local assets and liabilities to be noted, and the correct social diagnosis as well as the medical one to be made. With any luck the GP, social worker, health visitor, district nurse, or home-help may be present. Domiciliary assessment takes travel time but it is usually time well spent. Patients who need more detailed investigation without admission can be followed-up as day patients or outpatients.

If the patient requires admission a joint psychogeriatric assessment and short-stay treatment unit may best serve his various needs and promotes liaison between the psychiatric and geriatric services. Pitt and Silver (1980) have described one such unit. It is particularly useful for patients with delirium, those whose dementia needs investigation, those with significant physical *and* mental disorder, and those whose malaise, enfeeblement, anorexia, or incontinence is hard to ascribe clearly to a physical or a mental disease at a domiciliary visit. The psychiatrist and the geriatrician share a weekly multidisciplinary round and teach each other, their juniors, and the other staff their skills. The unit gives the psychogeriatric patient a place in the general hospital and enables psychiatric disorders such as transitory confusion or depression to be detected in those with predominantly physical symptoms. The collaboration necessary presents the community with the unified service advocated by Arie (1979). If there is no such unit a few beds on an acute geriatric ward may be set aside for joint appraisal (Arie and Dunn, 1973) or at least the psychiatrist and the geriatrician should consult regularly on each other's wards.

In the Nottingham unit described by Morton et al (1968) a senior social worker shared rights of admission and responsibility for arranging continuing care where necessary with the psychiatrist and the geriatrician. Unhappily, since the Seebohm revolution (Seebohm Committee, 1968) the separation of social work from the health services and the sacrifice of specialization to the concept of the generic worker have meant that such a happy arrangement is now rare indeed and the problem of a proper liaison with the Social Services is one of the biggest for psychogeriatrics. The need is obvious from the high psychiatric morbidity of the social worker's elderly clients (usually allocated to the least trained) and of the residents of local authority homes—Masterton et al (1979) found definite dementia in 27 per cent of these residents and some organic impairment in 66 per cent. However, Baker and Byrne (1977) worked hard at liaison by visiting area offices, sometimes social workers visit their clients in hospital and discuss them with the staff, and there are signs (Plank, 1979) that Social Service departments are starting to accept the need to do better for their elderly.

An alert and responsive psychogeriatric service encourages early diagnosis. The Edinburgh survey by Williamson et al (1964) demonstrated that GPs were unaware of 60 per cent of the cases of neurosis, 76 per cent of the cases of depression, and 87 per cent of the cases of slight to moderate dementia in their elderly patients. Barraclough's (1971) study of elderly suicides showed that many had seen their doctors shortly before their deaths but were not being treated for depression. Even the experts err, however. Roth (1979) commented on the Newcastle survey: "We are very poor at recognizing dementia in its early stages. In our own community studies we failed to recognize four fifths of those who were to present with unequivocal dementia 3–4 years later, but in other cases in which a positive diagnosis was made it was proved erroneous."

Nevertheless diagnosis is improved by education and motivation—the knowledge of which mental illnesses can befall the elderly and how to detect them, and the desire to treat them. The support of a psychogeriatric service should encourage the vigilance of the primary health care team. Depression is far more treatable if recognized within months rather than years, paranoia may be less entrenched if approached before all relationships have been terminated, and the vital support given by the families of the demented may continue indefinitely if regular relief and the sharing of care are offered early rather than late (Bergmann et al, 1978).

Apart from failure to find cases and refer them, misdiagnosis is all too common. This is partly because of the following: a mental set that expects dementia in the elderly, uncertainty about the range of normal behaviour in old age, the lack of a proper history (for which few tests, be they psychometric, biochemical, radiological, or physiological, are adequate substitutes), possible distortion of the clinical picture by premature medication, and the fact that the operation of more than one pathological process is not appreciated.

There are also some special diagnostic pitfalls; for example after perhaps 3 months the patient with subacute delirium may recover and demand to go home but because he was thought to be demented his flat would have been given up. Hare (1978) has pointed out the much better prognosis of confusional states if there are not parietal signs; patients whose problems are only with memory are far more likely to be discharged.

Depression too may be misdiagnosed as dementia when the patient is slow and vague; a previous or family history of depression, the onset of depressive symptoms before apparent memory impairment, the presence of malaise and querulousness if not frank nihilism and despair, early waking, diurnal variation in mood, weight loss, a failure to confabulate, and ultimately the response to antidepressant therapy or electroplexy are all helpful in reaching the correct conclusion. The attention-seeking agitated depressive may wrongly be labelled as hysterical by the brash or unwary and the severe anguish to which the perplexed patient is seeking to draw attention is missed. However, a far more common error is to overlook the masked atypical or moderate depression, either ascribing the condition to age without realizing how it has altered and limited the elderly person's life or investigating inexorably with successive tests at different clinics the depressive who presents only bodily symptoms.

Mania in old people sometimes presents as delirium. Long-established personality traits that cause difficulty such as cantankerousness, obstinacy, parsimony, hoarding, and reclusiveness are sometimes hopefully attributed to mental illness with the vague expectation that the psychiatrist will be able to remove the symptoms. And a behaviour disorder such as faecal incontinency or suicidal threats or gestures may wrongly be thought to indicate illness when in fact it may be an expression of disturbed relationships.

Treatment

After early and correct diagnosis the next principle of psychogeriatric treatment is to keep the patient at home as long as possible provided neither he nor those caring for him suffer unduly. Not only are institutional resources scarce but also old people fare best in familiar surroundings. This does not mean avoiding admission at all costs: often early treatment in hospital or a respite for the relatives by taking the old person into a residential home for a week or two means that long-term care can be avoided altogether. Although the proportion of middle-aged to elderly women has dropped and the proportion of the former out at work has increased from 10 per cent in 1921 to 50 per cent in 1971 (Moroney, 1976), families are still the mainstay of the elderly psychiatric patient at home. Of the demented elderly 80 per cent live in no kind of institution and Bergmann et al (1978) concluded from a study of patients with this disorder admitted to a day hospital that family support was the most important factor determining their continuing life in the community.

The psychogeriatric service can prescribe treatment to be taken at home, try to increase personal social services where appropriate, provide a community psychogeriatric nurse (for counselling and support, supervision, follow-up, and the administration of drugs), and arrange outpatient consultations, day hospital attendance, and short-term admission for holiday relief as a part of community care.

Outpatient clinics are useful when further investigations are needed as well as for psychotherapy and marital therapy and are an economical means of follow-up, but they work best where the patients do not require ambulance transport. Psychogeriatric patients are actually under-represented in outpatient clinics.

Day hospitals are unfortunately very dependent on ambulances which because of staff and oil shortages and industrial action have become less reliable lately while long distances and congested traffic have always meant that many of those attending take a considerable time getting to and from the centre. Nevertheless they are invaluable in providing an alternative to admission for treatment (Ford Robertson and Pitt, 1965) and accelerating the discharge of functional patients, and in containing large numbers of the demented awaiting continuing institutional care. These two functions are best kept separate in different wings of the day hospital or even different day hospitals. The DHSS (1972) recommended 0.65 day places/1000 elderly for the treatment of functional disorders (which is too few in view of the high prevalence, tendency to relapse, and chronicity) and 2–3 day places/1000 elderly for the demented. Baker and Byrne (1977) claimed that by increasing day care and community nursing the need for beds for the demented is much reduced but some, for example Jolley (1977), would contest this.

Relief admissions of the demented are most useful in enabling the key supporter to take a holiday. When used for respite, the supporter's tolerance may subsequently actually be reduced. Also the patient's confusion may be temporarily increased.

Relatives' support groups are not easy to convene but can provide powerful self-help for those facing the common problem of dementia (Fuller et al, 1979). Through these means or through personal support by the social worker, health visitor, GP, or sometimes the psychiatrist, the supporters are supported. Practical measures such as arranging an attendance allowance or a laundry service for the incontinent need to be complemented by help with such troubled and troublesome feelings as distress, bewilderment, overanxiety, anger, guilt, and scapegoating.

The numbers of the demented are so formidable and the effects of the disorder so devastating that every means of containing it within the community must be sought and energetically employed. Home-helps, paid "good neighbours", street and estate wardens, and sheltered housing and boarding-out are means of assisting or replacing family support. It is to be hoped that greater public awareness of the scale of the problems of mental infirmity in old age and the limitations of the service the State can provide will mean more voluntary work, especially by neighbourhood organizations and the fitter elderly.

A third principle of psychogeriatric treatment is neither to overtreat nor to undertreat. Overtreatment is apparent when a confused old person has been rendered drowsy, dehydrated, hypotensive, and ataxic through the administration of, say, chlorpromazine 100 mg intramuscularly for noisy restlessness on the night of admission to hospital. Incontinence, bed sores, fractures, and hypostatic pneumonia are other hazards of such overtreatment. Of course the other patients need their rest but such drastic drugging is rarely justified and talking to the patient until he has settled, nursing in a side room, or the use of a mild hypnotic like chlormethiazole of dichloralphenazone often suffices.

No drugs are of much use to the confused elderly. The tranquillizers (of which thioridazine and haloperidol are the most generally useful) may all cause sleepiness and immobility. The cerebrovascular dilators or activators have little effect on daily activities although they improve marginally some cognitive tests (*Drugs and*

Therapeutics Bulletin, 1975) and none of the substances intended to potentiate cholinergic mechanisms in Alzheimer's disease (for example choline chloride; Boyd et al, 1977) has proved its worth.

Overtreatment is probable when a formerly paranoid patient is admitted for falls, stiff with parkinsonism and perhaps drooling after 6 months on a depot preparation such as flupenthixol. Yet phenothiazines effectively control the delusions, auditory hallucinations and hostile behaviour of paraphrenia (Post, 1966) which can render an old person too difficult to remain in the community, and depot preparations ensure the necessary compliance. The dilemma is that the cure may be as bad as the disease. The best course is to treat only when the disorder is truly troublesome, to use the lowest effective dose possible and oral medication wherever compliance seems at all likely, to be especially cautious in the presence of confusion or physical infirmity, to use antiparkinsonian drugs at the first sign of side effects, to try occasional drug holidays, and to maintain close supervision during follow-up.

Examples of undertreatment are the overcautious prescription of antidepressants, not giving ECT when it is needed, not considering leucotomy for chronic severe agitated depression, and denying the elderly patient psychological treatments that take time and skill such as psychotherapy and behaviour therapy.

For true depressive illness most elderly patients require full adult dosages of antidepressant drugs, for example 75–150 mg dothiepin daily; monoamine oxidase inhibitors occasionally have their place, either alone or combined with tricyclics, in resistant cases. Lithium carbonate certainly has a place in the treatment of recurrent bipolar depressive illness in the elderly, but the risk of toxicity must be noted if there is renal impairment or diuretics are used.

Electroplexy came under fire recently from some people who are neither psychiatrists nor severe depressives (Kendell, 1978) but has withstood the attack and remains an honoured treatment in psychogeriatric practice. It can save the life of the nigh stuporose potentially dehydrated melancholic and avoid or reduce the stay in hospital of properly selected depressed patients, generally those with the more endogenous features. True, it is rarely a once and for all treatment but how many medical treatments are? It is remarkably safe and significant confusion after its use is far less common than is popularly feared, especially if a unilateral technique is used over the nondominant hemisphere and treatments are well spaced (for example weekly).

Leucotomy is in still worse odour but the modern techniques such as stereotactic tractotomy (Knight, 1969) are a far cry from the old cutting operations and can relieve the appalling anguish of chronic or frequently recurrent agitated depression that responds to no other remedies.

At the other end of the spectrum of psychiatric treatments are the psychological therapies—individual, marital, group and behaviour—which play too small a part in many psychogeriatric programmes because of the lack of skills, personnel, and the recognition that they have a proper place. They need adaptation to older patients but may be of value in dealing with the fear, resentment and hostility that may underlie symptoms and in lessening disturbed, disruptive, helpless, and hopeless behaviour.

Psychotherapy sessions may be shorter than for younger patients, with more enjoyment than interpretation of the transference and less pressure to terminate, although the intervals between sessions may be increased. Group therapy needs to be on hard chairs and before meals to combat somnolence. Among the objectives are freer expression of suppressed feelings and mutual support. Behaviour therapy includes operant conditioning (the reward for better behaviour commonly being staff time and attention) and assertive techniques to overcome "learned helpless-ness" (Seligman, 1975).

Institutional care is the lot of a minority of the elderly who are more likely to be isolated (by personality as well as circumstances), demented, and much older than those who remain at home. The provision of appropriate institutional care when it is needed is the major problem for psychogeriatrics today. When a demented old person living alone is seriously at risk or already suffering from self-neglect, despite the full use of community services or if the key supporter is intolerably strained, care should be arranged speedily. The inability always to achieve this is, frankly, scandalous and the need to appear to condone harrowing situations and to bear the brunt of the natural resentment of those who suffer is a challenge to the morale of those in the front line of psychogeriatrics.

Controversies about the respective roles of residential homes (Part III, volun-tary, and private) and geriatric or psychiatric wards can easily be resolved given goodwill and plenty of places by following the DHSS's (1972) guidelines: severely demented old people with a serious behaviour disturbance who are physically fit belong in psychiatric accommodation and those whose physical condition needs medical treatment (be they more or less severely demented) in geriatric accom-modation, while the rest are admitted to residential homes. In practice there is much acrimony about placements; criteria are modified according to circumstances and old people lodged unsuitably in one kind of accommodation may well have to await a swap to be better placed.

There is debate about the provision of special residential homes for the elderly mentally infirm. One view, for example that of the Group for the Psychiatry of Old Age of the Royal College of Psychiatrists (1976), supports them provided there is good liaison with the psychogeriatric service as well as trained staff, a high staff:resident ratio, and a special routine to meet these very disabled old people's special needs. Another view (for example Meacher, 1972) however, is that segregation and labelling confirm and increase the disability.

Morale on long-stay psychogeriatric wards needs to be sustained by an appropri-ate nurse-patient ratio (1:1.2 where the patients are heavily dependent), frequent and regular visits by the doctor, the senior staff, the physiotherapist, and the occupational therapist, and the staff's awareness of their particular role within the range of resources of the psychogeriatric team. Measures to combat institutional neurosis (Barton, 1966) should be promoted from the start for it is apparent often within a couple of days of admission after the elderly person has been processed for the institutional routine, disorientated by strange people and surroundings, bewil-dered by bizarre procedures, puzzled by the incongruous familiarity of very young nurses and their meaningless endearments, drugged into immobility and somno-lence, and deprived of personal clothing, possessions, occupation, and choice.

Giving the elderly patient his proper name and title, ensuring that he has the use of his glasses, hearing aid and false teeth, enabling him to have a locker, a wardrobe and personal clothing, communicating with him, and consulting his wishes as far as possible all help to preserve his personality and self-respect and a measure of independence.

Reality orientation therapy (Folsom, 1967) is a technique for teaching the patients some simple but useful facts by the regular and frequent reiteration of information about time, place, and person and the use of commonly encountered objects. Its value in improving the memory and social functioning of moderately demented subjects has been shown by Brook et al (1975) and Woods (1979). Keeping medication to the necessary minimum, a full programme of activities including exercise sessions, regular visits to accessible comfortable lavatories, and walks and excursions, as well as unrestricted visiting (which maintains bonds between patients and families and provides a valuable source of voluntary help) and cheerful surroundings with clear guides to orientation all help to sustain some quality of life in the final years. All this should not be regarded as an unattainable ideal but the least that should be provided as of right.

Psychogeriatric emergencies

To conclude I shall mention briefly the various problems that are presented as crises to a psychogeriatric service. The majority are, unfortunately, more social than medical (Arie, 1974) and represent desperate attempts to beat a frustrating system and to find quickly a safe place for a (usually) demented and difficult old person. The problem has probably been present for months if not years, but all of a sudden through death, sickness or rejection the key supporter is no longer available or the family, having visited after an interval of a few weeks, has woken up to the precariousness of the old person's existence. A last-straw incident of wandering, incontinence, burning the kettle, leaving the gas on unlit, or calling the doctor out once too often may precipitate a demand that something be done.

Before a crisis of intolerance has been reached and when no alternative to institutional care is brooked, the presence of an active psychogeriatric service with a full range of facilities and the identification of cases should reduce such referrals for which, otherwise, there is no simple satisfactory answer. A prompt visit by the psychogeriatric team may enable an appropriate short-term admission or intensification of day care and community supports to be arranged at once. If not, there is likely to be an emergency admission to a temporary place in a residential home or on some rather dubious medical pretext to an acute hospital bed, with animosity all round.

Genuine psychiatric emergencies in the elderly include the following:

1. The acute confusional state which presents with restless perplexed agitation and sometimes visual hallucinations and is most commonly due to a chest infection or a small stroke or is drug induced. The treatment is for the cause while the patient is carefully nursed without undue sedation usually in a general hospital ward, especially a joint geriatric/psychiatric ward if available. A clear history of confusion of recent onset should always suggest the diagnosis of an acute confusional state rather than dementia, although the former can complicate the latter.
2. Mania can start by resembling an acute confusional state, but the confusion passes and euphoric irritable hyperactivity remains. There is often a previous history of mania or depressed episodes. Treatment is usually with haloperidol 5–10 mg intramuscularly initially then 1–3 mg orally three times daily, with orphenadrine 50–100 mg three times daily if signs of parkinsonism develop. If there have been frequent recurrences lithium carbonate may be introduced. Compulsory admission (see below) may be warranted.
3. Severe depression causing overtly suicidal behaviour or failure to eat or drink requires prompt admission, rehydration where indicated, ECT (where there is

nigh stuporose negativism and low oral intake), sedation for severe agitation, and antidepressants.

4. Paranoia may arise from confusion, paraphrenia, or personality (see 5). Confusional paranoia results from the patient blaming others for difficulties arising from his forgetfulness which he fails to recognize. The paranoia takes the form of outbursts that pass quite quickly and are forgotten sooner by the patient than by those at whom they are directed. Medication is of little value and probably the best management is helping the accused to understand the pathology of the accusation, not to take it personally, and to respond constructively with tact rather than to argue or take umbrage.

   The sustained delusions, hallucinations, and hostility of the paraphrenic may erupt into violence towards neighbours (although this is rarely dangerous) or result in withdrawal into a state of siege with a serious risk of self-neglect and malnutrition. This again may necessitate compulsory admission. The pros and cons of phenothiazine therapy have been discussed above.

5. Personality clashes between husband and wife, parent and child or children, neighbours or helpers and helped are as common among the old as the young, but more likely in the former to lead to labelling as mentally ill. Difficult, paranoid, stubborn, uninhibited and eccentric old people have a greater tendency than more compliant, stable and sociable ones to clash with others, but it takes two to make a quarrel. The young and the untrained or inexperienced would-be helpers can ask for trouble by the brash, clumsy, officious or patronizing way in which they approach older relatives or clients, or by their hasty or offended reactions. Management involves taking a long unbiased look at the parties separately, placating them, removing the label if it is not applicable, and pointing out that since psychiatry cannot change personalities very much what cannot be remedied must be endured! Once endorsed, this can be the basis of an improved relationship in which the awkward old person is accepted for what he is rather than rejected for not being someone else.

Compulsory admission is used for perhaps 5 per cent of old people who come into psychiatric wards, usually when paranoid, manic, or dangerously depressed and less often when confused. The compulsion is, of course, on the patient whose mental illness endangers him (or others) or who is in serious need of treatment which because of the mental illness he is unwilling to accept; the compulsion is not on the hospital to take him if they do not think fit or if they do not have a bed. Sections 29 and 25 of the Mental Health Act, 1959, allow admission for 3 and 28 days, respectively. Application is made by the next of kin or a social worker, supported by the recommendation of one (Section 29) or of two (Section 25) doctors, one of whom must have special experience in mental illness. Sometimes the social worker is either unwilling to make an application or, out of office hours, unavailable. In this case, if the patient is disturbed and in a public place the police may be able to take him to hospital under Section 136.

Where there is no frank mental illness but an old person through eccentricity or infirmity is in a state of serious self-neglect or living in conditions so bad that they endanger health, Section 47 of the National Assistance Act, 1947, enables the community physician to apply to his local authority for compulsory removal to hospital or a residential home. A magistrate must make the order which is effective for 3 weeks or 3 months according to whether or not the person has been given a week's notice of the action intended. Except under those special circumstances, no old person can be compelled to go into a residential home.

Summary

Problems for psychogeriatrics include the large numbers of the elderly and their high morbidity for mental disorder, the lack of commitment to and training for specialization in the field, and ageist attitudes. A psychogeriatric team, assessment before admission, and active liaison are essential to a psychogeriatric service. Early diagnosis, keeping the patient at home as much as possible, and neither overtreating nor undertreating are important principles of therapy. Institutional care is vital for a minority of patients but less available than it should be. Most psychogeriatric emergencies are social and affect the demented. Others include acute confusional states, mania, severe depression, paranoia, and personality clashes. Compulsory admission may sometimes be justified in their management.

References

Arie, T (1971) *British Medical Journal*, iii, 166
— (1974) *in* Medicine in Old Age (edited by Ware, M). British Medical Journal Publications, Devonshire Press, Torquay
— (1979) *Bulletin of the Royal College of Psychiatrists*, November, 168
—, Dunn, T (1973) *Lancet*, ii, 1313
Baker, A A, Byrne, R J F (1977) *British Journal of Psychiatry*, **130**, 123
Barraclough, B (1971) *in* Recent Developments in Psychogeriatrics (edited by Kay, D W K, Walk, A). Headly Bros, Ashford. p.87
Barton, R (1966) Institutional Neurosis, 2nd edn. Wright, Bristol
Bergmann, K, Foster, E M, Justice, A W, Matthews, V (1978) *British Journal of Psychiatry*, **132**, 441
Boyd, W D, Graham White, J, Blackwood, G, Glen, I, McQueen, J (1977) *Lancet*, ii, 711
Brook, P, Degun, G, Mather, M (1975) *British Journal of Psychiatry*, **127**, 42
Butler, R N (1975) Why Survive Being Old in America? Harper and Row, New York
DHSS (1972) Services for Mental Illness Related to Old Age. HMSO (72)71
— (1978) A Happier Old Age. HMSO, London (Welsh Office)
Drugs and Therapeutics Bulletin (1975) **13**, 85
Folsom, J C (1967) *Current Psychiatric Therapeutics*, **7**, 209
Ford Robertson, W M, Pitt, B (1965) *British Journal of Psychiatry*, **111**, 635
Fuller, J, Ward, E, Evans, A, Masam, K, Gardner, A (1979) *British Medical Journal*, i, 1684
Group for the Psychiatry of Old Age of the Royal College of Psychiatrists (1976) *British Journal of Psychiatry*, September, 10
— (1978) *Bulletin of the Royal College of Psychiatrists*, January, 4
Hare, M (1978) *British Medical Journal*, ii, 266
Jolley, D J (1976) *Bulletin of the Royal College of Psychiatrists*, September
— (1977) *British Medical Journal*, i, 1335
Kay, D K W, Beamish, P, Roth, M (1964) *British Journal of Psychiatry*, **110**, 146
—, Bergmann, K, Foster, E M, McKechnie, A A, Roth, M (1970) *Comprehensive Psychiatry*, **11**, 1
Kendell, R E (1978) *Journal of the Royal Society of Medicine*, **71**, 319
Knight, G (1969) *British Journal of Psychiatry*, **115**, 257
Masterton, G, Holloway, E M, Timbury, G C (1979) *Age and Ageing*, **8**, 226
Meacher, M (1972) Taken for a Ride. Longman, London
Moroney, R M (1976) The Family and the State:Considerations for Social Policy. Longman, London
Morton, E, Barker, M, MacMillan, D (1968) *Gerontologia clinica*, **10**, 65
Pitt, B (1982) Psychogeriatrics: An Introduction to the Psychiatry of Old Age, 2nd edn. Churchill Livingstone, London and Edinburgh
— (1980) *Canadian Journal of Psychiatry*, **25**, 15
—, Silver, C P (1980) *Age and Ageing*, **9**, 33
Plank, D (1979) An Overview of the Position of Elderly People in Society. MIND, London
Portsmouth, O H D (1974) *Geriatrics*, **29**, No.6, 142
Post, F (1966) Persistent Persecutory States in the Elderly. Pergamon, London
Prinsley, D M (1973) *British Medical Journal*, iv, 169
Rawnsley, K, Kendell, R E (1979) *Bulletin of the Royal College of Psychiatrists*, July, 124

Roth, M (1979) Positive Approaches to Mental Infirmity in Old Age. 1978 Annual Conference Report. MIND, London

Seebohm Committee (1968) Report of the Committee on Local Authority and Allied Personal Social Services. Command Report No. 3703, HMSO, London

Seligman, M (1975) Helplessness: On Depression, Development and Death. W H Freeman, San Francisco

Wattis, J, Wattis, L and Aric, T (1981) *British Medical Journal*, **1**, 1529

White, D M D (1979) *Bulletin of the Royal College of Psychiatrists*, May, 77

Williamson, J et al (1964) *Lancet*, i, 1117

Woods, R T (1979) *British Journal of Psychiatry*, **134**, 502

Chapter 11

Toxic psychosis

Kenneth Davison, Newcastle General Hospital

Toxic psychosis is an imprecise and almost obsolete term which is still used somewhat loosely. To quote Lipowski (1980): "Toxic psychosis is a term most often used in reference to organic mental disorders caused by drugs and poisons. The use of this ambiguous term should be discouraged since it does not refer to any particular descriptive or etiologic class of disorders, but conceals several syndromes ..." The syndromes concerned are more precisely classified as follows (McClelland, 1981):

1. Behavioural toxicity (minimal or borderline reactions)
2. Delirium (confusional state, acute brain syndrome)
3. Affective reactions
   a. Depression
   b. Hypomania and mania
4. Paranoid and schizophrenia-like psychoses
5. Hallucinatory states
6. Dementia and pseudodementia
7. Neuropsychiatric states.

Behavioural toxicity

This term covers a number of symptoms and behavioural changes which can occur singly or in combination. These include drowsiness, insomnia, vivid dreams and nightmares, mild depression, mild excitement, anxiety, irritability, sensitivity to noise, listlessness, and restlessness (McClelland, 1981). Such symptoms hardly qualify for the epithet "psychosis" but they may be the precursors of more florid disturbances, particularly delirium.

Drowsiness

This is one of the commonest adverse drug effects (Martys, 1979). It is usually dose-dependent and is important because impaired concentration and prolonged reaction time may have adverse effects on driving ability (Skegg et al, 1979).

Behavioural changes

Such changes as irritability, aggressive outbursts, and general hostility are a component of many psychotic states but can also occur alone. More unusual behavioural disturbances include violence and hypersexuality from combined

TABLE 11.1. Drugs inducing behavioural toxicity (Davison, 1980)

Drowsiness	benzodiazepines
	phenothiazines
	antihistamines
	tricyclic antidepressants
	hypotensive drugs
Vivid dreams and nightmares	beta blockers
	methyldopa
	clonidine
	reserpine
	baclofen
	fenfluramine
	barbiturate or benzodiazepine withdrawal
Behavioural changes	benzodiazepines
	levodopa
	methyldopa + haloperidol
	levodopa + carbidopa
	lithium + neuroleptic drugs

levodopa–carbidopa therapy (Lin and Ziegler, 1976) and episodes of sleepwalking in patients taking lithium together with neuroleptic drugs (Charney et al, 1979).

The principal drugs concerned in the production of behavioural toxicity are listed in *Table 11.1*

Delirium

The cardinal feature of delirium (confusional state, acute brain syndrome) is a fluctuating impairment of consciousness resulting in diminished awareness of the self and the environment. This is manifested clinically as disorientation in time and space but, as the examination may coincide with a lucid interval, other evidence such as patchy amnesia and noisy restlessness at night must be taken into account. The patient's mood ranges from apathy through perplexity to excitement or panic and paranoid misinterpretation occurs. Hallucinations, predominantly visual, are frequently experienced and on recovery the patient usually has only a partial recollection of his experiences (Lipowski, 1980).

Delirium is common in the elderly, particularly in those with concurrent physical illness (Davison, 1971). There may be accompanying incontinence, ataxia and falls leading to fractures (Macdonald and Macdonald, 1977). Common offending drugs in this age-group are digoxin, benzodiazepine and barbiturate hypnotics, minor and major tranquillizers, antidepressants, antiparkinsonian agents, hypotensive drugs, and diuretics (Jarvis, 1981). The drugs implicated in all age-groups are listed in *Table 11.2*

Affective reactions

Depression

Depressive reactions to drugs vary from mild mood changes with weepiness, loss of interest and impaired concentration to severe psychoses with psychomotor retardation, suicidal thinking, anorexia, sleep disturbance and delusions of sin, disease,

TABLE 11.2. Drugs inducing delirium (Davison, 1980)

Tranquillizers and hypnotics	barbiturates benzodiazepines bromides phenothiazines
Cardiotherapeutic drugs	digitalis diuretics beta blockers
Anticholinergic drugs	atropine and homatropine hyoscine antiparkinsonian drugs tricyclic antidepressants
Dopamine agonists	levodopa bromocriptine amantadine
Antituberculous drugs	isoniazid cycloserine rifampicin
Antibiotics	penicillin streptomycin sulphonamides
Anticonvulsants	phenytoin sodium valproate
Miscellaneous drugs	disulfiram piperazine cimetidine chloroquine oral hypoglycaemic drugs
Drug withdrawal	barbiturates benzodiazepines chlormethiazole alcohol

TABLE 11.3. Drugs inducing depression

Hypotensive drugs	reserpine methyldopa clonidine

Major tranquillizers	chlorpromazine
	thioridazine
	haloperidol
	depot injections
	   fluphenazine
	   fluphenthixol

Analgesic drugs	pentazocine indomethacin
Miscellaneous drugs	levodopa corticosteroids oral contraceptives
Stimulant withdrawal	amphetamines fenfluramine

poverty, or nihilism. Drowsiness and lethargy alone should not be construed as depressive symptoms.

The principal drugs associated with depressive reactions are listed in *Table 11.3* and the commonest offenders are discussed below.

Hypotensive drugs   Reserpine was one of the first depression-inducing drugs to be recognized (Schroeder and Perry, 1955). The onset of depression is often delayed, insidious, and commoner with high doses (Freiss, 1954) and in patients with a depressive history (Muller et al, 1955). The depression has been attributed to the central noradrenaline-depleting effect of reserpine (Mendels and Fraser, 1974).

Reserpine has been largely superseded by other hypotensive drugs but some of these can also precipitate depression. An average incidence of 5.7 per cent was found in a review of 12 trials of methyldopa (Granville-Grossman, 1971); however, a recent paper from the Boston Collaborative Drug Surveillance Program, which is a survey of side effects attributed to drugs in hospitalized patients, reported an incidence of depression in only 0.5 per cent of 1067 patients receiving methyldopa (Lawson et al, 1978). It is often difficult to assess the role of drugs as opposed to other medical and psychosocial factors in the aetiology of depression in hypertensive patients (Bant, 1978).

Major tranquillizers   Neuroleptic drugs such as chlorpromazine, thioridazine, and haloperidol are thought to precipitate or aggravate depression (Kalinowsky and Hippius, 1969). Depression and suicide have also been reported in schizophrenic patients receiving depot injections of fluphenazine (Modecate; De Alarcon and Carney, 1969) and flupenthixol (Depixol; Carney and Sheffield, 1975), but it is not clear that it is the medication that is responsible rather than the inherent features of the disorder (Forrest, 1969).

Analgesic drugs   Depression is the commonest reaction to pentazocine (Kane and Pokorny, 1975) and it occurs in association with headache in patients receiving indomethacin (Boardman and Hart, 1967).

Miscellaneous drugs   Levodopa: The association of parkinsonism with depression tends to obscure the possible depressing effects of levodopa. This probably accounts for the wide variation in the reported incidence (0–11 per cent) in different series (Goodwin, 1971).
Corticosteroids: In the 1971 report of the Boston Collaborative Drug Surveillance Program, prednisone was the commonest cause of serious psychiatric reactions in medical wards. These occurred in 5 per cent of patients receiving steroids and depression was the most frequent reaction.
Oral contraceptives: The relationship of oral contraceptives to depression is controversial but a recent review concluded that 6–10 per cent of women taking these preparations become significantly depressed (McClelland, 1981).

Stimulant withdrawal   Amphetamine withdrawal often leads to drowsiness and depression and this is one of the factors contributing to the development of psychological dependence. Withdrawal depression has also occurred with fenfluramine (Steel and Briggs, 1972).

Hypomania and mania

Some degree of euphoria is common in behavioural toxicity but specific manic or hypomanic reactions are rare. In hypomania there is elevated mood, often with accompanying excitement, arrogant hostility, overactivity, insomnia, pressure of speech, and boastful overconfidence. Mania is a more extreme form, frequently with grandiose or paranoid delusions.

Corticosteroids and ACTH are probably the commonest agents to induce euphoria amounting to hypomania, particularly in high doses (Michael and Gibbons, 1963). Levodopa induces this state in 1.5 per cent of patients (Goodwin, 1971) and associated hypersexuality may lead to socially embarrassing behaviour (Goodwin et al, 1971). The euphoriant effect of opiates is one reason for their dependence-inducing properties and similar reactions occur with pentazocine (Kane and Pokorny, 1975), cyclizine, aspirin, amantadine, and aminophylline (McClelland, 1981), although outright mania or hypomania is rare.

Mania has occurred in the puerperium after suppression of lactation by bromo-criptine (Brooke and Cookson, 1978; Vlissides et al, 1978).

The precipitation of mania by tricyclic or monoamine oxidase inhibitor anti-depressants is probably a reflection of an underlying bipolar psychosis rather than an adverse drug reaction. High doses of euphoriant drugs such as amphetamines induce paranoid psychoses rather than mania (see below).

Paranoid and schizophrenia-like psychoses

Paranoid psychoses are characterized by delusions of persecution in the absence of clouding of consciousness; these may occur either with or without auditory hallucinations. The additional presence of primary delusions, incoherence of thought, or emotional withdrawal, blunting, or incongruity warrants the description "schizophrenia-like psychoses". The clinical resemblance to natural schizophrenia can be close (Davison, 1976).

A wide spectrum of drugs and other exogenous toxins has been associated with the occurrence of these psychoses (*Table 11.4*). The more important examples are discussed below.

Hallucinogenic drugs

These include lysergide (LSD), mescaline, DOM (STP; Davison, 1976), psilocybin (in certain mushrooms; Hyde et al, 1978), phencyclidine (angel dust; Allen and Young, 1978), cannabis (Davison and Wilson, 1972), and volatile hydrocarbons contained in various solvents, glues (Merry and Zachariadis, 1962), and petrol (Tolan and Lingle, 1964). Such drugs are widely abused and are liable to precipitate psychotic reactions of the following types (Davison, 1976).

Acute drug reaction

This condition (hallucinatory "trip") is distinguished from natural schizophrenia by the preponderance of visual hallucinations and retention of insight. However, some features resemble those of acute schizophreniform psychoses. The reaction usually lasts only a few hours and occurs after a single exposure.

TABLE 11.4. Drugs and toxins inducing paranoid or schizophrenia-like psychoses (Davison, 1976)

Hallucinogens	lysergide
	mescaline
	psilocybin
	phenylcyclidine
	DOM
	cannabis
CNS stimulants	amphetamines
	appetite suppressants
	nasal decongestants
	cocaine
CNS depressants	ethyl alcohol
	barbiturates
	bromides
	chloral
	antihistamines
	anticonvulsants
Anti-infective agents	antituberculous drugs
	antimalarial drugs
	antibiotics
	sulphonamides
Cardiovascular drugs	digitalis
	stramonium
	hydrallazine
	disopyramide
	methyldopa
Antiparkinsonian drugs	levodopa
	bromocriptine
	anticholinergic drugs
Miscellaneous drugs	corticosteroids, ACTH
	indomethacin
	disulfiram
Metallic poisons	lead
	arsenic
	thallium
Vegetable poisons	mushrooms
	ergot
	lathyrus

Prolonged psychotic reaction

This is defined as being over 48 hours in duration. It resembles natural schizophrenia more closely than the acute drug reaction and can also occur after a single exposure.

Chronic psychosis

This state resembles chronic undifferentiated or simple schizophrenia and occurs after a prolonged period of drug exposure.

Spontaneous recurrence (flashback)

This is identical to the acute drug reaction but occurs spontaneously some time after the original drug exposure.

The psychotogenic effect of these drugs is probably related to their antiserotonin properties (Brawley and Duffield, 1972); serotonin (5-hydroxytryptamine) is an important neurotransmitter at cerebral synapses.

Amphetamine psychosis

This condition is met less frequently now that doctors prescribe fewer amphetamines and related compounds. It occasionally develops in someone who is taking an amphetamine for a legitimate reason such as narcolepsy (Young and Scoville, 1938) but is more likely to occur in a drug abuser. Related compounds such as methylphenidate, diethylpropion, phenmetrazine, ephedrine and propylhexedrine are occasionally responsible (Davison, 1976).

Connell (1958) described the clinical picture of amphetamine psychosis as "primarily a paranoid psychosis with ideas of reference, delusion of persecution, auditory and visual hallucinations in a setting of clear consciousness". He emphasized the absence of diagnostic physical signs and pointed out that the mental picture may be indistinguishable from paranoid schizophrenia and so often diagnosed as such. Van Praag (1968) proposed two diagnostic criteria:

1. The finding of amphetamine derivatives in the urine
2. Spontaneous recovery within 2 weeks of abstinence from the offending drug.

However, there are reports of recovery taking weeks or months (Davison, 1976).

The psychotogenic effect of amphetamines is thought to be related to their action in releasing increased amounts of dopamine and noradrenaline at cerebral synapses (Snyder, 1973).

Alcoholic hallucinosis

Ethyl alcohol is a CNS depressant which is associated with several psychiatric syndromes including a specific form of withdrawal delirium, delirium tremens. Whereas in the latter consciousness is clouded and visual hallucinations predominate, in alcoholic hallucinosis the hallucinations are auditory and consciousness and memory are unaffected (Gross et al, 1967). Characteristically the affected person becomes aware of unformed auditory hallucinations, such as clicks, knocks and bells which gradually develop into voices that criticize, threaten, or command (Saravay and Pardes, 1967). These experiences are interpreted in delusional fashion so that the sufferer feels surrounded by enemies, watched, or·spied upon and often acts on these beliefs. Comparisons with natural schizophrenia are reviewed by Davison (1976).

Hallucinatory states

The hallucinations involved are usually visual but occur alone, without other features of delirium or psychosis. They can be extremely vivid, are often in colour, and are frequently of animals. Sometimes they take a microptic or lilliputian form (Harper and Knothe, 1973). The commonest drugs implicated in this reaction are listed in *Table 11.5.*

TABLE 11.5. Drugs inducing isolated hallucinations (Davison, 1980)

Psychotropic drugs	tricyclic antidepressants benzodiazepines bromides
Antiparkinsonian drugs	levodopa bromocriptine anticholinergic drugs
Cardiovascular drugs	digitalis beta blockers disopyramide
Analgesic drugs	pentazocine indomethacin salicylates

Dementia and pseudodementia

Dementia is a deterioration, usually irreversible, of intellect, memory, and personality and is normally secondary to organic cerebral disease. Although this syndrome has been reported in patients receiving levodopa (Hunter et al, 1973), isoniazid (*British Medical Journal*, 1969), or lithium salts alone (Ghose, 1977) or combined with haloperidol (Thomas, 1979), most examples turn out to be chronic delirious states which are reversible (pseudodementia). These occur particularly in the elderly (Jarvis, 1981) and the drugs most often responsible are barbiturate and benzodiazepine hypnotics, major tranquillizers, hypotensive drugs, diuretics, tricyclic antidepressants, antiparkinsonian drugs, and digoxin (Jarvis, 1981). Overdosage of anticonvulsants in some epileptics (Trimble and Reynolds, 1976) and of oral hypoglycaemic drugs (Seltzer, 1979) or insulin (Schwandt et al, 1979) in diabetics can produce a similar picture. Bromides are still occasionally involved (Raskind et al, 1978).

Neuropsychiatric states

These are combinations of psychiatric and neurological symptoms and signs. A newly recognized example is bismuth encephalopathy secondary to the ingestion of bismuth salts for gastric disorders. This is particularly prevalent in France, Belgium and Australia, presumably reflecting the consumption of bismuth in those countries. Collignon et al (1979) analysed 99 case reports and added seven of their own. Typically, a prodromal stage of headache, insomnia, asthenia and mental sluggishness is followed by a confusional state with visual, auditory and gustatory hallucinations, hostility, and excitement often progressing to coma. At the same time myoclonic jerks, ataxia, dysarthria and convulsions develop. Although several deaths have occurred, a gradual recovery on cessation of bismuth ingestion is usual.

Phenytoin can induce a paranoid-hallucinatory psychosis or delirium accompanied by cerebellar signs and symptoms (Logan and Freeman, 1969).

The extrapyramidal syndrome induced by neuroleptic drugs is well known but it may be accompanied by symptoms resembling catatonia, including negativism, autism, posturing, and waxy flexibility (Gelenberg and Mandel, 1977). A few develop pyrexia, cyanosis and dyspnoea as in the "lethal catatonia" syndrome (Weinberg and Kelly, 1977).

Predisposing factors (Prescott, 1979)

In addition to drug-related factors such as dose, duration of therapy, and drug interaction, nondrug factors such as placebo effects (Loranger et al, 1961) and adverse environments such as ITUs (Tomlin, 1977) are often contributory. Both the very young and the elderly are particularly vulnerable (Prescott, 1979) and concurrent physical disease increases the risk of adverse drug reactions (James, 1975). Inherited differences in drug metabolism (Rawlins, 1975) may play a part but less than in somatic drug reactions.

Although depressive reactions, for example to reserpine, appear to occur in susceptible individuals (Muller et al, 1955), no personality or genetic predisposition to natural schizophrenia has been identified in those who develop a paranoid or schizophrenia-like psychosis in response to drugs (Davison, 1976).

Diagnosis

Some of the difficulties have already been described. The sudden development of an unexpected psychiatric condition shortly after the exhibition of a drug should certainly arouse suspicion. Insidiously developing disorders in patients with a constant drug intake over a long period are more difficult to recognize. Any drug, no matter how harmless it usually is, should be suspected. If in doubt a therapeutic test by reducing or withdrawing the suspect drug may clarify the situation.

Management

Whenever possible the offending drug should be discontinued. If medication is necessary a different drug should be used, but if this is not practicable the offending drug may be used in reduced dosage.

Behavioural toxicity, hallucinosis, and delirium usually subside quickly after drug withdrawal. Specific psychiatric syndromes may persist and then require treatment in their own right, for example with antidepressants or ECT for depression or with neuroleptic drugs for schizophrenia-like psychoses. It should, however, be remembered that psychotropic drugs are themselves a source of psychiatric morbidity.

The prognosis is good and specific treatment can usually be withdrawn within 2 weeks of the resolution of the syndrome.

Prevention (George and Kingscombe, 1980)

Adherence to the following simple guidelines minimizes the occurrence of adverse drug reactions, both somatic and psychiatric.

1. Question whether drug therapy is really needed
2. Use appropriately reduced doses for children and the elderly
3. Avoid polypharmacy as far as possible
4. Introduce and withdraw drugs gradually
5. Avoid known toxic drugs if at all possible.

The wider use of plasma drug level estimation may help in both diagnosis and prevention (Mucklow, 1978).

Summary

Adverse drug reactions account for an appreciable amount of psychiatric morbidity which is likely to increase as new and more potent drugs are evolved. Doctors should be alert to this possibility because it is an area of psychiatric illness that often responds with gratifying rapidity to relatively simple measures.

References

Allen, R M, Young, S J (1978) *American Journal of Psychiatry*, **135**, 1081
Bant, W P (1978) *Psychological Medicine*, **8**, 275
Boardman, P L, Hart, F D (1967) *Annals of Rheumatic Diseases*, **26**, 127
Boston Collaborative Drug Surveillance Program (1971) *Seminars in Psychiatry*, **3**, 406
Brawley, P, Duffield, J C (1972) *Pharmacology Review*, **24**, 31
British Medical Journal (1969) i, 461
Brooke, N M, Cookson, I B (1978) *British Medical Journal*, i, 790
Carney, M W P, Sheffield, B F (1975) *Current Medical Research and Opinion*, **3**, 447
Charney, D S, Kales, A, Soldatos, C R, Nelson, J C (1979) *British Journal of Psychiatry*, **135**, 418
Collignon, R, Bruyer, R, Rectem, D, Indekeu, P, Laterre, E C (1979) *Acta neurologica Belgica*, **79**, 73
Connell, P H (1958) Maudsley Monograph No.5: Amphetamine Psychosis. Chapman and Hall, London
Davison, K (1976) *in* Schizophrenia Today (edited by Kemali, D, Bartholini, G, Richter, D). Pergamon Press, Oxford. p.105
— (1980) *Medicine (3rd series)*, **35**, 1823
—, Wilson, C H (1972) *British Journal of Addiction*, **67**, 225
Davison, W (1971) *British Journal of Hospital Medicine*, **6**, 83
De Alarcon, R, Carney, M W P (1969) *British Medical Journal*, iii, 564
Forrest, A D (1969) *ibid*, iv, 169
Freiss, E D (1954) *New England Journal of Medicine*, **251**, 1006
Gelenberg, A J, Mandel, M R (1977) *Archives of General Psychiatry*, **34**, 947
George, C F, Kingscombe, P M (1980) *Adverse Drug Reaction Bulletin*, **80**, 288
Ghose, K (1977) *British Journal of Hospital Medicine*, **18**, 578
Goodwin, F K (1971) *Journal of the American Medical Association*, **218**, 1915
—, Murphy, D L, Brodie, H K H, Bunney, E W (1971) *Clinical Pharmacology and Therapeutics*, **12**, 383
Granville-Grossman (1971) Recent Advances in Clinical Psychiatry. Churchill Livingstone, London. p.199
Gross, M M, Halpert, E, Sabot, L (1967) *Journal of Nervous and Mental Diseases*, **145**, 500
Harper, R W, Knothe, B A U C (1973) *Medical Journal of Australia*, i, 444
Hunter, K R, Shaw, K M, Laurence, D R, Stern, G M (1973) *Lancet*, ii, 929
Hyde, C, Glancy, G, Omerod, P, Hall, D, Taylor, G S (1978) *British Journal of Psychiatry*, **132**, 602
James, I M (1975) *Adverse Drug Reaction Bulletin*, **51**, 172
Jarvis, E H (1981) *ibid*. **86**, 312
Kalinowsky, L B, Hippius, H (1969) Pharmacological, Convulsive and Other Somatic Treatments in Psychiatry, 4th edn. Grune and Stratton, New York. p.137
Kane, F J, Pokorny, A (1975) *Southern Medical Journal*, **68**, 808
Lawson, D H, Gloss, D, Jick, H (1978) *American Heart Journal*, **96**, 572
Lin, J T Y, Ziegler, D K (1976) *Neurology*, **26**, 699
Lipowski, Z J (1980) Delirium. Thomas, Springfield, Illinois. p.38
Logan, W, Freeman, J (1969) *Archives of Neurology*, **21**, 631
Loranger, A W, Prout, C T, White, M A (1961) *Journal of the American Medical Association*, **176**, 920
McClelland, H A (1981) *in* Textbook of Adverse Drug Reactions (edited by Davies, D M). University Press, Oxford. p.479
Macdonald, J B, Macdonald, E T (1977) *British Medical Journal*, ii, 483
Martys, C R (1979) *ibid. ii, 1194*
Mendels, J, Fraser, A (1974) *Archives of General Psychiatry*, **30**, 447
Merry, J, Zachariadis, N (1962) *British Medical Journal*, ii, 1448
Michael, R P, Gibbons, J L (1963) *International Review of Neurobiology*, **5**, 243
Mucklow, J C (1978) *Adverse Drug Reaction Bulletin*, **73**, 260

110   Toxic psychosis

Muller, J C, Pryor, W W, Gibbons, J E, Orgain, E S (1955) *Journal of the American Medical Association*, **159**, 836
Prescott, L F (1979) *Adverse Drug Reaction Bulletin*, **78**, 280
Raskind, M A, Kitchell, M, Alverez, C (1978) *Journal of the American Geriatric Society*, **26**, 222
Rawlins, M D (1975) *Adverse Drug Reaction Bulletin*, **53**, 180
Saravay, S M, Pardes, H (1967) *Archives of General Psychiatry*, **16**, 652
Schroeder, H A, Perry, H M (1955) *Journal of the American Medical Association*, **159**, 839
Schwandt, P, Richter, W, Wilkening, J (1979) *Lancet*, ii, 261
Seltzer, H S (1979) *Comprehensive Therapy*, **5**, 21
Skegg, D C G, Richards, S M, Doll, R (1979) *British Medical Journal,* i, 917
Snyder, S H (1973) *American Journal of Psychiatry*, **130**, 61
Steel, J M, Briggs, M (1972) *British Medical Journal*, iii, 26
Thomas, C J (1979) *British Journal of Psychiatry*, **134**, 552
Tolan, E J, Lingle, F A (1964) *American Journal of Psychiatry*, **126**, 757
Tomlin, P J (1977) *British Medical Journal*, ii, 441
Trimble, M R, Reynolds, E H (1976) *Psychological Medicine*, **6**, 169
Van Praag, H M (1968) *in* Drug-induced Diseases, Vol. 3 (edited by Meyler, L, Peek, H M). Excerpta Medica, Amsterdam. p.281
Vlissides, D N, Gill, D, Castelow, J (1978) *British Medical Journal*, i, 510
Weinberg, D R, Kelly, M J (1977) *Journal of Nervous and Mental Disease*, **165**, 263
Young, D, Scoville, W B (1938) *Medical Clinics of North America*, **22**, 637

Chapter 12

Neuropsychiatric aspects of tics and spasms

R W Tibbetts, United Birmingham Hospitals and Midland Centre for Neurosurgery

The understanding of disorders of movement has been obscured for many years by difficulties of classification. These in turn have been based on the apparently inconsistent and improbable nature of some of the disorders, their intimate relationship with emotional upset, scant evidence of a plausible pathology, and the influence of fashionable doctrinaire theories notably those of psychoanalysis.

An improved situation has arisen from the fact that some abnormal movements such as spasmodic torticollis and tardive dyskinesia have unwittingly been reproduced by modern drugs. In addition there has been the stimulus of biochemical research, particularly research on dopamine metabolism, which goes some way to explain the intimate link between emotion and disorder of movement.

Definitions

A tic is a purposeless, stereotyped, and repetitive jerky movement. Such movements are most commonly found in the head and neck and the incidence decreases with descent to the periphery.

A spasm is an involuntary movement, sometimes clonic but often sustained. It is due to accesses of increased muscular tone in related groups of muscles.

History

Descriptions of these disorders certainly go back to Hippocrates. A peak of interest occurred late in the 19th century with the Salpêtrière as a focus. Such familiar names as Babinski and Trousseau were prominent. Brissaud (1895) considered a spasm to be due to stimuli in a reflex arc whereas tics were based on corticospinal pathways. He referred to "torticollis mental", thereby echoing the views of Rabelais. An authoritative treatise by Meige and Feindel (1907) was translated by Kinnier Wilson.

Failure to distinguish between tics and Sydenham's chorea was common, especially as the movements of chorea often give way to tic-like jerks. Many a child spent months in bed for no good reason, particularly if a systolic murmur was detected. By the same token many tonsils were sacrificed on the altar of focal sepsis. Abnormal movement lent itself to psychoanalytical interpretation and the idea of a twitching phallus in various parts of the body was not without its champions.

In recent decades aetiological theories have had more substance and both behavioural therapy and chemotherapy have shown some promise, even if the extent of this is still far from established.

Tics

These are most commonly found in children. The incidence is about 12 per cent (Lapouse and Monk, 1964) and there are three or four times more boys than girls with tics (Pasamanick and Kawi, 1956; Corbett et al, 1969). The mean age of onset is about 7 years, with blinking as the commonest manifestation. Facial movements, including those of the nose and mouth, are common while below the shoulder tics are infrequent. Onset may at times relate to emotional provocation or to an irritant stimulus such as a rough collar (now an anachronism). The practice outlives the stimulus and so in some cases justifies the older term "habit tic". Almost invariably the movements are aggravated by emotional upset and self-consciousness and are relieved by distraction. They disappear in sleep. It is important to stress that these characteristics are also features of movements of extrapyramidal origin. Voluntary effort may inhibit a tic temporarily but does so at the expense of increased inner tension.

In their study of 112 cases, Corbett et al (1969) compared their group of tiqueurs with a control group of disturbed (but not psychotic) children. Intelligence and symptoms of emotional disturbance were much the same in the two groups but obsessional symptoms were found more significantly in the tiqueurs. In the disturbed children the family history of tics was insignificant, but there was a much higher family history of psychiatric illness (31 per cent) in one or both parents.

Two reliable follow-up studies (Torup, 1962; Corbett et al, 1969) showed improvement in 80–90 per cent of the children over about 5 years, and of those total remission occurred in nearly half. However, there was a residual tendency to restlessness, anxiety, and depression. Childhood tics of acute onset are essentially benign; the emphasis is on the repercussions of the tic on vulnerable children and parents and on teachers, some of whom were only too ready to refer to St Vitus' dance. Bullying or unfriendly mimicry is likely to prejudice improvement and achievement at school. Occasionally the tics are dramatic in onset and may involve a sudden leap in the air and if this occurs in a public place it invites reaction from those around varying from gross indulgence to condemnation of the parents.

In the small minority in whom tics persist it seems likely that mismanagement, parental involvement, and unhappiness at school play their part. In a few patients there is a hint of hysterical prolongation of a manipulative kind and obsessional features in the personality tend to favour the persistence of habitual manifestations, whether of thought or movement. Tics of the face, head, and shoulder are less persistent and vocal tics are the most stubborn (Corbett et al, 1969).

Multiple tics

These also occur in childhood but usually disappear before adolescence is complete. A few persist, sometimes indefinitely, and if the multiple tics are linked with explosive vocal utterances the condition is known as Gilles de la Tourette's syndrome. Eponymous, euphonious, and exotic, this syndrome has invited a degree of interest justified more by the academic challenge than by the incidence.

The condition was first described by Itard (1825) and elaborated by Gilles de la

Tourette (1885), a pupil of Charcot. The essential features are multiple tics beginning before the age of 16 and including vocal ejaculations which frequently involve coprolalia (obscene utterances) and less often echolalia. The mean age of onset is about 7 years. The explosions may occur quite out of context and are often resisted to little effect. Compulsive acts may be associated with them but psychotic features are not seen, nor does the condition deteriorate into schizophrenia as was once thought. The course is fluctuant but where remission occurs there is a strong liability to recurrence and eventual chronicity, although one hopes that this statement may have to be modified in the light of modern treatment. Shapiro et al (1978) described a subgroup with actions suggestive of abortive dystonic movement.

The male:female ratio is similar to that of simple tics, that is 3:1 (Fernando, 1967; Shapiro et al, 1978). The condition occurs in all social classes and many ethnic groups and the range of intelligence is normal. With simple tics Shapiro et al (1978) found a family history of over 30 per cent, while the family history of Gilles de la Tourette's syndrome was 2.8 per cent in a series of 145 patients.

Treatment

With simple tics which affect mostly children management should be as restrained as possible. Sources of stress at home or in school should receive attention and a dependable relationship with a psychiatrist or a social worker is helpful. A relatively common finding is an overexacting father making excessive demands on a male child.

Hypnosis, relaxation techniques and behavioural therapy should be reserved for severe cases. The younger the subject the greater should be the reluctance to prescribe drugs and particularly butyrophenones.

Multiple tics have enjoyed a liberal range of treatment over the years. Tics are not very placebo responsive but an improvement rate of 30 per cent for any treatment should not be taken to indicate a meaningful response.

Behavioural therapy with, for instance, relaxation techniques or massed practice has recently enjoyed a vogue, but Shapiro et al (1978) are no more impressed by these than by psychoanalysis. However, they are powerful advocates of haloperidol and claim significant improvement in 90 per cent of their patients with a 4-year follow-up. Other butyrophenones, for example pimozide and trifluperidol, are effective but phenothiazines are less so. There is little place for tranquillizers, anticonvulsants, or antiparkinsonian drugs.

Butyrophenones are particularly liable to produce unwelcome side effects, the most alarming being an acute dystonic reaction and in the longer term tardive dyskinesia. The liability may be reduced by antiparkinsonian drugs such as benztropine which some doctors prescribe routinely.

It is wise to start with a small dose of haloperidol, for instance 1.5 mg three times daily. Tolerance varies greatly and an average maintenance dose of 5 mg three times a day may be greatly exceeded. There is no doubt that haloperidol is the treatment of choice but the high response rate claimed by Shapiro et al (1978) is not universal and where improvement is uncertain empiricism is justified.

Aetiology

The evidence is sufficiently equivocal to allow for interpretation according to personal bias.

Shapiro et al (1978) stated that family history of tics was high but twin studies were inconclusive. There was no significant history of complicated pregnancy or delivery. A high rate of minimal brain dysfunction was suggestive but required confirmation. Minor abnormalities such as motor asymmetries and nonspecific EEG changes pointed inconclusively to an organic factor. The author himself has two patients who have developed extrapyramidal signs on personal follow-up. The few autopsy studies add little to our understanding.

Involuntary movements and vocalizations found after the epidemic of encephalitis lethargica had much in common with Gilles de la Tourette's syndrome but there were distinctions, especially the coprolalia. The dopamine hypothesis is highly relevant. This refers to the evidence, mostly inferential, that neurotransmitters play a part in the dyskinesias. The issue is complex and full of apparent pradoxes. Among the variables are the neurotransmitters concerned and their concentrations, the point of action of the agonists and antagonists, and which nuclei in the basal ganglia are involved. The suggestion is that there is a dopaminergic excess in the multiple tic syndrome and that haloperidol acts by postsynaptic blockade of dopamine (Shapiro et al, 1978). Haloperidol can provoke parkinsonian symptoms, tardive dyskinesia, and dystonic reactions, and in all likelihood the mechanism is catecholamine depletion. Depression also occurs with serotonin depletion (as after reserpine) and it should be remembered that striatal disorders and temporal lobe epilepsy are both liable to be linked with personality change and disorders of mood and that structurally both conditions involve the limbic system.

Those who favour psychogenesis draw attention to the impressive family histories of psychiatric disorders, the anxious restlessness of tiqueurs, associated disorders such as enuresis, and the unconcealed fluctuations in intensity with stress. The issue is complicated by neurotic attitudes secondary to the socially disruptive symptomatology. Although Shapiro et al (1978) tended to play down the psychiatric implications, some of us may recall multiple tic patients in whom the diagnosis was not in doubt but whose motor disorder intermitted with frankly exhibitionistic behaviour. Enoch and Trethowan (1979) challenged the view that response to butyrophenones necessarily implies an organic aetiology.

Finally there are the obscenities that give the disorder its peculiar distinction. No organicist has gone so far as to postulate a "porn centre" in the brain. It is a common experience to treat patients with obsessional neuroses who have conformist dispositions but are plagued by obscene or sadistic thoughts which, although contained, cause great feelings of guilt. Morphew and Sim (1969) were impressed by the similarity to a certain form of stammering, finding common ground in symbolic sexuality, inhibited hostility, and an obsessional component.

Simple tics have received less elaborate investigation. The aetiological arguments are essentially similar, but the pointers to a physical cause are less impressive and the high remission rate and the link with neurotic symptoms tip the balance towards psychogenesis. The conclusion must be that the cause of tics is not known but is probably multifactorial. The most satisfying explanation at present is that there is a structural and biochemical vulnerability, almost certainly involving the extrapyramidal system and due to damage or to islands of immature development. Emotion is prominent among the elements that cause a latent disorder to declare itself or a manifest disorder to be exacerbated. The sex ratio and other factors make it very likely that the multiple tic and simple tic syndromes enjoy no sharp distinction and that the organic deficit occurs on a sliding scale, being most impressive in Gilles de la Tourette's syndrome.

Spasms

These differ from tics in so far as the movements are less sharply circumscribed and as the tone gradually increases the distortion of movement follows. The increased tone may be sustained or may intermit with or be replaced by repetitive clonic movements. Distribution may be wide as with dystonia musculorum deformans but the focal dystonias, for example spasmodic torticollis, usually involve the same muscle groups particularly those of the head and neck.

There has been a strong change of opinion towards an organic cause with structural or neurophysiological abnormalities, probably in the corpus striatum.

A diagnosis of hysteria should be resisted since follow-up will seldom support it. However, there are hysterical disorders that mimic focal dystonias. Typically the subjects are young and female, the movements inconsistent, and the motivation more apparent. Psychiatric treatment, especially suggestion, often effects unstable remission.

Writer's cramp

This is rare but nevertheless the commonest form of the occupational cramps. There is a muscular spasm of the fingers and hand often spreading to the shoulder girdle. The fingers assume abnormal writing positions; as writing continues there is more and more pressure on the pen and the writing becomes small and illegible. There is associated discomfort but seldom unbearable pain and there may be tremor and coarse jerking. Attempts to work with the good hand usually come to involve it as well. The disorder is commoner in males than females and the wide range of age of onset clusters between 30 and 50 years.

Aetiology The abnormal motor pattern is very consistent and this, together with age of onset and male predominance, hints at an organic factor. The personalities of the subjects do not favour hysterical conversion. Writer's cramp and facial spasm do occur exceptionally in association with spasmodic torticollis (Meares, 1973). There are forms of hysterical dysgraphia with distinguishing features as outlined above.

In true writer's cramp there is commonly a combination of factors that makes it unwise to discount psychogenesis entirely. The author's findings (Bindman and Tibbetts, 1977) concur closely with those of Crisp and Moldofsky (1965). Typically the patients have constructive obsessional personalities hampered by difficulty in expressing feelings of resentment. Their work frequently involves writing and a characteristic precipitating event would be unventilated anger caused by the promotion of a junior over the patient in spite of his years of devoted service. Writer's cramp can be regarded as a true psychosomatic disorder. It has much in common with stammering; like speech, writing involves a complex manipulation of symbols and cortical function, so that emotion and self-awareness are likely to disrupt the smooth functioning of synergistic activity.

Treatment Writer's cramp is a stubborn disorder. Antiparkinsonian drugs and others have no specific role. Re-education starting with a broad nib and large writing is worthwhile. Crisp and Moldofsky (1965) combined this with relaxation techniques and psychotherapy and found that a "strong positive transference"

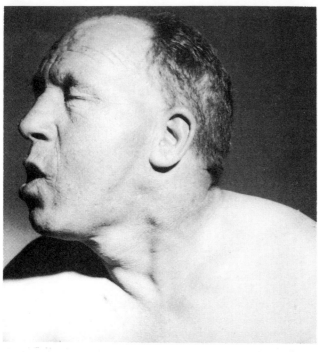

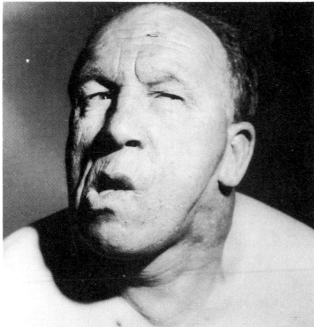

Figure 12.1 At the age of 51 this patient was referred by a consultant ophthalmologist with a diagnosis of hysterical blepharospasm. He is a man of modest intelligence but robust personality. Congenital cataracts, mild diabetes, short spatulate hands, and epicanthic folds suggest a genetic factor. On follow-up he developed retrocollic movements and facial dyskinesia unrelated to drugs.

favoured response. Six of their seven patients were distinctly if precariously improved.

Behavioural therapy in some form has been tried for many years. Liversedge and Sylvester (1955) developed aversion techniques with a pen that produced an electric shock if it strayed from its appointed path. More recently Bindman and Tibbetts (1977) described 10 patients, six of whom were treated by biofeedback. The degree of muscle tension was recorded electromyographically and made apparent to the patient by increasing intensity of sound. One patient remitted and three enjoyed modest improvement.

Blepharospasm

This is due to sustained spasm of the orbicularis oculi muscles (*Figure 12.1*). There is a hysterical form in which there appears to be more volition and less spasm, but a diagnosis of hysteria should be entertained with great reserve as true blepharospasm may herald the onset of parkinsonism or other extrapyramidal disorders.

Orofacial (tardive) dyskinesia

This involves movements of different types but mainly buccolinguomasticatory ones with chewing, lip-smacking, and a darting protrusion of the tongue (*Figures 12.1 and 12.3c*). It is not considered here in detail. Suffice it to say that it is of special concern to the psychiatrist who is the main source of the disorder by virtue of his prescribing of phenothiazines and butyrophenones (Crane, 1973). If these drugs are stopped there is often exacerbation before possible improvement. The mechanism is thought to be increased dopaminergic activity due to increased dopamine receptor blockade.

Hemifacial spasm

Usually this starts with a twitching of one eye and then the spasm spreads to the rest of that side of the face. It does not affect young people but does not readily remit. The basis for it may be peripheral and there are no psychiatric implications.

Spasmodic torticollis

This may be defined as "a condition in which there are repeated purposeless movements of the head and neck or sustained abnormal postures or both. There is always an element of spasm" (*Figures 12.1, 12.2 and 12.3*). There is wide involvement of muscles on both sides, mainly the sternomastoids. Both sexes are equally affected and the typical age of onset is 30–45 years. The family history is of a very low order but is almost certainly significant for subgroups. Vulnerable personalities, often obsessional, are reported in about half the patients (Herz and Glaser, 1949; Tibbetts, 1971; Meares, 1973) but Paterson (1945) found neuroticism in 80 per cent while Cockburn (1971) reported a normal sample. Spasmodic torticollis is aggravated by emotion and idiosyncratic factors and it disappears in sleep. There is varying emphasis on pain and after some years serious pathology of the cervical spine occurs. Natural remission is seen in a quarter of the patients and others reach a plateau after 5–10 years. Dementia does not normally develop.

118

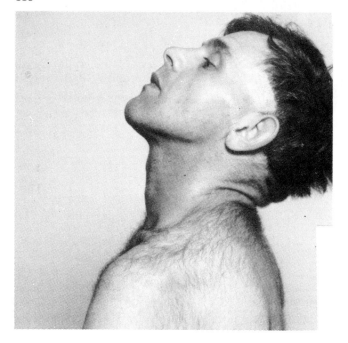

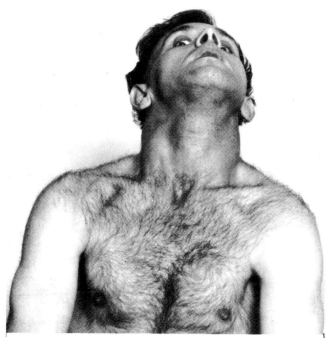

Figure 12.2a and 12.2b At the time of referral.

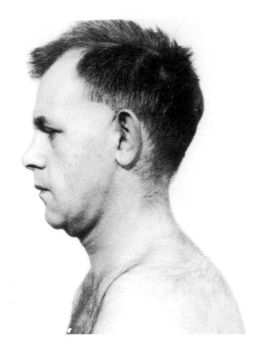

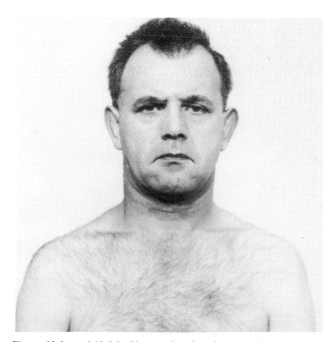

Figure 12.2c and 12.2d　Six months after the operation.

Figure 12.2　This patient suffered from severe persistent retrocollis at the age of 36, but his morale was excellent. After a two-stage bilateral thalamotomy in 1970 he has worked regularly and is in excellent form apart from a mild dysarthria and a mild disturbance of gait attributable to the operation.

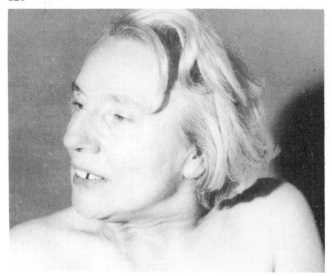

Figure 12.3a Contraction and hypertrophy of the left sternomastoid.

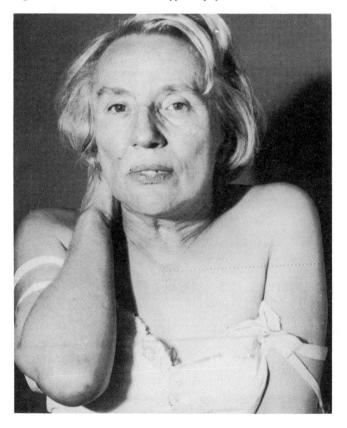

Figure 12.3b The "geste antagoniste efficace" in which support, even of token strength, brings temporary relief supposedly by some reflex action.

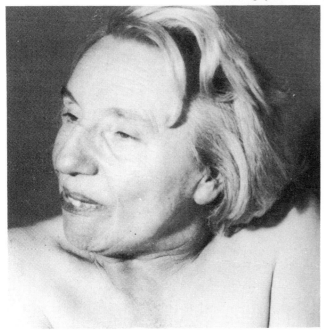

Figure 12.3c   Facial dyskinesia, not drug induced, which developed later.

Figure 12.3   This patient was referred at the age of 48 and has had a follow-up of 22 years (the photographs shown were taken at the age of 56). A stereotactic operation was considered but deferred because the severity was not extreme. A tolerable plateau has now been reached.

Historically there has been much dispute about aetiology but a big switch to an organic emphasis has occurred in the last two decades.

Factors to be considered are as follows:

1. Likely causative events, for example head injury, encephalitis, and multiple sclerosis, are reported in a significant minority
2. Associated neurological abnormalities are not in frequent, varying from minor irregularities in tone to generalized dystonia musculorum deformans; many cases are almost certainly a segmental torsion dystonia (Marsden and Parkes, 1973) which occasionally becomes diffuse
3. Exact reproduction of torticollis with phenothiazines and butryophenones
4. Autopsy studies make little contribution
5. A significant family history of dystonia has been found in Ashkenazi Jews in whom it is inherited as an autosomal recessive trait (Eldridge, 1970); Shapiro et al (1978) also noted a significant family history of Gilles de la Tourette's syndrome in Eastern European Jews
6. Link with depression: Tibbetts (1971) found, admittedly in retrospect, a history of an abnormal mental state in nearly half his patients at the time of onset and in a quarter of them he witnessed at first hand the development of depression which in no way correlated with the severity of the torticollis; in this context it is

relevant to mention that biological depression commonly occurs in Huntington's chorea and significantly in parkinsonism as mentioned above

7. Follow-up: the author's own interest began with a ballerina from Balham whose face turned away from her partner in a pas de deux—this plainly invited a hysterical interpretation but follow-up proved otherwise.

The author studied over 100 patients for more than 20 years. Some atypical cases were deliberately included and most of these later developed unequivocal evidence of an organic basis. On the strength of this follow-up he feels able to give certain guidelines:

1. A diagnosis of hysteria should not be entertained if the movements involve spasm (especially retrocollic), if there is the characteristic combination of tonic and clonic elements and recoil, or if there is a change of muscular tone elsewhere or any other motor abnormality, be it only a darting movement of the tongue
2. Natural remission, apparent response to suggestion, a neurotic personality, or associated depression should invite an open mind, but nothing approaching certainty of psychogenesis
3. A minority of truly hysterical patients display aversion or tilting without real spasm (for this reason they should not strictly be included) and show the features already outlined.

Treatment   Spasm is a distressing disorder and support in an atmosphere of qualified optimism is appreciated, as is an inflatable collar which does not rub. Drugs such as tetrabenazine, thiopropazate or benzhexol are worth a trial but expectations should be modest. Tenotomy and cervical root section are better avoided. Bilateral thalamotomy (*Figure 12.2*) can produce spectacular results but the operation, being something of a gamble, should be reserved for severe cases treated in very expert hands (Cooper, 1964). Where the aetiology is uncertain it is justifiable, if unscientific, to combine physically orientated measures and psychological techniques such as behavioural therapy or psychotherapy.

Differential diagnosis of tics and spasms

Disorders of the middle ear and ophthalmological abnormalities may cause a tilting of the head but not spasm. Wry-neck of infancy may be congenital or acquired, such as by haemorrhage into the sternomastoid. This causes confusion especially in orthopaedic circles but has no link with spasmodic torticollis.

Grimacing is seen in schizophrenia but the movements are more casual and the context is usually obvious.

A range of relevant neurological conditions is reviewed by Marsden and Parkes (1973) so only a passing reference is made here to Sydenham's and Huntington's choreas, myoclonic disorders, and Wilson's disease.

It has been stressed throughout that a diagnosis of hysteria calls for great caution but on the other hand a readily treatable patient may be neglected if a diagnosis of hysteria is not sometimes made on positive psychiatric evidence.

I am indebted to Mr Dee of the Department of Clinical Photography, Queen Elizabeth Hospital, Birmingham, and to the patients concerned for permission to use the photographs.

References

Bindman, E, Tibbetts, R W (1977) *British Journal of Psychiatry*, **131**, 143

Brissaud, E (1895) Leçons sur les Maladies Nerveuses. Henry Meige, Paris

Cockburn, J J (1971) *Journal of Psychosomatic Research*, **15**, 471

Cooper, I S (1964) *New England Journal of Medicine*, **270**, 967

Corbett, J A, Mathews, A M, Connell, P H, Shapiro, D A (1969) *British Journal of Psychiatry*, **115**, 1229

Crane, G E (1973) *ibid.* **122**, 395

Crisp, A H, Moldofsky, H (1965) *ibid.* **111**, 841

Eldridge, R (1970) *Neurology*, **20**, No. 11. p.1

Enoch, D, Trethowan, W H (1979) Uncommon Psychiatric Syndromes. John Wright, Bristol

Fernando, S J M (1967) *British Journal of Psychiatry*, **113**, 607

Gilles de la Tourette, G (1885) *Archives of Neurology*, **9**, 19

Herz, E, Glaser, G H (1949) *Archives of Neurology and Psychiatry*, **61**, 227

Itard, J M G (1825) *Archives of General Medicine*, **8**, 385

Lapouse, R, Monk, M (1964) *American Journal of Orthopsychiatry*, **34**, 436

Liversedge, L A, Sylvester, J D (1955) *Lancet*, i, 1147

Marsden, C D, Parkes, J D (1973) *British Journal of Hospital Medicine*, **10**, 428

Meares, R (1973) *ibid.* **9**, 235

Meige, H, Feindel, E (1907) Tics and Their Treatment. Sidney Appleton. London

Morphew, J A, Sim, M (1969) *British Journal of Medical Psychology*, **42**, 293

Pasamanick, B, Kawi, A (1956) *Journal of Pediatrics*, **48**, 596

Paterson, M T (1945) *Lancet*, ii, 556

Shapiro, A K, Shapiro, E S, Bruun, R D, Sweet, R D (1978) Gilles de la Tourette Syndrome. Raven Press, New York

Tibbetts, R W (1971) *Journal of Psychosomatic Research*, **15**, 461

Torup, E (1962) *Acta paediatrica Scandinavica*, **51**, 261

Chapter 13

Supportive psychotherapy

Sidney Bloch, University of Oxford and Warneford Hospital, Oxford

Supportive psychotherapy is probably the commonest form of psychotherapy used in medical practice. Yet a perusal of psychiatric texts reveals that it is usually mentioned only sketchily, if at all, and my discussions with colleagues show that they differ widely in their conceptualization of it. In this article an attempt is made to define supportive psychotherapy and to consider its goals, indications, format, and chief side effect.

Definition

A good definition of supportive therapy is hard to come by. Most texts on psychiatry either do not define the term or ignore it entirely. Exclusion criteria are usually used to describe it; thus it is a form of psychotherapy that does *not* involve exploration of the unconscious, a focus on transference, and an understanding by the patient of his characteristic defences.

More direct definition is problematic. One could use the derivation of the word itself: supportare, sup = sub + portare = to carry (Onions, 1970). The obvious implication is that the therapist's task is to "hold up" the patient, in other words to lend him a hand. Instead of struggling to define the term directly, it may be more useful to consider the goals which are intrinsic to the treatment.

Goals

What are the goals of supportive therapy? As with the definition, there is a tendency for psychiatric texts not to deal with this question. When goals are mentioned the authorities cover more or less the same ground, for example "reinforce the person's existing personality structure and defence mechanisms and assist him in managing his current reality problems" (Kleeman and Solomon, 1974); "restoring or strengthening the defences and integrative capacities which have been impaired" (Stewart and Levine, 1967); and "to reduce the tensions of anxiety or of other incapacitating tensions (and) help the patient to maintain or improve his ability to face and handle his reality at his best integrative level" (Kolb, 1973).

A common thread running through these objectives is the restoration of the patient to his former state. The therapist's goal is to retrieve the status quo and enable the patient to achieve once again a level of psychological equilibrium. There are assumptions that treatment is palliative rather than radical and that no major life or personality changes are intended. Indeed care is taken not to disrupt reasonable defences. the generation of conflict is avoided, and critical feedback to the patient is kept to a minimum.

Indications

If supportive therapy does not aim to change personality traits or defence mechanisms but rather to stabilize them, in whom is it indicated? There are two potential groups of patients:

1. Those experienceing stressful circumstances such as bereavement, divorce, loss of job, the menopause, physical illness, and academic difficulties. The degree of tension and the resultant distress prove too much and the coping abilities are insufficient.
2. Those who are severely handicapped emotionally and/or interpersonally because of chronic schizophrenia, a chronic affective disorder, or some extreme form of personality disorder. The therapist sees no prospect of fundamental improvement in these patients, but a continuing need exists to help them achieve the best adaptation possible. Furthermore the severity of the disorder and the fragile quality of this personality preclude the use of any radical form of psychotherapy that is apt to provoke anxiety and other unfavourable reactions.

Format

What are the components of the treatment? Probably the most important factor is the relationship that develops between therapist and patient. In adopting the role of a benevolent professional the former manifests a willingness to help, concern, understanding, warmth, acceptance, and interest. Within this relationship the patient feels increasing trust in the therapist both as a person and as a healer, and his hopes and positive expectations of relief are reinforced.

To a large extent the relationship resembles the bond between parent and child as described by Strupp (1973). In many forms of psychotherapy, notably the variety traditionally designated supportive, the major leverage is the helping relationship that the therapist creates and maintains; he is the good parent, warm and empathic. He provides the security, shelter, and caring on which the patient depends. By assuming a role of responsibility he permits the patient to relinquish all or some of his self-reliance. This total or partial dependency is legitimized on the premise that the effects of the stress or severe personality handicap have incapacitated the patient and rendered him unfit to sustain himself independently. Because the dependent role is sanctioned, the patient need not feel shame or embarrassment about occupying it.

In addition to this relationship, various therapeutic techniques come into play such as active listening, reassurance, explanation, advice, persuasion, suggestion, encouragement, permission for catharsis (so that the patient can openly express previously suppressed problems and feelings), and environmental manipulation which involves altering aspects of the patient's lifestyle, for instance his job or accommodation.

The chief side effect—dependency

At first sight it seems surprising that supportive therapy has undesirable effects. After all it mainly involves a benevolent therapist entering into a caring relationship with a patient who is in need of help. Yet every clinician must have frequently encountered patients who have become overly dependent on him and incapable without the provision of continuing support. The dependency needs of even the well-integrated personality increase in the face of stress and the individual who tends towards dependency is likely to display this trait all the more in a relationship that permits or even encourages it. The chronically handicapped patient, like the chronic schizophrenic, may well bask under the protective mantle offered by the therapist. Whatever the personality pattern and situational factors associated with the onset of supportive therapy, the prospect exists that dependency (which is intrinsic to the treatment) will both escalate and persist in a way that is not necessarily in the patient's long-term interests.

Thus Kolb (1973) cautions: "In employing supportive therapy, the physician should bear in mind the danger that he may thereby encourage dependence and a regressive passivity in the patient". Alexander's (1964) comment, although referring to psychoanalysis, applies to supportive therapy as well: "Psychotherapeutic treatment must aim to bring the patient to the point where his natural growth can be resumed. Treatment beyond this point—or infantilization—interferes with the natural growth potential and tempts the patient's ego to take the easy path of continuing dependency on parental figures. This dependency is exactly what the therapy tries to overcome."

In what way is the development of dependency harmful? Once a patient has sampled the advantages of dependency—the security embodied by the therapist's support, particularly when he feels overwhelmed or perplexed—there is not surprisingly an inclination to indulge himself further. It could be argued that provided a therapist is willing to support a patient in need no problem arises; a mutually satisfying complementary relationship is created. But its success may not be matched by the patient's coping behaviour outside therapy where he may hibitually become dependent on everyone but himself and reluctant to relinquish his "secure" role.

One therefore has a treatment that inherently calls for a degree of dependency but carries the risk that this may become overly intense and/or prolonged. Balint (1964) regards dependency as inevitable in every doctor–patient relationship. "The only question is how much dependence is desirable" or, put another way, "How much dependence constitutes a good starting point for a successful therapy and when does it turn into an obstacle?"

Most therapists are prepared to fulfil a supportive role on initial clinical contact and to maintain it thereafter for a period that they consider reasonable (based on clinical appraisal, previous experience of similar patients, the therapist's value system, and so on). Beyond this point many therapists encounter difficulty as they grapple with both the patient's entrenched dependency behaviour and their own discomfort in trying to modify their clinical role. They frequently try to interrupt the system by setting limits or "retreating" from the patient. The relationship inevitably sours and becomes strained, and any therapeutic benefit that has accrued is either lost or jeopardized.

Another common difficulty concerning dependency arises due to the pragmatic job requirements of the therapist, who may move to another position either in the same institution or elsewhere. When the therapist attempts to transfer a patient to a colleague or to discharge him the results are predictable: the patient is distressed at losing his agent of protection and reluctant to adopt a more independent stance. The most expedient solution for both patient and departing therapist (assuaging the latter's guilt is an important motive here) is the perpetuation of the patient's dependency; henceforth the institution, represented by the substitute therapist, maintains the supportive framework. Inevitably, the patient leaves behind him a trail of several therapists, is never formally discharged, becomes a chronic attender, and acquires or has reinforced a sense of helplessness.

Another factor that may contribute to excessive dependency resides more deeply within the therapist. This is the need to prove to himself and others that, first, he does play an important role in helping patients and, secondly, even in "incurable" cases he can be useful.

In many psychological disorders evidence that the therapist's efforts actually result in improvement is still lacking, and the controversy over the effectiveness of psychotherapy in general remains unresolved. I suspect that therapists unknowingly counter the uncertainty of whether or not they are really effective by relying on the concept of support (I recognize this pattern repeatedly in myself). Because supportive therapy by definition denotes the therapist's active protective role in the clinical relationship, even if the efficacy of his intervention remains unproven he can derive comfort from the notion that for the patient *he* is a significant figure through his role as a benevolent authoritative provider of support.

In the case of the incurable patient, when the therapist is by and large impotent in changing the patient in any substantial fashion he may provide unduly excessive supportive therapy to satisfy himself that he is doing something. A comparable situation in general medicine is the heroic effort made by some physicians and surgeons in their treatment of the terminally ill. They may resort to such an approach, which does not contribute to the patient's welfare, when they have difficulty in conceding that they can no longer play an active health-restoring role (Bloch, 1976).

An approach to the use of supportive therapy

Perhaps the most important factor in the use of supportive therapy is that one has a clear idea of the goals of treatment. One helpful approach is to examine the distinction between the use of supportive therapy for the patient in crisis and for the chronically handicapped patient.

The patient in crisis

This patient is a reasonably well-integrated personality who is overwhelmed by some major stress. The concepts of crisis and crisis intervention which have come into wide use in recent years are particularly relevant in this context. Two types of crisis can be identified—developmental and accidental. The former are those traumatic transitional periods between the phases of the life-cycle, such as early adolescence, the menopause, and the onset of old age, which are commonly marked by psychological distress (Erikson, 1965). Accidental crises occur as a result of specific incidents, for instance divorce, bereavement, loss of job, physical illness, and so on.

No matter which form the crisis takes the patient's customary methods of coping prove ineffective (Caplan, 1964). His distress, whether it be expressed as anxiety, depression, guilt, or irritability, rises to an uncomfortable level and he fails to function adequately. In an attempt to gain relief he summons the assistance of a medical professional with the message "Help me deal with the problem which seems to have got the better of me". The therapist should respond unambiguously to provide a supportive framework within which his transiently disabled patient can acquire a breathing space, feel expectant of obtaining help, and receive guidance and reassurance.

A contract is established between therapist and patient at the outset. Their joint objectives are alleviation of the distress, improved functioning, and better adaptive coping with the stress. There is agreement on a collaborative endeavour in which the patient is an *active* participant even while leaning on the therapist.

The treatment programme is spelt out as clearly as possible to indicate the duration (in most cases a period of weeks), the frequency of contact (weekly or twice weekly), the length of each session (30–60 minutes), the possible involvement of others (one or more family members, employer, university tutor, schoolteacher, and so on), and an explanation of the reason for medication if prescribed.

Both patient and therapist are now aware of the objectives and format of treatment, and (importantly) both recognize and accept their respective roles and tasks. The patient's temporary need to forgo some measure of his independence is emphasized, but there is a concensus that as he gradually feels and functions better he will assume a greater degree of responsibility for himself.

"Working through" a crisis need not mean merely the patient's return to his former state. Caplan (1964) asserts that the experience can bring benefits by leading to the development of new effective methods of coping and problem-solving; the individual acquires a wider and richer psychological repertoire to call upon in the event of future stress.

The chronically handicapped patient

This patient is handicapped by an enduring condition that is not amenable to fundamental change such as some forms of schizophrenia and marked personality disorders. As a result he is impaired socially and either lacks intimate relationships or is unable to maintain them; his work record is often poor. Commonly he has been hospitalized on one or more occasions. His overall adjustment may be marginal and his is prone to decompensate even under mild stress.

The supportive therapy in this case differs from that given in the context of crisis. Because of the chronic nature of his condition, the individual requires help for several years if not for life. (A medical parallel is the chronic diabetic who, due to the condition's incurability and association with severe complications, requires professional supervision throughout his life.) The therapist is largely directive and undertakes an active role in helping the patient to achieve the best adjustment possible. Through being aware of the patient's strengths and limitations, the therapist encourages him to capitalize on the former but is careful not to push him beyond his capabilities. A delicate balance is sought which enables the patient both to achieve some measure of autonomy and to receive the benefits of the therapist's protection such as advice on day-to-day issues, environmental manipulation, encouragement, and so on.

By contrast with the patient in crisis, the therapist allows for the maintenance of a dependent relationship. Treatment is geared to the provision of support on a regular continuing basis. The frequency of contact varies according to the patient's circumstances from monthly to 3-monthly and the duration inevitably extends over several years at least. A family member may be involved in therapy and prescription of medication is necessary in the schizophrenic patient.

The therapist's caseload increases as new patients are admitted and only a neglibible number are discharged (some may of course require prolonged hospitalization, some may move away, and some may live permanently in a "supportive institution" such as a hostel or community home). Not only the clinic's eventual size but also the responsibility that the therapist is required to assume and the lack of any fundamental improvement in the patients make this form of supportive therapy somewhat demanding and wearisome.

One way of lessening the difficulty is for the therapist to establish with the patient from the outset that the institution or helping agency with its various resources, and not he alone, will provide the necessary support. The patient thus relies on a team made up of GPs, psychiatrists, psychologists, social workers, occupational therapists, nurses, fellow patients, and family members. He can also depend on different parts of the institution such as the occupational therapy workshop, the day hospital, the outpatient clinic, the social club, and so on. The departure of any one member of the team is not a threat to the patient since his supportive framework remains otherwise intact. For the therapist, the support derived from colleagues helps to prevent this type of work from becoming too arduous.

I have included fellow patients and relatives in the supportive team. The resource of patients with similar needs has been used effectively as a means of providing mutual support. The efficacy of patient groups of this kind (Alcoholics Anonymous is a good example) relies on such therapeutic factors as cohesiveness (the solidarity that group members feel together), universality (patients learning that their situation is not unique), altruism (the satisfaction of helping others), hope, and the sharing of information. Mobilizing the support of the family and other informal helpers for instance friends, co-workers, and neighbours can also be an effective adjunct to the supportive therapy given by the specialist and his colleagues. However, these other sources may need professional guidance on how to fulfil their role.

An expansion of many of the points made in this article is to be found in 'Supportive Psychotherapy', in An Introduction to the Psychotherapies, edited by Bloch, S, Oxford University Press, 1979.

References

Alexander, F. (1964) *in* Psychoanalysis and the Human Situation (edited by Marmorston, J., Stainbrook, E.). Vantage Press, New York. p. 82
Balint, M. (1964) The Doctor, his Patient and the Illness. 2nd edn. Pitman Medical, London
Bloch, S. (1976) *Medical Education*, **10**, 269
Caplan, G. (1964) Principles of Preventive Psychiatry. Tavistock, London
Erikson, E H. (1965) Childhood and Society. Penguin, Harmondsworth
Kleeman, S T, Solomon, P. (1974) *in* Handbook of Psychiatry (edited by Solomon, P, Patch, V D). Lange Medical, Los Altos. p.353
Kolb, L C (1973) Modern Clinical Psychiatry. Saunders, Philadelphia
Onions, C T (1970) Editor. Shorter Oxford English Dictionary, 3rd edn. University Press, Oxford
Stewart, R L, Levine, M (1967) *in* Comprehensive Textbook of Psychiatry (edited by Freedman, A, Kaplan, H). Williams and Wilkins, Baltimore. p. 1212
Strupp, H H (1973) *Journal of Consulting and Clinical Psychology*, **41**, 1

Chapter 14

Action techniques in psychotherapy

Mark Aveline, Mapperley Hospital, Nottingham

Although man has always been fascinated by the nature of his existence and the ways in which he could and should lead his life, the history of therapeutic concern with the individual and his problems in personal relationships begins with Sigmund Freud at the turn of the last century. Freud, faithful to his early neurophysiological training and subject to the prevailing belief in determinism and the expectation that the ultimate rules of science would soon be discovered, propounded a view of man expressed in the language of biology.

Paradoxically, Freud's essential contribution was not biological but psychological; his biological theory was a semantic one in which the language was one of metaphor and meaning rather than causality (Rycroft, 1968). He saw himself as an expert helping the patient to unravel troublesome aspects of himself that were not plain (conscious) to him. His approach was verbal and employed the techniques of free association and analysis of behaviour and attitudes derived from unconscious sources and displayed towards the therapist (transference). His was a hopeful message, that by thought one could counter the determinates from the past operating in the present. As a result, Freud's emphasis on self-reflection and verbal analysis for many years dominated the practice of British psychotherapy.

Elsewhere, particularly in the USA, other ideas originating from diverse sources were emerging and have now led to the elaboration of action techniques. In the hands of some these have supplanted classical practice, but I believe they are better seen as useful, powerful adjuncts in the exploration of a person's psychological existence alone and with others. The key concepts are a desire for brevity and immediacy, a reaction against words and professional expertise, a preference for feeling rather than thought, a drive towards authenticity and learning from interaction, and an assertion of personal responsibility and choice (Gendlin, 1975). In this article I set out the origin, form, and use of these techniques.

By action techniques I mean predominantly nonverbal approaches that draw upon our ability to think symbolically and dramatically. Through their use an area of personal conflict such as lack of trust may be manifested and explored. The conflict may be within the person or with other people who may or may not be present in the therapy session. The course of therapy has two elements: by enaction of the conflict its reality is directly experienced and understood by the participants, and by acting through the difficulties in a safe space new resolutions may be reached, tested, rehearsed, and adopted. While some of these approaches may be

130

used in individual therapy, they are most appropriate to a group setting of between eight and 20 people and it is in this context that I describe them. Art, music, and dance therapy come within this definition, but the first is the only one mentioned here.

Origins

Psychodrama

To Jacob Levy Moreno, born in Rumania in 1892, must go much of the credit for evolving these techniques. He studied first philosophy then medicine and while in Vienna (1921–23) developed the Theatre of Spontaneity. He went to the USA in 1925 and practised there as a therapist until his death in 1974. From observations that the dramatization of personally difficult situations leads to their resolution he evolved psychodrama.

In formal psychodrama the dramatic overtones may be highlighted by the use of a stage, props and an audience. The therapy is focused on one individual at a time, a protagonist who is helped by the director to recreate his problems using members of the audience to represent aspects of himself (auxiliary egos) or important people in his life. Attention is given to making the recreation of a psychologically significant incident as accurate as possible and then playing it out as if it is happening here and now, allowing new associations or ideas to arise spontaneously and alter the direction of the drama. Such an enactment evokes strong feelings the expression of which can be cathartic. A drama would be preceded by a warm-up phase and followed by feedback from each of the participants speaking in his role.

The approach allows the individual to explore in a safe situation various aspects of his personality and the attitudes of others to him, try out alternative courses of action, learn the likely consequences, and chart the hindrances to free expression of new strategies within both himself and others (Davies, 1976). Although the release of feeling and increase in inner awareness overlap with Freud's model, the dramatization of reality and emphasis on enquiry and experiment now and in the future stand in contrast.

Special techniques used by the director, such as the auxiliary ego, role reversal, doubling, and mirroring, can be employed in other settings and are discussed later.

The T-group and human growth movement

The psychoanalysts who broke away from orthodoxy in the 1920s and emigrated to the USA were influenced by the American ethic of self-reliance, autonomy, and industry which rewards those who best personify these characteristics. Sandor Ferenczi emphasized reality in his therapy and Karen Horney the consequences for the individual of his behaviour, while Harry Stack Sullivan sought to identify with the patient his characteristic style placing it firmly in the context of relationships with others.

In the late 1940s interest burgeoned in developing personal maturation through interaction between group members with little reference to past events. Building on the pioneering work of Kurt Lewin, a social psychologist and founder of vector psychology, the National Training Laboratories (NTL) developed which provided essentially an educative service in the form of training groups for normal people who were not mentally disordered. Lewin had noticed that people defined themselves through assumptions that were often unrealistic but when held by those about them were restrictive to change. By providing an environment that did not rely on past self-definition the individual was "unfrozen" and through self-disclosure, interpersonal honesty, and feedback led to greater self-actualization (an inelegant word meaning fulfilling one's own human potential).

Carl Rogers has been the chief advocate of there being a potential for personal growth resident in every person. In the climate of unconditional positive regard, genuineness, and empathy from the therapist, an atmosphere of trust develops and in it the individual's potential unfolds. The therapist relates to the person as he is, confident in his belief that the other's inner goodness which is at present obscured is soon to be revealed. Analysis, categorization and interpretation are eschewed. The person is helped to become more aware of his here-and-now feelings as they relate to current events. The central process in therapy is the *encounter* between two people, a true meeting. Rogers (1961, 1973) began with individual therapy but is now committed to applying the same approach in groups. Encounter groups (which are seen by some as an antidote to the alienation of modern life) provide for their members, often through the use of action techniques that erode the boundaries between people, an experience that is immediate, often exhilarating, occasionally facilitating, and not without risks.

The use of body contact is taken further in bioenergetics, a system of therapy derived from the theories of Wilhelm Reich. Reich (1949) drew attention to the significance of posture as communication, a way of indicating a person's attitude to himself and his world. By altering posture or translating areas of muscular tension into direct expression of the underlying feelings such as rage or fear, the individual is able to free himself from his inhibiting "character armour". In an extreme form (Rolfing), deep massage and painful rearrangement by others of one's body as it should be is employed (Rolf, 1958).

In gestalt therapy, as developed by Fritz Perls, the aim is to integrate aspects of the personality that are alienated or function separately from the whole. The individual is encouraged to personify various parts of his body and mind and then have a dialogue between them in order to elucidate and resolve conflicts. In addition the therapist may make use of the "empty chair", one that is literally empty but in which the person may imagine someone important to him with whom he can engage in fantasized conversation. In this approach little use is made of group interaction, the others present serving merely as an audience (Perls, 1969). Gestalt therapists rarely acknowledge their indebtedness to Carl Jung who long before had illuminatingly subdivided the self into persona, animus or anima, and shadow, and had amplified the meaning of dreams by encouraging the patient to associate to each element in the dream in turn (Jung, 1934).

It should be borne in mind that the human growth movement arose in response to the wish of essentially normal people to deepen their self-awareness and improve their relationships. In contrast, the slower less confronting methods of classical psychotherapy were adapted to the overriding need to survive of patients with greater handicaps in their personalities.

Philosophy

Three of the key concepts underlying action techniques, namely purpose, responsibility, and authenticity, have been expounded in the philosophical writings of therapists subscribing to the existential and humanist schools. Having survived the horrors of a German concentration camp, Viktor Frankl knew at first hand the vital imperative of finding some meaning in life—some purpose to live for that would transcend the impossibility of the present moment. When he is with his patients he tries to help them discover their own particular purpose now and in the remainder of their time (Frankl, 1969). In this he may use an interesting technique of "paradoxical intention" whereby the patient is instructed to be the person he fears he is, for example by experimenting with being even more timid and without opinions than usual. Dialectically a greater certainty of what he would like to be is reached.

Rollo May (1970) asserts the old-fashioned virtues of responsibility, that we will what we are, and that we have choice in what we do. A capacity for self-responsibility and choice is assumed by most of the newer psychotherapies.

Martin Buber, the Austrian theologian, reacted against the then ascendant scientific view of people as machines as being dehumanizing and urged that if relationships were to be meaningful they had to be personal—"I-thou" not "I-it" (Buber, 1957). Jourard, a psychologist, has argued persuasively for authenticity in the meeting between therapist and patient as both a uniquely valuable experience in itself and a paradigm for ideal relationships (Jourard, 1964). It follows that the therapeutic relationship should be immediate, without pretence, nondistancing, and an end in itself.

Behaviour therapy

Behavioural psychologists have in recent years made important contributions to the study of how interpersonal learning happens. They have articulated the premise that psychotherapy is a process whereby the individual *learns* to be more effective. We learn to manifest the behaviours that are rewarded (reinforced) by important people in our world (contingencies) and avoid those that are responded to negatively. In this operant conditioning reward is more effective than punishment. We also learn from the successful behaviour *modelled* by others which we *rehearse* until it becomes part of our own repertoire (Lazarus, 1971). It is a matter of common experience that people are conservative by nature, preferring to talk about doing something new rather than doing it. In an action session risks can be seen to be taken and survived and the opportunity for practice is there to be used.

Cognitive psychology, based on the work of George Kelly, attends to the personal world of meaning that each of us inhabits and that determines how we perceive any situation. This approach serves as a timely reminder of the importance of thought and may prove to be the bridge between the dynamic and behavioural therapies, which are too often polarized as incompatible opposites (Ryle, 1978). The technique of fixed role is noteworthy: within the safety of the session the patient experiments by displaying those characteristics that he would like to possess in greater abundance, for example an overcompliant man could disagree with everything the therapist said and thereby achieve a new view of what is possible for him (Bannister, 1975).

Play

There is a close parallel between the play of children and action techniques. In play, children may recapitulate aspects of recent experience, anticipate roles to come, make good what is unsatisfactory in their external lives, learn to communicate, and simply enjoy themselves (Kahn, 1971). The mixture of reality and unreality in play allows a child to tackle creatively issues important to his emotional growth. Winnicott (1974) in his psychotherapeutic work would not raise areas of conflict until he had established a safe play-area between himself and the child.

Peter Brook (1968) as a theatre director has the same theme: before his actors can be creative he has to set them free to play. In a theatre we suspend disbelief so as to unite with the dramas of others (and the reflection of our own dramas in them) without the dangers of personally experiencing those lives. In an action session adults are encouraged to play and through a common external experience explore individual inner realities.

Action techniques

There are hundreds of games for therapy of which only a few are mentioned here. Each leader adapts these and improvizes many more. As a source book I recommend Lewis and Streitfield (1970). Schutz (1967), Stevens (1971), Blatner (1973), Blumberg and Golembiewski (1976; on T-groups), Yalom (1976; on group psychotherapy), and Barker (1977) are also useful.

Although action techniques may be used singly, a normal sequence in a 1½-hour session is a series of warm-up exercises lasting 10–20 minutes, focused play for 30–45 minutes, and the remaining time devoted to reflection and winding down, possibly aided by further exercises.

General instructions

The success of these techniques depends as much on the leader's personality, his way of presenting them, and his sense of timing and appropriateness as on the strengths of the conflicts being explored. The leader should follow these general instructions:

1. The room ought to be comfortable and preferably carpeted, with plenty of space and no interruptions
2. The participants should wear comfortable clothes, be on their feet, and not smoke
3. Explain the ground rules: it is a pleasurable way to learn; no one will get hurt; individuals are free not to participate in any given exercise; the optimum attitude is to concentrate on feelings, be adventurous, take risks, and avoid censoring spontaneous reactions and thoughts—be prepared to share these with others
4. Make instructions simple, vivid, and intriguing and check that they are understood; exude confidence (however ill felt) and, at least to begin with, be decisive
5. Go at a pace the group can tolerate; do not force or humiliate anyone; approach difficult issues slowly; and focus on what is relevant and vital to members—their agenda not the leader's
6. Be ready to change direction if anxieties become too great or any unforeseen conflict emerges; intervene if someone is getting hurt and the group is not helping.

Warm-up

This should be fun, noisy, and somewhat ridiculous. Its purpose is to develop an imaginative spontaneous mood and strengthen group cohesiveness. In a nonex-plorative setting the warm-up may be used alone.

Start quietly. Mill about the room exploring the space. When you come across someone stop and see that person freshly. Move on and meet more people. Continue with your eyes closed. When you bump into someone reach up and slowly explore his face. With eyes open find a comfortable place. Explore it. Are there people in it? Make contact. Be a tree growing, a flower opening, or a stand of wheat rippled by the wind. Get as far away from others as you can—experience distance. Slowly come together into a heap—experience closeness.

Start more noisily. Make a circle. Turn half right. Shake the shoulders of the person in front, then reverse. Form pairs and one be a shadow following the other exactly about the room, then reverse. Make a machine: one person begins moving a limb while making an appropriate noise, another joins on with a different movement and noise and so on. Form two teams and take it in turn for one to sculpt the other into a contorted impossible structure. Construct a fantasy object, for example a train with noises and actions. Lying down, form a chain with each person's head on another's stomach and laugh. Act out a melodrama or fairy tale, hamming up each role.

Introductions: in a circle throw a cushion about, the recipient shouting out his own name. Introduce variants by shouting an appropriate month, animal, or colour, your Walter Mitty self. Going on first impressions the thrower shouts out one characteristic he likes and one he dislikes about the receiver. In pairs, in turn, tell of two good and two bad things that have happened in the last week.

Focused play

The focus may be directed towards one or two members aided by the rest or everyone can work singly or in small groups and come together for discussion at the end.

To explore intimacy, trust exercises can be used. In pairs, fall backwards to be caught by the other, then reverse. Alternatively lie on the floor and allow the other passively to move your arms and head, be cared for. Lie down and be patted or stroked by the group as you direct or be lifted up and swayed and rocked. In pairs, in turn, seek out areas of tension in the other's body and massage it away or with your eyes shut explore each other's faces. Lying on the floor, hold hands with two people and choose one. In threes two talk silently together excluding the third, then welcome in the outsider.

To explore boundaries there are other exercises. In pairs, approach the other person to the limit of comfortable closeness, retreat to the point of losing contact, then reverse and repeat, now getting too close and then too remote. In pairs, standing face to face, a few inches apart, in turn mirror the arm movements of the other person, then reverse, finally trying to move as one with neither leading nor following.

To explore control and aggression, form a circle. One person is in the middle and has to break out or outside having to break in and is resisted by the group. In pairs or two teams, command as puppets the others by finger gestures to advance, retreat, bow down, and so on. In pairs, in turn, press the other to the ground with your hands on his shoulders, help him up, arm wrestle, or use ritual fighting.

To work through fantasy the magic shop can be used. Members in turn barter with a shopkeeper (usually the leader) for personality attributes they would like to have and that are for sale, offering in exchange qualities they already possess. Once the sale is completed the new self is tried out. Guided fantasy is another technique, either as a group or with two members who have a difficult relationship. Lie on the floor with heads together and eyes shut. The leader starts off with an image such as entering a cave or a house, going on a train, or something relevant to a conflict within the group. The participants voice images that spontaneously come to them. The leader guides the fantasy to a close after 30–45 minutes.

Often it is too difficult for people to express directly how they feel about others. Modelling clay or manhandling a pillow, which at one remove substitutes for the object of wrath or fear, may help a person to begin. Similarly, representing in paint oneself and one's family as they are and how one would like them to be opens up the problem for all to see.

In sculpting, a versatile and vivid technique much used by family therapists, the relationships between family members are expressed through posture and distance. One member chooses people from the group to stand for his relatives and chronicles his life by placing them so as to represent his experience throughout his lifetime. Speaking in role the participants add their reactions to the scene (Skinner, 1976). Another way to represent personal characteristics is by taking figures of speech literally and giving them physical form.

Once a problem has been manifested the opportunity for change exists. A game may be repeated allowing a new outcome to emerge and a new role to be rehearsed (incidentally providing a natural opportunity for training in social skills). The meaning may be amplified by the person exchanging his role to see the event from the other's viewpoint (role reversal) or having another speak for him (doubling) or even substitute for him (mirroring). Polarized aspects of his conflict such as tender versus defensive self may be voiced by others acting as auxiliary egos.

Reflection and wind-down

Each game and element in it has multiple meanings depending on the individual, the emphasis given by the leader, and the group context. For example face exploring may be experienced as an invasion, a violation, a loss of individuality, or a fusing and calming experience. It is often erotic, which may lead to anxiety or pleasure. These reactions may occur in combination or sequence. Meanings and feelings should be explored through discussion either at the end of a sequence or after each game, which then provides a stimulus for shaping the subsequent focus. It is important to share reactions so that issues may be known and worked on later and also to return to normality anyone who has been playing a role.

It is customary for participants individually to take their leave of each other. Before this some more games may be appropriate, for example a group hug or tangles (stand in a circle holding hands, interweave until unable to move, then untangle without letting go).

Hazards and precautions

To call a technique a game should not obscure its power. Particularly when used on the handicapped population treated by psychiatrists it is easy to overstep the bounds of tolerance, overintrude on the schizoid, or provoke persecutory ideas in the paranoid and fear of loss of control in the obsessional. Lieberman et al (1973) studied 204 Stanford undergraduates 8 months after they had participated in encounter groups. A positive change was shown by 39 per cent compared with 17 per cent in the control group. There was an unusually high number of casualties of the group process—7.5 per cent. Individuals with low self-esteem and unrealistically high expectations of help who were members of groups with aggressive, stimulating, and charismatic leaders were most at risk.

Action techniques are easy to learn, but the leader should be experienced in their use and sufficiently skilled in group psychotherapy and psychodynamic theory to anticipate the likely reactions of both the individual and the group. Being excluded or pushed too far too quickly is threatening, especially for the newcomer. The leader has a responsibility to look after anyone to whom this is likely to happen and may himself choose whom to pair in order to ensure a positive experience. Usually the leader participates in the warm-up but is an observer/assistant in the focused play. It is sensible to work with a cotherapist who can take a more dispassionate view of how the session is progressing and intervene if necessary, as when transference or countertransference feelings get out of hand.

Applications

The main application is in brief focal psychotherapy in a group setting with patients who have interactional problems arising from their personalities. Action techniques do not fit into leader-centered transference-analysing groups but are easily integrated into member-centered ones. In my department a conventional group meeting is followed by an action session concentrating on the themes raised earlier. These techniques are widely used in therapeutic communities, adolescent units, community meetings on admission wards, and day hospitals. Patients with poor verbal ability are assisted (thereby extending the range of utility of psychotherapy), those who overintellectualize have their major defence undercut, and the inhibited are prompted to take risks. Long-stay patients and those with mental handicap benefit from warm-ups used alone.

A fruitful use of action techniques is in staff training as part of regular sensitivity meetings. The greater resilience of the professional worker allows the techniques to be used to the full, provided the focus is on the work of the unit rather than the personal deficiencies of team members.

Evaluation

There has been little evaluative research on action techniques in psychotherapy. This is in part because the methodological problems are so great (small numbers, heterogeneous conflicts and treatment variables, uncontrollable external variables, and inherently imprecise measures of outcome) but equally because the techniques were developed outside the arena of therapy and addressed to a nonpatient population. By their nature they are powerful, immediate, and involving, factors that correlate with positive outcome. What needs to be established is whether their use furthers the course of psychotherapy. Clinical experience suggests that they are effective in initiating change but this still requires time and good fortune to become established.

The use of action techniques has certain disadvantages. It is more difficult for the therapist to be nondisclosing, to maintain psychological distance, and to resist being swept away by the impetus of the moment; at times the first two of these may prove to be advantages. Since the techniques are directive, groups tend to be leader-centered with the risk of stifling autonomy in members and promoting only the leader's solutions. In an established group familiar with these techniques the risk is minimal because the members themselves decide the content and direction of the session. Finally, people can learn to simulate involvement, although this rarely happens in clinical practice. Action techniques engage people's ability to think creatively and symbolically. They affirm the individual's capacity to be responsible, make choices, and assist others. By enaction the problem is manifested in an immediate visible way. By acting through in a safe space, new more effective responses may be reached, rehearsed, and adopted into the individual's repertoire.

I should like to acknowledge the helpful comments of colleagues in preparing this paper.

References

Bannister, D (1975) Issues and Approaches in the Psychological Therapies. John Wiley, Chichester. p.127

Barker, C (1977) Theatre Games. Eyre Methuen, London

Blatner, H A (1973) Acting-In: Practical Applications of Psycho-dramatic Methods. Springer-Verlag, New York

Blumberg, A, Golembiewski, R T (1976) Learning and Change in Groups. Penguin, Harmondsworth

Brook, P (1968) The Empty Space. MacGibbon and Kee, London

Buber, M (1957) *Psychiatry*, **20**, 95

Davies, M H (1976) *British Journal of Psychiatry*, **129**, 201

Frankl, V E (1969) The Will to Meaning. World Publishing, New York

Gendlin, E T (1975) American Handbook of Psychiatry, Vol. 5, 2nd edn (edited by Freedman, D X, Drynd, J E). Basic Books, New York. p. 269

Jourard, S M (1964) The Transparent Self. Van Nostrand Reinhold, New York

Jung, C G (1934) The Practical Use of Dream Analysis. Collected Works, Vol. 16. Routledge and Kegan Paul, London

Kahn, J (1971) Human Growth and the Growth of Personality. Pergamon Press, Oxford

Lazarus, A A (1971) Behaviour Therapy and Beyond. McGraw-Hill, New York

Lewis, H R, Streitfield, H S (1970) Growth Games. Harcourt, Brace and Jovanovich, New York

Lieberman, M A, Yalom, I D, Miles, M B (1973) Encounter Groups: First Facts. Basic Books, New York

May, R (1970) Love and Will. Souvenir Press, London

Perls, F (1969) Gestalt Therapy Verbatim. Real People Press, Lafayette, California

Reich, W (1949) Character-Analysis, 3rd edn. Orgone Institute Press, New York

Rogers, C R (1961) On Becoming a Person. Houghton Mifflin, Boston

— (1973) Encounter Groups. Pelican, Harmondsworth

Rolf, I (1958) Structural Integration. The Guild for Structural Integration, San Francisco

Rycroft, C (1968) Causes and Meaning in Psychoanalysis Observed. Pelican, Harmondsworth

Ryle, A (1978) *British Journal of Psychiatry*, **132**, 585

Schutz, W C (1967) Joy: Expanding Human Awareness. Pelican, Harmondsworth

Skinner, S W (1976) Family Therapy—The Treatment of Natural Systems. Routledge and Kegan Paul, London

Stevens, J O (1971) Awareness—Exploring, Experimenting, Experiencing. Real People Press, Lafayette, California

Winnicott, D W (1974) Playing and Reality. Pelican, Harmondsworth

Yalom, I D (1976) Theory and Practice of Group Psychotherapy, 2nd edn. Basic Books, New York

Chapter 15

Psychological aspects and management of obesity

E M Mitchell, St George's Hospital, London

Obesity is a well researched field encompassing a great deal of creative work on different aspects of overeating. Most researchers would probably accept the view that obesity is a complex multidetermined phenomenon, requiring concerted multidisciplinary collaborative investigation. There have been many theories attempting to account for obesity, ranging from those that stress physiological and metabolic factors as paramount to those that emphasize the importance of the role of psychological factors in the genesis and maintenance of obesity. Indeed, Pudel (1976) writes: "Man's relation to his diet is so complex that it is difficult to evaluate the network of vast overlay of nonphysiological factors".

Externality versus internality

The main psychological hypotheses relating to overeating can best be subsumed under the psychosomatic and externality theories of obesity. Both accept as a basic premise that obesity itself is caused by a defect in energy balance and is the result of an excessive intake of calories beyond an individual's requirements.

The psychosomatic theory of obesity was first summarized by Kaplan and Kaplan (1957) who postulated that "psychic cortical factors in addition to or in spite of certain of the automatic somatic regulatory mechanisms produce a disturbance in the activity of the hypothalamic eating centre: this causes an abnormal appetite which may result in an abnormal increase in food intake". They went on to suggest the possibility that hunger is a learned drive, being conditioned to a variety of cognitive, visual, olfactory, and auditory stimuli and provoked by feelings of fear, loneliness, and unworthiness. They also suggested that eating is an act that is incompatible with intense anxiety or fear rather than serving to reduce it.

Atkinson and Ringuette (1967) supported Kaplan and Kaplan's (1957) psychosomatic theory in a survey of psychological features of the massively obese. Their study is one of the few that look at the psychological aspects of eating in the massively obese patient and they found that of 20 patients (both men and women) evaluated on the Minnesota Multiphasic Personality Inventory two thirds reported that emotional factors triggered their overeating.

Bruch's (1969) hypothesis on the excessive intake of the obese individual can also be incorporated into the psychosomatic theory of obesity. She discusses the importance of the relationship between mother and child, in particular their interactions concerning the nature of food, in the development of obesity. She states that as a result of the ambivalence between mother and child food comes to take precedence over other forms of comfort in relieving distress. Ultimately this leads to an inability in the child to differentiate between hunger and emotional stress. Bruch hypothesizes that overeating becomes a nonspecific passive response to any affective or aroused state.

Following Bruch's (1969) hypothesis that obese people fail to discriminate between hunger and emotional states there was a flood of experimental studies examining the responsivity of such individuals to internal and external cues. Although many of these findings conflict and the studies differ widely in their methodology and subject population, the result of such studies have added greatly to an understanding of the relevant psychological variables governing eating behaviour in both normal and obese subjects. Emotional arousal is one of the main internal variables that have been studied in relation to food intake.

Emotional arousal and eating

Stunkard and Koch's (1964) classic experiments involved a comparison of self-reported hunger and gastric motility in obese and normal subjects. While they found that the concordance between these was only 47.6 per cent for those who were obese compared with 71 per cent for normal subjects, obese women showed a response bias generally towards denying hunger. They also found no relationship between hunger responses and scores on the Taylor Manifest Anxiety Scale. More recent studies suggest that there is no clear-cut distinction between correlations of self-reported hunger and gastric contractions. It would seem that both normal and obese individuals are equally poor discriminators. However, there is a good deal of evidence to show that there does appear to be a relationship between emotionality and eating.

Perhaps the most sophisticated studies in this area are by Pudel (1977) whose extensive work with obese, normal, and underweight subjects of all ages led him to conclude that the relationship between emotional arousal and eating follows an inverted-U curve as shown in *Figure 15.1*. Thus moderate arousal is most effective in producing an increase in eating behaviour in obese people. Using stressors such as irregular noise, insoluble anagrams and monotonous sound, he found that the obese increased their intake of fluid above their individual baseline means in response to these. All subjects regardless of weight had difficulty estimating the amount of fluid that they consumed. Obese subjects were also more likely to be responsive to the arousal manipulations used, confirming the work of Rodin (1970) which showed that the obese are more responsive to emotional stimuli.

Slochower (1976) using false feedback of heart rate as the anxiety variable, also manipulated attribution in her experiment on stress and concluded that where arousal is unlabelled or where there is no immediate explanation for physiological symptoms or anxiety there is more likely to be large increases in eating in obese subjects. In her study some subjects were led to believe that their heart rate was being monitored with auditory feedback given. In fact they were artificially fed a high or low heart rate, and whereas one group received an explanation for their high heart rate the other did not. Slochower found that the obese subjects in the no-explanation group ate more, suggesting that labelling or attribution is likely to affect perception of stress and hence eating behaviour. Despite some difficulties in this study, it is important in that it stresses the role of cognitions as a relevant

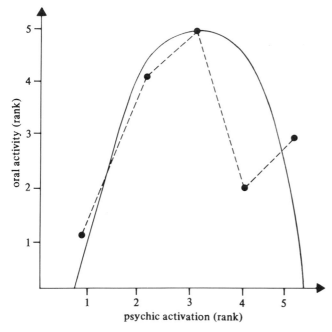

Figure 15.1 The relationship between the degree of psychic activation (pulse-rate ranking) and oral activity (ingestion plus non-nutritive sucking). The inverted-U function demonstrates that a low degree of induced stress and a high degree of induced stress lead to a decrease in oral activity in children. (From Pudel, 1977).

variable for assessment. The results of home diaries, self-report records of the eating behaviour of obese subjects, and mood states also suggest that obese subjects who fail to maintain weight losses eat in relation to a wide variety of emotional states (Leon and Chamberlain, 1973) although eating does not necessarily reduce anxiety.

These studies are in disagreement with Schachter's (1971) externality model of obesity which postulates that excessive eating is primarily due to an increased responsiveness to external cues such as time of day, availability of food, amount of effort required to obtain food, and palatability of the food.

In his early work, Schachter (Schachter et al, 1968) found no significant increase in the amount consumed by obese patients under stress, in this case the threat of electric shock. While the normal subjects ate less when anxious, the obese subjects showed only a nonsignificant trend towards greater consumption. From this, and a series of ingeniously devised experiments measuring the eating behaviour of obese individuals in both naturalistic and experimental settings, he concluded that the obese are more influenced by environmental cues than by the state of their emotions. His conclusions, in particular that obese subjects are more likely to choose the easiest way to eat, to be finicky about their food, to be found in good restaurants, and to be more responsive to good-tasting food, were often based on studies with limited generalizability (that is mildly obese college students) and have not been substantiated by further research. Even when the results are consistent, for example that obese people expend less effort to obtain food and may be more responsive to visually prominent food cues, the studies can be criticized. While the amount of food bought by the obese in supermarkets may eventually be eaten, it may also relate to financial state, number per family, and so on. Many anorectic patients, especially abstainers, hoard vast quantities of food but do not consume it. In addition, when taste ratings are used to induce eating in experimental situations the amount of food consumed is influenced by the type of food given, awareness of being monitored, and confidence regarding ratings. Taste responsiveness too appears to be a complex variable influenced by level of deprivation, type of food consumed previously, and individual preferences.

Perhaps the most interesting results obtained from studies on externality were those showing that compared with lean individuals obese subjects are more distractible, more responsive to emotional stimuli, and more responsive to time manipulations, and have less tolerance and feel that time passes more slowly when they are exposed to boring tapes than to interesting ones.

Despite equivocal results the externality theory has had an enormous influence on the treatment of obese patients, leading directly to the design and implementation of group and individual treatment strategies intended to minimize external influences on eating behaviour and to promote self-control.

However, even Rodin, a prominent researcher in externality, now concludes that those who are truly obese (50 per cent above ideal body weight) are relatively unresponsive to external cues and that externality may be a more generalized trait occurring in varying degrees across a wide variety of weights (Rodin, 1978). Moreover, the vast majority of observational studies on the eating behaviour of obese individuals in naturalistic settings have failed to confirm that existence of an eating style that is specific to them, for example whether they eat more quickly and take fewer bites than normal people. However, there is still little evidence related to periods of weight gain and amount of food consumed because most studies assume that the obese are static in weight, neither increasing nor decreasing.

Perhaps, then, Schachter's (1971) rejection of the psychosomatic hypothesis was premature. As Pudel (1977) has shown, level of arousal is critical in determining whether eating rates increase. In addition, previous exposure to or experience of the stressor influences the results obtained. In a recent experiment with hyperobese patients presenting for bypass operation, subjects shown both high-anxiety and low-anxiety films in the context of presurgical preparation did not display heightened arousal as measured by increased heart rate and skin conductance. It was also reported that previous experience of hospitals and operations and expectations regarding outcome affected their perception of the material presented and consequently their eating behaviour (Mitchell, 1980).

So, given the available evidence, what conclusions can be drawn about the eating behaviour of the obese? First, there is no specific eating style among the obese as was previously believed to be the case. Secondly, while there is some debate as to whether obese individuals eat more than those who are normal they do eat more than their requirements, and both external and internal cues such as emotions and cognitions which were previously considered unimportant produce an effect on eating behaviour and need to be considered in treatment. Other relevant factors governing food intake in the obese are still being explored and it seems unlikely that any one theory could account for all the findings. Rodin (1978) herself concludes that "overeating in the short-term is controlled by external and social factors but responsiveness to external cues may be a reflection of internal physiological cues" (Cabanac and Duclaux, 1970; Wooley et al, 1979). Thus cues such as palatability could be influenced by factors such as level of deprivation or hunger. Similarly, Robbins and Fray (1980) attempted to reconcile external and internal theories of eating by postulating that internal variables, including stress, may increase responsivity to external stimuli, such as type of food, by producing increased activation or arousal. This increase in responsivity then affects internal stimuli, such as insulin secretion, which enhance activation and lead to further eating. Since their work was largely on animals it remains to be seen whether these results hold true for humans.

Personality characteristics of the obese

Parallel with attempts to devise explanatory theories of obesity and the search of variables predictive of food intake, success in treatment, and so on, there have been many studies suggesting that obese people share certain personality traits. In general the results of these studies have been disappointing. Hyperphagia does appear to be correlated with high neuroticism scores on the Eysenck Personality Questionnaire but on the whole, as in other areas, personality attributes tend to be poor predictors of future behaviour.

Psychological treatments

Psychotherapy

It is beyond the scope of this article to review in detail the numerous studies on individual and group procedures aimed at effecting weight loss through insight into the emotional problems assumed to be underlying weight gain. Many of these studies have been case reports and in general neither group nor individual studies appear to be associated with successful weight reduction in the long term.

Behavioural therapy

Behavioural psychologists were initially attracted to the treatment of obesity since it was thought to offer a clear-cut outcome measure of the effectiveness of behavioural intervention. However, the literature shows clearly that weight loss is the result of a complex interaction between physiological and psychological factors, not all of which are within the individual's control. Even when he complies fully with treatment he may still be unsuccessful at sustaining adequate weight loss. Individual differences in metabolic rate and energy intake and expenditure are considerable and affect the rate of weight loss. At least for some fat patients the resting metabolic rate has been shown to decrease with weight loss (Apfelbaum et al, 1973). Behavioural therapy is most commonly used at the beginning of treatment when weight loss is most likely to occur and is more often initially a reflection of fluid loss rather than fat loss.

Notwithstanding, all behavioural treatments of obesity aim primarily to reduce calorie intake by focusing on external factors that are associated with increased food consumption. Although behavioural therapy appears to be effective in the short term, with participants losing up to 5 kg in weight on average, long-term outcome studies are disappointing. The debate outlined above as to the relevance of internal versus external influences and eating behaviour challenges many of the assumptions on which behavioural treatments are based.

TABLE 15.1. Antecedents; specific recommendations abstracted from Stuart and Davis (1972)

TABLE 15.1a. Elimination

		Specific recommendations	Rationale
Basic assumptions	Eating behaviour is elicited by certain antecedent stimuli		
	Reduction of these cues results in an overall reduction of eating		
Step 1		Arrange to eat in only one room and to eat in only one place in that room Do not engage in any other activity while eating	Respondent conditioning — situational cues acquire eating-response-eliciting properties Situational control of hunger — obese people are more vulnerable to external stimulation of hunger and eating responses than the nonobese (Schachter, 1971)
Step 2		Avoid the purchase of problematic foods; shop only from a list and take only enough money to cover the cost	Situational control of hunger by putting temptation out of reach — obese people are more vulnerable to the sight and taste of palatable food
Step 3		Avoid contact with problematic foods that must be kept, that is do not serve high calorie condiments at meals Allow children and spouse to help themselves to dessert Clear plates directly into the garbage	As steps 1 and 2
Step 4		Make problematic eating as difficult as possible: buy foods that need elaborate preparation; toast bread; return loaf to storage after taking one slice	Obese individuals tend not to emit complex or difficult responses to obtain food (Schachter, 1971) A long chain of responses provides three aids: it increases the response cost of eating; it interrupts a process in which automatic eating can occur; and it creates a number of choice points at which an individual may choose not to eat

TABLE 15.1b. Suppression (recommended when elimination is not possible, that is social cues)

	Specific recommendations	*Rationale*
Step 1	Reprogramme the social environment to render the use of food as constructive as possible Provide for positive cueing of desirable behaviours Provide positive reinforcement for acceptable eating, *not* negative reinforcement for overeating	Significant others play a large part in the production of the cues and consequences previously referred to
Step 2	Have other people monitor eating patterns	"When people are alone their social behaviour is often more crude than when they are in social situations" (Stuart and Davis, 1972); they found that fewer cookies were eaten during an experiment when the number was monitored, especially by others
Step 3	Minimize contact with food Serve food on plates in measured small quantities Leave the table soon after finishing the meal	Many calories are consumed in picking at food while slower eaters finish their meal Escape when you cannot avoid problematic food
Step 4	Make small portions of food appear as large as possible — serve on smaller plates	By extrapolation from Schachter's (1971) finding of the influence of the appearance of food one can assume the influence of the appearance of the quantity of food — 70 per cent of women reported greater satisfaction from food on salad plates even though it was self-served (Stuart and Davis, 1972)
Step 5	Control states of deprivation, that is control food deprivation by regular meals, energy deprivation by adequate sleep, and stimulus deprivation by keeping interesting activities available	Food deprivation increases the reinforcement value of food — overeaters frequently eat when fatigued or when bored if more reinforcing activities are not being engaged in

Little evidence exists that differentiates an eating style among the obese from the normal pattern and Wooley et al (1975) suggest that there is not much to show that the stereotyped view of obese people as gluttons is accurate. The bulk of behavioural treatment methods emphasize stimulus-control procedures which focus primarily on modifying the availability of food and the manner in which it is consumed. Perhaps the most widespread recommendations for treatment are those of Stuart and Davis (1972) shown in *Tables 15.1, 15.2, and 15.3*. This programme includes self-monitoring of food intake (either pre-intake or post-intake), self-reinforcement for weight loss and change in eating behaviour, and strategies for overeating based on controlling environmental cues. While some programmes are individualized, the majority are group based and may include contracts for participants as a means of reducing high attrition rates (Hall and Hall, 1974) which

TABLE 15.1c. Strengthening

		Specific recommendations	Rationale
Basic assumptions	Responses that compete with inappropriate eating are elicited by certain antecedent stimuli		
	Increases in these cues result in an overall increase in these responses		
	There is a decrease in inappropriate eating		
Step 1		Provide a reasonable array of acceptable food choices, that is a flexible diet guide	Knowledge of quality and quantity of food provides a cue for appropriate eating
		Provide feedback about the amount that can be eaten by keeping a cumulative record of intake	
Step 2		Save allowable foods from meals for snacks	"Snacking is a treacherous act for overeaters" so save part of the allowed meal in case the desire for a snack arises later
Step 3		Make acceptable foods as attractive as possible by using low-calorie garnishes	Obese people are influenced by the appearance of food but low-calorie food can look as attractive as problematic food

vary from 0 to 83 per cent, and increasing the subjects' compliance. Unfortunately there are very few predictors of good outcome in therapy and many studies confound their results by differing in methodology. Type of subject population, degree of overweight, therapist expertise, and outcome measures used all affect the nature of the results.

Although it would now also appear that externality is a trait that is not specific to the obese, it may well be that high externalizing obese subjects could benefit from these programmes. Similarly, although food consumption by the obese may not be as high as previously thought, food intake is still excessive in respect of their individual energy requirements and it may be useful to elicit situations that provoke excessive uncontrolled eating. The pattern of food intake as well as the amount consumed has been shown to differ, with grossly obese subjects consuming the majority of their daily intake in the evening and little or no breakfast or lunch.

TABLE 15.2. Behaviour; specific recommendations abstracted for Stuart and Davis (1972)

		Specific recommendations	Rationale
Basic assumptions	Obese people have a different eating style from those who are not obese		
	Eating like nonobese people results in weight loss		
Step 1		Slow the pace of eating by: interposing a delay shortly after the start of the meal and as often afterwards as is helpful; swallowing food that is already in the mouth before more food is added and putting cutlery down between mouthfuls; using cutlery at all times for all foods; and counting mouthfuls per minute if necessary	This limits the amount that can be consumed in the available time

Symbolic value provides an early experience of control

Many obese individuals complain of difficulty in controlling what they term their compulsive eating behaviour

When the eating response is given a deviance label and set aside, the individual is not encouraged to undertake changes necessary for its appropriate management |

One promising line of research for treatment of obese patients is the examination of restraint as a variable that more accurately predicts eating behaviour than weight alone. This was first developed in the form of a questionnaire by Herman and Mack (1975) and it reinforces the importance of cognitive factors in food intake. Thus, restraint refers to the restrictions placed by individuals on themselves to curtail their food intake and individuals may be high or low in restraint whatever their weight.

In experimental studies Herman and Polivy (1975) found that subjects high in restraint consumed more following what they imagined to be a high-calorie drink than after a low-calorie drink, regardless of the actual calories involved. In addition, restrained individuals were hyperemotional and failed to consume less when anxious. Although Beinart (1978) in a series of individual case studies did not support this counter-regulation effect, she found that binges were triggered by feelings of guilt and failure. Wardle (1980) concludes that bingeing occurs across a wide range of populations of differing weights and that anxiety and excessive eating as determined by the individuals themselves are likely to result in such behaviour. Thus treatment should focus on reducing restraint and preoccupation with continual dieting. It is interesting that this coincides with the treatment of obese

TABLE 15.3. Consequences: starting with the basic assumption that eating, like other human behaviour, is controlled by its consequences; specific recommendations abstracted from Stuart and Davis (1972)

TABLE 15.3a. Decelerating

	Specific recommendations	*Rationale*
Step 1	Social monitors should respond neutrally to all negative deviations from a weight-control plan	The attention usually given to "bad" behaviour may reinforce it
		This procedure reduces eating — eliciting tension produced by negative interactions
		This potentiates the importance of social reinforcement for adherence to the programme
Step 2	Bring into focus the ultimate aversive consequences of overeating, that is make an individualized list including embarrassment and health risks	Ferster's agreement regarding the long delay of aversive consequences of overeating as opposed to the immediate positive reinforcement (Ferster et al, 1962)

TABLE 15.3b. Accelerating, a more constructive approach

	Specific recommendations	*Rationale*
Step 1	Update eating, exercise, and weight, changing graphs daily	Provides immediate feedback and opportunity for reinforcement — both self and social
Step 2	Arrange for the provision of material reinforcement following completion of eating and exercise requirement and/or weight loss	Material reinforcement promotes high rates of human behaviour and provides opportunity for social reinforcement
		Compliance to the programme must be reinforced as well as weight loss for more immediate reinforcement
Step 3	Social monitors should provide social reinforcement for all constructive efforts to modify weight-relevant behaviours	This adds to the other reinforcers
	Subjects should discuss slimming only with those sympathetic to their objectives	As Stuart and Davis (1972) found: "This is in keeping with the general requirement that an effective weight-control programme must lead to a general reorganization of the role of energy intake and output in the life of an individual and broad changes of this character are likely to be reflected in general philosophical beliefs about what constitutes a 'good life'. For the person effectively controlling his weight, the good life must be expanded to include intelligent decisions with respect to the energy balance and must be narrowed to exclude the pursuit of opportunities to overeat and underexercise."

patients suggested by Orbach (1978) who, while emphasizing the role of society and group pressure to remain slim, could be viewed as facilitating self-monitoring introspection about food consumed as well as reducing guilt and self-blame for failure.

Classical conditioning techniques

The results of aversion therapy, covert desensitization, and covert reinforcement alone have been disappointing in that the weight losses obtained are often minimal and not maintained. In these procedures attempts to associate eating specific foods with negative stimuli such as shock, nausea and noxious odours have met with little success, and in covert desensitization the main finding of interest is that subjects who show the highest arousal are more likely to show the greatest weight loss (Janda and Rimm, 1972).

Summary of behavioural treatments

The failure of psychological treatments to produce consistent long-term weight loss in obese subjects has led directly to a re-examination of the nature of their eating behaviour and, as stated above, to the development of new theoretical models of obesity. While behavioural therapy techniques have succeeded in producing weight losses in the region of 5 kg on average, and in the short term may be more cost-effective than drug therapy when the patients are seen in groups and by paraprofessionals, many of these subjects regain the weight lost. The majority of treatment methods involve a reduction in food intake most commonly by self-control procedures. Since recent evidence implies that the use of these techniques may derive from false assumptions, a return to individually designed treatments is perhaps the optimum strategy to maximize long-term weight loss (Wooley et al, 1979). It may be necessary to focus on relevant areas involving the wider application of behavioural therapy methods such as anxiety-management training including cue exposure and response prevention. As is most commonly suggested, a change of responses leading inevitably to overeating can be identified.

The development of innovative treatment methods for obesity will require an increased understanding by therapists of the role of physiological factors in weight loss and maintenance of target weight and of the limitations these place on the outcome. Perhaps one neglected area in treatment is helping the individual during the following weight loss towards a greater understanding of the factors that for him are likely to be associated with weight gain. Self-reinforcement for maintaining weight and the role of the family in promoting, facilitating and maintaining weight loss may also be useful. However, the acknowledgement of the role of cognitive factors may eventually lead towards the development of more sophisticated treatment methodologies encompassing physiological aspects of obesity and based on social psychological theories of attitude change.

References

Apfelbaum, M, Bostsarron, J, Lacatis, D (1973) in Energy Balance in Man. (edited by Apfelbaum, M). Masson, Paris. p. 71
Atkinson, R M, Ringuette, E L (1967) Psychosomatic Medicine, 29, 121
Beinart, H (1978) unpublished MPhil Thesis, University of London

Bruch, H (1969) *Journal of Nervous and Mental Disease*, **149**, 91
Cabanac, M, Duclaux, R (1970) *Science*, **168**, 496
Ferster, C B, Nurnberger, J I, Levitt, E B (1962) *Journal of Mathetics*, **I**, 87
Hall, S M, Hall, R G (1974) *Behaviour Therapy*, **5**, 352
—, —, Hanson, R W, Borden, B L (1974) *Journal of Consulting and Clinical Psychology*, **42**, 781
Herman, C P, Mack, D (1975) *Journal of Personality*, **43**, 647
—, Polivy, J (1975) *Journal of Abnormal Psychology*, **84**, 666
Janda, L H, Rimm, D C (1972) *ibid.* **80**, 37
Kaplan, H I, Kaplan, M S (1957) *Journal of Nervous and Mental Disease*, **125**, 181
Leon, G R, Chamberlain, K (1973) *Journal of Consulting and Clinical Psychology*, **40**, 474
Mitchell, E (1980) unpublished
Orbach, S (1978) Fat is a Feminist Issue. Hamlyn, Middlesex
Pudel, V E (1976) *in* Appetite and Food Intake (edited by Silverstone, T). Abakon Verbag Gesellschaft, Berlin.
—(1977) *International Journal of Obesity*, **1**, 369
Robbins, T W, Fray, P J (1980) *Appetite*, **1**, 103
Rodin, J (1970) unpublished Doctoral dissertation, University of Columbia
—(1978) *in* Recent Advances in Obesity Research (edited by Bray, G A). Newman, London. p. 75
Schachter, S (1971) Emotion, Obesity, and Crime. Academic Press, London
—, Goldman, R, Gordon, A (1968) *Journal of Personality and Social Psychology*, **10**, 91
Slochower, J A (1976) *Psychosomatic Medicine*, **38**, 131
Stuart, R B, Davis, B (1972) Slim Chance in a Fat World: Behavioural Control of Obesity. Research Press, Illinois
Stunkard, A J, Koch, C (1964) *Archives of General Psychiatry*, **11**, 74
Wardle, J (1980) *Journal of Consulting and Clinical Psychology*
Wooley, O W, Wooley, S C, Woods, W A (1975) *Journal of Comparative and Physiological Psychology*, **89**, 619
Wooley, S C, Wooley, O W, Dyrenforth, S W (1979) *Journal of Applied Behaviour Analysis*, **12**, 3

Further reading
Bruch, H (1973) Eating Disorders. New York Basic Books, New York

Chapter 16

Psychotherapy research today

Sidney Crown, The London Hospital

Psychotherapy research, while remaining self-critical, enters the 1980s in an optimistic frame of mind. Achievements are admirably presented in the critical reviews forming Garfield and Bergin's (1978) fine handbook. This book combines a searching critical attitude together with a sense of solid achievement. It should surely impress all except critics whose approach to psychotherapy, sadly, seems unalterably negative.

Psychotherapists, both psychodynamic and behavioural, recognize the need for objective research using sound basic methodology. They are also on the lookout for new and worthwhile problems to investigate and aware of the need for fresh investigative approaches.

In this paper I wish to discuss some researches relating mostly to psychodynamic individual psychotherapy which strike me as promising and original and which might spark off ideas for research in others. I have not attempted to cover research in group, marital, family, or behavioural therapy or the specific sex therapies.

This paper forms a pair with another (Crown, 1980) in which I attempted to outline the future of the psychotherapies in a more formal way, concentrating on basic research problems, the need for control or comparison groups, the assessment of results, follow-up, and so on.

"Spontaneous" recovery revisited

Careful sifting of the evidence led Bergin and Lambert (1978) to suggest that 43 per cent of clients recover without psychotherapy ("spontaneously"); the overall figure for recovery with psychotherapy is 65 per cent. These quantitative considerations raise several important points for outcome research, considered here and in the next section.

First, what constitutes therapy? Patients report both positive help and negative consequences from human interactions as varying in intensity and structure from a single line in a play to 15 years of psychoanalysis. Life events affected people's psychological development for better or worse long before the area was documented as life-events research.

The nearest we can approach to the untreated patient—to the systematic investigation of spontaneous change—and the related question of what constitutes therapy is to document the changes following, catalysed by, or achieved by a minimal but systematically recorded interaction with a psychiatrist as in a psychotherapeutic consultation. This might also help with another important question: what is the quality of spontaneous remission?

The only research known to the writer to record these issues systematically and in depth, combining an appropriately rigorous method with rich clinical documentation, is that of Malan et al (1975). This team's sample consisted of 45 patients seen for consultation at the Tavistock Centre who, for various reasons, never received treatment and were followed-up for a minimum period of 2 years. Of these, 23 (51 per cent) were judged to be "improved" at least symptomatically and 11 (24 per cent) psychodynamically. It is interesting, in view of the catchment area served by the Tavistock Centre (a middle-class area of London with a high intellectual attainment), that a slightly higher figure than Bergin and Lambert's (1978) overall 43 per cent spontaneous recovery was achieved.

In this paper, however, I focus attention upon the analysis and description of the 11 patients judged by Malan et al (1975) to be improved on psychodynamic criteria. The information in the case notes was used, before seeing the patient for follow-up, to make an explanatory hypothesis of the subject's disturbances together with criteria, taking into account his situation as a whole, that must be met if he is to be regarded as altered psychodynamically. Systematic study was also made of the qualitative information and of the comments of patient and therapist initially and at follow-up. Two distinct therapeutic factors were discovered: insight and bringing the patient face to face with the necessity of taking responsibility for his own life.

These findings fit interestingly into what I would see as a general concordance of view among psychotherapists of varied backgrounds and approaches as to the importance of both self-knowledge (insight) and the need for self-determination in order to shift personal responsibility from others (including the psychotherapist) to the patient himself. This approach finds parallel interest in social psychology as the "locus of control" theory. It has also long been expounded by J D Frank (for example Frank, 1974) as an important therapeutic component of psychotherapy.

These considerations are of value because of the light they throw on spontaneous change and what constitutes therapy and also on the possibility of spontaneous change being truly psychodynamic rather than restricted to symptomatic change. They are relevant not only to the as yet underinvestigated area of the possibility of designing and using a minimal treatment technique such as one or two psychotherapy interviews to effect change in psychoneurotic, psychosocial, and psychosexual problems, but also in the field of liaison psychiatry with colleagues in medicine, surgery, and primary care. There is already some evidence of the effects of minimal psychotherapy on the utilization of medical and surgical services, as discussed below (Schlesinger et al, 1981).

Fresh approaches to psychotherapy outcome

Good rather than bad effects are the aim of psychotherapy. Thus, of the two fundamental areas of psychotherapy research, outcome (or what happens) is even more basic than process, which is concerned with how psychotherapy causes change. Outcome and process are, however, intricately interrelated and this relationship has been emphasized in the constant question asked of clinicians and researchers: which psychotherapy, by which therapist, for which sort of client?

Here I only want to note in passing the need for systematic small-scale, carefully constructed, and controlled studies of the effects of alternative therapies or of therapy and no-treatment control because this approach was stressed in my companion paper (Crown, 1980). Let me turn instead to an indication of fresh approaches to outcome research.

Amateurs versus professionals

In the last few years there has been an invasion into psychotherapy of essentially amateur therapists—often anti-Establishment, pragmatic, and atheoretical. These persons are represented partly in the self-help movement and partly in the so-called third force (after psychoanalysis and behaviourism) of the humanist–existential therapies. Doubts and fears about standards and training have been voiced by Strupp (1976).

It is, however, Strupp himself with his team in the Vanderbilt Psychotherapy Project who have initiated a series of fascinating experiments. Strupp and Hadley (1981) compared therapeutic outcome and therapeutic process in 15 patients (referred to a student health service and suffering from neurotic depression anxiety, and personality disorders) given psychotherapy by trained psychotherapists with a comparable patient group treated by college professors chosen for their ability to form understanding and empathic relationships and for their interest in students but with no formal psychotherapeutic training.

The overall improvement of patients in the two groups was comparable. There was, however, considerable individual variability in therapeutic benefit or deterioration. Professional therapists appeared particularly effective with patients who were well motivated for therapy and whose resistance to change was low. In contrast, patient involvement was less important to nonprofessional therapists who on average were moderately successful regardless of such involvement.

This paradox will not be news to trained psychotherapists who tend to have a negative attitude to patients who fail to fulfil requirements such as high motivation, whereas the less well trained or untrained person may have fewer inhibitions about treating an apparently unsuitable client.

This research design should be replicated. If confirmed it should help to throw light on how far psychotherapeutic results are obtained by training and specific techniques over and above the qualities inherent in any good human relationship. It might, for example, be shown that the professional as compared with the untrained therapist may achieve more uniform results; isolated brilliant results or therapeutic miracles can be achieved by anyone, but not consistently! Higher general outcome level and less variability would, of itself, be a convincing argument for formal psychotherapy training.

Therapeutic success and failure in the same therapist

Every psychotherapist has both therapeutic successes and therapeutic failures and it is often difficult to know why one or the other. This area extends into the problem of the negative effects and dangers of psychotherapy which are considered below.

Strupp (1980a) hit on the interesting but obvious-when-you-think-about-it idea of actually comparing details of therapeutic success and failure by individual therapists. He systematically compared two patients treated by the same therapist for apparently similar problems under comparable conditions. Criteria for classifying the patient as successfully treated or unsuccessfully treated were extensive and comprehensive and included psychometric tests, rating scales, and video observation.

A careful examination of pretreatment, and of treatment, and post-treatment follow-up data underlined the overriding importance of the patient's antecedent personality make-up to the success or otherwise of therapy. While both patients had seemed clinically and psychometrically similar, it became apparent that they were in fact very different individuals in a number of ways. The successfully treated patient was reasonably mature, competent, and assertive; he had relatively specific difficulties and was highly motivated for help and willing to work towards solution of his problems. The unsuccessfully treated patient was immature, passive dependent, timid, and ambivalent about psychotherapy.

The systematic comparison of patients successfully treated and unsuccessfully treated by the same therapist was repeated with other patient–therapist dyads (Strupp, 1980b, c); in one of these comparisons (Strupp, 1980d) the performance of one of the nonprofessional lay counsellors mentioned above (Strupp and Hadley, 1981) was investigated. All comparisons of success and nonsuccess led to the importance of the patient's basic personality and how this affected the patient–therapist interaction.

These papers confirmed the clinically strongly held view of the overriding relevance of the patient's personality (ego strength, maturity, motivation, ability to involve himself in the therapy, and so on) to the outcome of psychotherapy. It is important to note, however, that such findings are not in accord with one currently influential view that *therapist-provided conditions* such as empathy, warmth, and genuineness are the crucial factors in successful psychotherapy. This point is considered below in the discussion of the psychotherapeutic process.

Dangers of psychotherapy

Any active medical treatment has potential dangers and psychotherapy is no exception. For many psychotherapists it was Bergin's (1971) review that made them face up to the problem of deterioration effects, both in clinical practice and as a research problem. In connection with the assessment of outcome Bergin (1971) suggested that averaging the effects of psychotherapy was not necessarily the most appropriate mode of assessment because there was a considerable range of outcome and good might be counterbalanced by bad.

In a systematic investigation Hadley and Strupp (1976) asked 150 psychotherapists of all major approaches whether they acknowledged the existence of negative effects of psychotherapy—that is permanent effects attributable to the psychotherapy—and what were the likely sources of such effects. Seventy therapists replied and the existence of negative effects was agreed virtually unanimously. These included personal repercussions (for example severe breakdown, dropping out of therapy, and substituting undesirable personality traits for symptoms), as well as repercussions on important aspects of the patient's life such as work, friendships, spouse, or children.

Many possible causes were adduced for such negative effects. These included faults in the therapist such as personality deficiencies, poor clinical judgement, or deficiencies in training and skills; incompatibility between the patient's and therapist's personalities and deficiencies in the patient such as poor motivation or inadequate personality resources for therapy as well as inaccurate or deficient assessment of the patient so as to fail to reveal these deficiencies. The goals of therapy may be vague or unrealistically high. There may be technical faults such as the misuse of interpretations, the therapist's consciously or unconsciously encouraging dependency in the patient and sometimes producing a "therapy addict", or the handling of countertransference problems—especially hostile ones—badly.

The negative effects of psychotherapy are an area of clinical salience and further research needs to be aimed at the anticipation and avoidance of such effects and at developing methods for their alleviation if they arise.

Psychotherapy and medical utilization

Psychotherapy research has almost universally focused on the patient, the therapist, and their interaction. The effect of these on outcome is usually defined in terms of alteration in symptoms or "target" complaints and on work, social, family, and sexual adjustment.

Utilization studies form an important methodological contribution from social medicine. Attempts are made to establish the impact of a given intervention, whether a screening programme or treatment, on the utilization of services— medical, surgical, or social. This focus is relevant both as a practical contribution in times of economic stringency and as an alternative research strategy to the direct study of patients.

Schlesinger et al (1981) reviewed two different kinds of research evidence in order to assess the impact of psychotherapy on medical utilization: "archival" studies and controlled experimental studies. Archival studies are retrospective quasi-experiments, making use of existing clinical records in which the patient's use of medical services before, during, and after psychotherapy is documented. Some studies had comparison groups who did not receive psychotherapy and others used patients as their own controls. While the method is far from rigorous because a number of the component studies are methodologically flawed, the findings suggest that patients who have psychotherapy subsequently use medical services less than those in the comparison group who do not have psychotherapy. Expressed numerically the psychotherapy group showed an average reduction in subsequent medical utilization of up to 14 per cent.

Controlled experiments are of course superior in evidential quality to archival studies. Such studies were carried out in three areas: the treatment of alcoholism and of asthma and the recovery from medical and surgical crises. The effects on alcoholism were unimpressive in that, although an initial treatment effect could be demonstrated, results for treated cases and controls were identical within one year of follow-up. With asthma the results were comparable with those for psychotherapy in general. There was a demonstrable effect on outcome indicators having direct medical relevance, for example the use of medicine, hospitalization, and visits to the emergency room. Studies of "psychologically informed intervention" on patients facing surgery showed that fewer than 10 per cent of 82 outcome indicator comparisons favoured the control group. Studies that used duration of postsurgery hospitalization as an outcome indicator demonstrated that psychotherapy patients had hospital stays almost 2 days shorter than controls.

This methodology is interesting and promising; it has been neglected in the UK but deserves our further attention.

Statistical meta-analysis of effectiveness of psychotherapy

In an influential paper Smith and Glass (1977) made what they called a meta-analysis of psychotherapy outcome studies, introducing what appears to be a useful method of statistical analysis to quantify the general effectiveness of psychotherapy. This method involves a statistic called the effect size (ES). Published data are first evaluated for the adequacy of their basic methodology, in particular that a psychotherapy treatment group should be compared with a comparison or control group. ES involves a type of statistical significance effect.

ES is the mean difference between the treated and the control subjects divided by the standard deviation of the control group. It may be calculated on any outcome variable the researcher chooses to measure, for instance anxiety, self-esteem, and work achievement.

In Smith and Glass's (1977) paper, nearly 400 controlled evaluations of psychotherapy and counselling were considered. On average the therapy client is better off than 75 per cent of untreated individuals. No differences in effectiveness were discovered between all broadly behavioural and all broadly nonbehavioural (including psychodynamic) approaches. What makes the method especially interesting is, first, the care with which studies are examined and rated for detailed methodology before being included in the statistical meta-analysis and, secondly, that large numbers of both studies and patients are included in the analysis.

The ES method therefore buttresses the analysis of Bergin and Lambert (1978) in showing, albeit in a quantitative rather "blanket" way, that psychotherapy is effective. We are still left with the need to plan and execute smaller-scale studies designed to investigate particular aspects of psychotherapy in detail so as to establish qualitatively as well as quantitatively exactly what is achieved with whom and by whom.

The psychotherapeutic process: patient–therapist interaction

Second only to whether psychotherapy gets results—now surely established beyond reasonable doubt—is how these results are achieved, that is the psychotherapeutic process. There has been a tendency up until recently to adopt an attitude to process whereby the principal actors—patient and therapist—as well as their social situation were pictured as somewhat static and unchangeable. Thus if a patient's "personality" is assessed by a given method as "unsuitable" for psychotherapy there is grave danger in assuming not only that this patient "cannot work" in interpretative therapy but also *will never be able to do so*. However, in various areas of psychotherapy, such as marital and family therapy and therapy for psychosexual dysfunctions, contemporary emphasis has become, rightly in my view, interactional. This implies that one key to the psychotherapeutic process may lie not in what is present at the beginning of therapy between patient and therapist but in what develops and transpires between them. Thus what we may properly be concerned with is a detailed analysis of the patient–therapist interaction rather than with supposedly fixed personality qualities or with an immutable environment.

I would therefore like to focus on some examples of research in which the interaction between patient and therapist is of major concern. I include studies that seem to provide fresh approaches to process, several of which strike me as particularly imaginative, interesting in themselves, or potentially fruitful for research.

Therapist interpersonal skills, transference, and other process factors

Therapist interpersonal skills   The search for *the* factors basic to change in psychotherapy received a fillip from the formulation by Truax and Carkhuff (1967) of necessary and sufficient conditions for change in psychotherapy: accurate empathy, nonpossessive warmth, and genuineness. These ideas sparked off considerable therapeutic enthusiasm. Although seemingly an oversimple formulation to many, counsellors especially and many psychotherapists leapt prematurely on this Rogerian bandwagon as if an acquaintance with these therapist variables was the answer to how to become an effective psychotherapist.

Considerable research followed and inevitably came the reaction when this research was looked at critically. A review by Lambert et al (1978) is trenchant in its marshalling of the facts and their evaluation. Empathy, warmth and genuineness are difficult to define operationally and difficult to measure—different measures correlate very poorly with one another—and seem to have only a modest individual relationship to therapeutic outcome. If they are relevant to outcome it is important to establish *when* they are or are not relevant. Thus it may not be the empathy, warmth and genuineness *as such* that are important process variables but *when* in the therapy these therapist interpersonal skills are likely to be productive.

The matter rests at the moment polarized but with the probability that if these therapist variables are important considerable further refined analysis and research will be needed.

Transference   In psychoanalysis the interpretation of how the patient puts onto the therapist ways of relating to important figures in the past has been a basic contribution to what would now be called the psychotherapeutic process. The need to objectify the concept and refine its investigation arose. Malan (1963, 1976) in replicated studies with statistically reliable techniques showed that a good therapeutic outcome tended to be related to a therapist–parent transference link occurring and to the interpretation being made early in the course of therapy.

Luborsky et al (1979) studied objectively the preconditions and consequences of transference interpretations in three patients using a methodology that involved independent judges taking 250 word samples before and after an interpretation and then rating these. Each patient was shown to have an individual response to interpretation which was typical for him. There was also a clear parallel between the amount of immediate response to interpretation and the therapeutic outcome.

Transference is a key area of the dynamic psychotherapies and this type of objective research is to be welcomed.

Readiness to change—attitude or set, arousal, motivation, and locus of control   Accumulating clinical and research experience consistently underlines the relation to psychotherapeutic effectiveness of a group of complex cognitive-motivational factors which might loosely be described as readiness to change. Although related in part to the patient's initial personality characteristics, these factors also seem to develop within the patient–therapist interaction and their development may be associated with outcome. The immediate response to interpretation mentioned in the previous section (Luborsky et al, 1979) may represent one facet of these complex factors. Certainly readiness to change seems to have components of attitude or set, of arousal, of motivation, and of the desire for inner rather than outer directedness.

That emotional arousal might lead patients to be more susceptible to persuasive communications was suggested by Frank (1974) who carried out mildly confirmatory experiments using drugs such as ether or adrenaline. Sifneos (1979) is also of the view that anxiety-provoking questions stimulate patients to look at areas of conflict; witness the name for his therapy—short-term anxiety-provoking psychotherapy (STAPP). The relation of arousal and tension to optimal performance is frequently represented by an inverted U-shaped curve: too little or too much is detrimental. The research problem remaining in relation to psychotherapy seems to be to establish this relationship more precisely.

Motivation to change in terms of willingness to allow basic personality adjustments has for long been thought of as crucial for successful psychotherapy. It also seems an element likely to be related partly to personality factors in the client at the outset of therapy and partly to developments within the ongoing psychotherapeutic process. Sifneos (1979) emphasizes that the client should show high motivation for change and not only for symptom relief. He specifies criteria for judging motivation. These include the ability to recognize symptoms as psychological in nature, to introspect, to give an honest account of emotional difficulties, and to participate actively in treatment.

Keithly et al (1980) objectified their intake interview, the assessment of process, and the outcome measures. A motivation scale was elaborated from Sifneos' (1979) criteria. The reliability between judges was assessed. The results not only showed good motivation to be related to outcome but also emphasized the interactional aspects of patient motivation: that its presence may influence the *therapist's behaviour* towards the client during treatment.

Inner-directedness versus outer-directedness, locus of control, feeling of self-directedness rather than other-directedness, and self-responsibility—these all express an area of interest felt by many psychotherapists of different approaches to be of increasing importance. In accounting for spontaneous positive change Malan et al (1975) suggested that the clients who showed positive change seemed to take some responsibility for themselves and their problems together with developing insight during the diagnostic interview.

This is a genuinely intriguing area in need of further objective evaluation.

Personal values and attitudes

That the process of psychotherapy might be influenced by personal values and attitudes of therapist and client is not a new idea. In one sense it seems obvious in terms of personal friendships and enmities. Where psychotherapists have perhaps been too naive is in supposing that factors such as the training of the therapist or his personal insight can eliminate this important variable. The opposite view is expressed by the suggestion that success in psychotherapy may be achieved in proportion to the gradually converging values of therapist and client.

The issue has been raised in more eloquent form by Bergin (1980), a distinguished psychotherapist, innovative researcher, and influential synthesizer. He takes up the problem from the viewpoint of religious values and attitudes, noting that in the USA 90 per cent of the population express religious belief and 30 per cent strong conviction. These figures are likely to be significantly discrepant with the therapist's religious involvement which tends to a religious liberalism compared with the general population. Bergin quotes studies showing that other values of mental health professionals with respect to such topics as sexuality, aggression, and authority also contrast with the values held by a large proportion of their clients.

Psychotherapy with the socially disadvantaged

In his classic essay Goffman (1963) defines stigmatized people as those who, for whatever (and many) reasons, are not afforded full social recognition. In this sense he instances the blind, the deaf, and the physically handicapped. The concept of stigma can be usefully extended to the psychotherapy field where patients who are young, intelligent and basically effective (despite their symptoms) have, perhaps understandably, always been enthusiastically considered for psychotherapy. Sifneos (1979), for example, representing an influential approach to brief psychotherapy, tends to restrict therapy to persons whose psychosexual development is relatively adult (oedipal problems) and who are highly motivated as described in the previous section. Thus he perpetuates an elitist tradition. Given the caseload of the average NHS psychiatric outpatient department, it is of major importance to see how far psychotherapy can be effective with less privileged clients.

Three groups of clients may be taken as an example: those of lower social class, the middle-aged and elderly, and ethnic subgroups.

Social class   The evidence on social class suggests that it is verbal-educational status that is important rather than social class as such and this would agree with the clinical experience of the writer working in East London. As a general principle, with lower class clients the balance between a dynamic-interpretative approach and a behaviourally orientated one should be shifted towards the latter. Further research in the UK is needed.

Age   Age as such is probably a far less important factor than conventionally thought for success in insight-orientated psychotherapy. Emotional flexibility, motivation, desire to change, and ability to establish a trusting relationship are what are important and there is no evidence that these qualities are age-related.

This general point may be underlined in relation to a specific area: sexuality. Pfeiffer (1974) points out that at 68 years of age about 70 per cent of men with previously active sex lives have regular sexual activity and at 78 years about 25 per cent are sexually active. Nor is there any biological limitation to sexual capacity in the ageing female. For a long time ageing persons have been considered not to have any sexual feelings. But what follows from the recognition of the sexual needs of the elderly is that, just as with younger persons, sexual problems arise that trouble older people and psychotherapy can and should be extended to cover these and other problems of living of the older person. Again further research is needed.

Ethnicity   The other parameter of psychotherapeutic nonacceptance and stigma relates to ethnicity: can psychotherapy be successfully carried out with persons from a different culture? This is a salient problem in the UK.

The bulk of research has come from the USA and concerns concordant and nonconcordant matching of black or white clients with black or white therapists. Early research suggested that concordant matching achieved the best results. However, a recent elaborate and extremely impressive piece of research by Jones (1980), himself black, suggests from an elaborately balanced design such that all ethnic combinations of therapist and client were studied that the factor of ethnic matching had little relationship to outcome.

It must be remembered, however, that in the USA both black and white client and therapist speak the same language. In the UK we have many ethnic groups whose language and culture are likely to be different from those of the psychotherapist.

Eliminating the therapist: how far can we go?

It is right not to take previously held, accepted, or even hallowed views about psychotherapy without question. In this sense, while for certain psychotherapists and certain patients the importance of the therapist may be paramount, there are some therapeutic contexts in which the therapist may be less important or even contraindicated. Lieberman et al (1973), for example, in their comprehensive investigation of many different forms of encounter group included two groups led by tape recorder.

Packaged therapies

Clients not infrequently ask for books to read and often seem to find their reading helpful to their therapy. So do students as part of the educational process and there is reason to regard psychotherapy, at least in part, as educational in its mode of operation. A natural extension of this line of reasoning is to experiment with how far certain therapies might be packaged, especially those dealing with the relatively circumscribed areas such as specific phobias or psychosexual problems. It is in the latter area that there is some objective information.

Matthews et al (1976), in an investigation of the behavioural treatment of sexual inadequacy, included a treatment modality described as directed practice with minimal counselling. Couples were seen only three times during treatment and instructions about directed practice were sent weekly through the post. This and two other treatment procedures involving greater contact with the therapist were randomly allocated. Thirty-six couples were involved including mainly male erectile impotency or premature ejaculation or female low sexual interest, arousal, or anorgasmia. There were no significant differences between the results of these three treatments either post-treatment or at follow-up 3 months later.

In a different context Currey (1970) used a questionnaire to assess sexual difficulties in a group of 121 persons suffering from osteoarthrosis of the hip. Two thirds experienced some degree of sexual difficulty. The author assessed the number of patients who would have been grateful for advice on sexual problems and the form they would have preferred this advice-giving to follow. Just under one half (48 per cent) of 81 of the group favoured a booklet—a far higher proportion than those who favoured their family doctor (16 per cent), a hospital doctor (21 per cent), or a medical social worker (6 per cent). Even taking into account that this is essentially a middle-aged group (the majority 40–60 years old), this desire for a distance approach to sexual counselling is striking. The finding relates too to the need expressed in the previous section for counsellors and psychotherapists to cater for the middle-aged and elderly.

Group practice of psychotherapy

Cummings and Vanden Bos (1981) suggest (and give supporting case material) the idea, taken from group general practice (primary care), that several psychotherapists, each expert in a different modality of brief psychotherapy, should work from a centre. A client over the course of years in a particular district and attending a particular practice may present with different problems needing varying approaches. Thus at separate times a client might be treated by different experts according to the problem. Therefore, although the therapist *as such* would not be eliminated, a specific client-therapist relationship between two people would not be regarded as unique in its quality or indispensability.

Summary

If, as Popper's apt title suggests, science consists of conjectures and refutations, then in addition to sound methodology bright ideas are needed. I have outlined some ideas and directions within psychotherapy research which I describe as intriguing. Thus the qualitative nature of spontaneous change is being established as a baseline with which to compare therapeutic change. Of the basic problem of psychotherapy research improving outcome remains paramount and, on the other side of the coin, the recognition and elimination of negative effects.

Attempts are being made to determine in what ways training in psychotherapy helps effectiveness over and above being a concerned "other person". To advance further the understanding of an elusive issue a given therapist's outstanding successes have been compared with his humiliating failures to try to determine why one and why the other. There are new attempts at evaluating psychotherapy such as its effect on medical and surgical utilization. A new statistic, Effect Size (ES), appears useful to demonstrate psychotherapeutic effectiveness over and above a control or comparison treatment.

Process studies have been re-evaluating the importance of therapist interpersonal skills such as empathy, warmth, and genuineness. Interactional aspects are also being explored: *when* should therapists optimally show empathy? Transference, a hallmark of the analytic psychotherapist, is being subjected to objective analysis as is motivation, a much emphasized selection variable. Many therapists stress the need for clients to acquire the capacity for inner directedness rather than the passive acceptance of help. The goodness or badness of fit between the personal values and attitudes of therapist and patient are coming under increasing scrutiny. There is a need to determine how far psychotherapeutic techniques in general or which technique in particular is appropriate to the socially disadvantaged. Exploration is also being directed to how far hallowed psychotherapeutic assumptions, such as the need for a therapist or for a particular therapist, are actually justified.

References

Bergin, A E (1971) *in* Handbook of Psychotherapy and Behavior Change: An Empirical Analysis (edited by Bergin, A E, Garfield, S L). John Wiley, New York
—(1980) *Journal of Consulting Clinical Psychology*, **48**, 95
—. Lambert, M J (1978) *in* Handbook of Psychotherapy and Behavior Change: An Empirical Analysis, 2nd edn (edited by Garfield, S L, Bergin, A E). John Wiley, New York. p. 139
Crown, S (1980) *in* Priorities in Psychiatric Research (edited by Lader, M). John Wiley, New York. p. 129
Cummings, N, Vanden Bos. G (1981) *Professional Psychology*
Currey, H L F (1970) *Annals of Rheumatic Disease*, **29**, 488
Frank, J D (1974) *Journal of Nervous and Mental Disease*, **159**, 325
Garfield, S L, Bergin, A E (1978) Editors. Handbook of Psychotherapy and Behavior Change: An Empirical Analysis, 2nd edn. Wiley, New York
Goffman, E (1963) Stigma. Penguin, Harmondsworth
Jones, E E (1980) Paper read at Society for Psychotherapy Research, Oxford
Hadley, S W, Strupp, H H (1976) *Archives of General Psychiatry*, **33**, 1291
Keithly, L J, Samples, S J, Strupp, H H (1980) *Psychotherapy and Psychosomatics*, **33**, 87
Lambert, M, DeJulio, S, Stein, D (1978) *Psychological Bulletin*, **85**, 467

Lieberman, M A, Yalom, I D, Miles, M B (1973) Encounter Groups: First Facts. Basic Books, New York

Luborsky, L, Bachrach, H, Graff, H, Pulver, S, Christoph, P (1979) *Journal of Nervous and Mental Disease*, **167**, 391

Malan, D H (1963) A Study of Brief Psychotherapy. Tavistock Publications, London

—(1976) The Frontier of Brief Psychotherapy: An Example of the Convergence of Research and Clinical Practice. Plenum, New York

—, Heath, E S, Bacal, H A, Balfour, FHG (1975) *Archives of General Psychiatry*, **32**, 110

Matthews, A et al (1976) *Behaviour Research and Therapy*, **14**, 427

Pfeiffer, E (1974) *Journal of the American Geriatrics Society*, **22**, 481

Schlesinger, H J, Mumford, E, Glass, G V (1981) *in* Sage Annual Reviews of Community Mental Health, Vol. 2: Psychotherapy—Practice. Research, Policy (edited by Vanden Bos, G R). Sage, London

Sifneos, P E (1979) Short-Term Dynamic Psychotherapy. Plenum, London

Smith, M L, Glass, G V (1977) *American Psychologist*, September, p. 752

Strupp, H H (1976) *ibid*, **31**, 561

—(1980a) *Archives of General Psychiatry*, **37**, 595

—(1980b) *ibid*, **37**, 708

—(1980c) *ibid*, **37**, 947

—(1980d) *ibid*, **37**, 837

—, Hadley, S W (1981) *ibid*, **36**, 1125

Truax, C B, Carkhuff, R R (1967) Towards Effective Counselling and Psychotherapy. Aldine, Chicago

Chapter 17

Coping with schizophrenia

Hugh L Freeman, Hope Hospital, Salford

This title might be taken to imply that doctors do most of the coping with people suffering from schizophrenia, but in fact relatives bear the greatest part of this burden in spite of social and demographic changes that make it increasingly difficult for them to do so. Although only the minority of schizophrenics in hospitals and hostels are coped with primarily by nurses or residential care staff, the medical function is still essential; however, it is intermittent and does not require the stress of living in close contact with these patients. In exercising their skills in diagnosis, prescription and administration of services, doctors can easily overlook the continued patience and dedication that others have to show in caring, as well as the risk of this deteriorating into neglect. Better psychiatric training has improved the medical understanding of schizophrenia, but voluntary organizations—particularly the National Schizophrenia Fellowship—have also contributed greatly to this and to the mutual support of affected families.

Nature of the problem

With the conquest of infectious diseases schizophrenia has become the major public health problem of developed societies, not so much as a result of its prevalence— Cooper (1978) reports a mean annual incidence of 3.3 per 1000—but because it usually begins in adolescence or early adulthood. Since schizophrenics have a life expectancy little different from that of the general population they may be chronically ill or susceptible to further relapse for up to 50 years. Such lengths of time constitute the real size of the problem and should govern the pattern of services, for instance in trying to reduce the discontinuities resulting from constant changes of professional staff.

The Office of Health Economics (1979) estimates that 300 000 people in the UK have had a diagnosis of schizophrenia at some point in their lives and 150 000 are affected at any one time. More people of working age (in hospital or disabled in the community) suffer from it than from any other condition. The annual cost of health and social care for schizophrenics is some £200 million—most of it for staff and less than 4 per cent for neuroleptics, which therefore seems very cost-effective. With all public spending under scrutiny the management of schizophrenia should be a special concern of social policy, although there is little sign of it being so.

While an association has long been noted between schizophrenia and low social class, it is now generally accepted that this is not causal but the result of drift. Cooper (1978) describes "a pattern in which early timidity and shyness, loss of peer relationships in adolescence, poor school performance and early work record, reduction in social status and, finally, migration into a decaying, disorganized urban area" occurs in those with an inherent vulnerability, often combined with environmental stress. Their migration takes place "along with many others who show reduced economic effectiveness and reduced social-network cohesiveness" (Levy and Rowitz, 1973). The result is an excess of schizophrenics (as of alcoholics and persons with severe personality disorders) in inner-city districts; they are often unmarried and detached from family or other social networks.

Schizophrenics are a considerable problem for mental health services, not only because of the severity of their conditions but also because social isolation and often poverty increase their demands. It would follow that a higher level of service provision is needed in inner-city areas, yet the opposite is often the case. National planning ought to take account of the movements of schizophrenics and there is a special need to integrate medical, social, and voluntary services for them. By no means all are socially isolated, but Cooper (1961) found that patients who had been living alone at the time of admission had a much worse outcome than those from a family setting, probably because of a lack of social support.

The overall problem of schizophrenia is also related to prognosis, yet its prediction is often problematic. The international follow-up study by the WHO (1979) found great variability in outcome over 2 years, even among patients who showed the same initial clinical picture. The results supported the previously accepted predictors of good outcome (affective symptomatology, acute onset, good premorbid personality, and married status). However, there was also a marked difference between developed and developing countries—outcome being much better in the latter—although most of the variance could not be related to any known factors. Brown et al (1966) followed up 111 patients first admitted to three hospitals in 1956 and found that after 5 years 56 per cent had recovered socially, while another 34 per cent were socially disabled but out of hospital. Overall outcome is unlikely to have changed significantly since then, so there are many schizophrenics with moderate to severe chronic disability who need care.

Although hospitalization is not necessarily directly related to clinical status, the most handicapped are likely to be chronic inpatients. Cunningham Owens and Johnstone (1980) examined all long-stay schizophrenics in a large mental hospital and found them in general to be extremely impaired in terms of mental state, cognitive abilities, motor functioning, and capacity to satisfy physical and social needs. Each of the various abnormalities showed a strong correlation with the others so that only hospital care could cope adequately with the general degree of disability. Although these patients represent one end of the spectrum of prognosis, their numbers are significant. The National Schizophrenia Fellowship (1979) has described the past 20 years' run-down in mental hospital beds as "a dangerous mixture of idealism and expediency" since one third of schizophrenics require "continuous treatment, protection and support in hospital or equivalent sheltered surroundings". Many severely handicapped patients are looked after for years by devoted relatives but are likely to need alternative care sooner or later.

The most frequent behaviour problems at home reported by relatives to Creer and Wing (1974) were social withdrawal, underactivity, lack of conversation, absence of interests, slowness, restless overactivity, odd ideas and behaviour, depression, and neglect of appearance. Since the incidence of their seeking help had generally been discouraging, it was surprising that so many had managed to find a way of living with their situation. However, an acceptance that a low level of performance or disturbed behaviour is "normal" for a schizophrenic may be required. In a survey of chronic schizophrenics living outside hospital in Salford (Cheadle et al, 1978; Korer et al, 1978) 41 per cent showed no sign of psychosis, but almost all of these were taking neuroleptics mostly in depot form. On the other hand, neurotic symptoms were frequent and showed a strong association with social handicaps.

Pattern of services

The philosophy behind the present pattern of services is contained in the White Paper *Better Services for the Mentall Ill* (DHSS, 1975). This derived from the discovery of effective physical treatments, developments in social psychiatry, the 1957 Royal Commission's emphasis on movement from institutional to community-based care, the concept of the district general hospital, and the unification of social services. It has resulted in a partial reversal of the process of concentrating the mentally ill in public asylums which began early in the last century as a reaction against the "community care" of prisons, workhouses, and private exploitation (Wing, 1978a); however, the process was never completed. Social factors are always important; for example, Mills (1962) found in East London in the late 1950s that admission was unlikely if there was a female relative in the home who was available to care for the psychotic patient.

The move to community-based care, however, rested on the assumption that a network of alternative facilities would be set up, mainly by local authorities. Since no government would make them mandatory or earmark funds for them, provision has remained patchy and far below official targets. In Surrey the number of places for day care is 557 below the recommended guidelines (Priestley, 1979) and there are still authorities providing neither day care nor hostels. Acute hospital care has been taking place increasingly within the district general hospital, but very unevenly: over two thirds of schizophrenic admissions are still to mental hospitals, which are also responsible for most long-term care. While the psychiatric hospital population has fallen dramatically in the last 25 years, new long-stay patients continue to accumulate and most are schizophrenics. Mann and Cree (1975) in their national sample of this group found that only 15 per cent were suitable to live outside the hospital without supervision; 33 per cent needed further hospital care and 20 per cent required a supervised residential setting.

Hospital services for schizophrenics are generally satisfactory, although admission arrangements may need to be quicker and smoother in acute episodes; these are best dealt with on an inpatient basis unless a combination of day care and family support can provide an effective substitute. However, organized programmes of supervised accommodation remain scanty and the right degree of social pressure can only be applied if there is a continuum of residential settings (National Schizophrenia Fellowship, 1979). It is not only the lack of facilities but also the different styles of management within them that hamper the patient's progress and assessment; the National Schizophrenia Fellowship's proposed solution is a "campus community" in which accommodation with varying degrees of supervision would be on a single site with a common staff.

In a survey of hostel residents Hewett and Ryan (1975) found them mostly working and with few behaviour problems, but tending to see the hostel more as a long-term home than as transitional accommodation. However, staffed hostels are very expensive and the group home has emerged as a much cheaper alternative, with visiting supervision by nurses and social workers (Soni et al, 1978). Sympathetic landladies can also make a valuable contribution but are difficult to find, and all forms of sheltered accommodation, including that provided by patients' families, require day care as an essential complement. Better integration of the activities of existing services would in fact lead to all of them working more effectively.

The roles of professional staff

Schizophrenia causes special difficulties in the roles of professional staff because of the complexity of its effects. As a long-term disease with most sufferers outside hospital, its management should be the responsibility of GPs (Parkes et al, 1962; Freeman, 1968). A sympathetic and informed GP can be very helpful, yet most patients have a very different experience and "The concept of the 'primary health care team'...remains largely a mythical ideal" (Priestley, 1979). As a result specialist secondary care workers must often take over continued responsibility, but since no individual is constantly available for the lengths of time involved this has to be a *team* commitment. The psychiatrist generally has the function of coordinating relevant services; however, a development in the USA is the nonprofessional "case manager" (a member of the Community Support Systems programme) who has the responsibility of ensuring that the treatment plan is carried out (Turner, 1978).

Priestley (1979) also found that relatives of schizophrenics are very unlikely to seek help from social services. However, an experienced social worker with psychiatric knowledge can support and counsel these families, for example by devising with them more effective ways of handling difficult behaviour (Creer, 1978). An informative, nonjudgemental, and readily available counselling service is one of the overwhelming needs of relatives, but social services very rarely provide it. Not only is mental health generally of low priority but psychiatric expertise has also been seriously affected by the Seebohm reorganization. Yet the psychiatric social worker is just as essential as the doctor or nurse with specialist training.

To some extent the gap has been filled by the remarkable recent growth of community psychiatric nursing. Clearly, a nurse is not the same as a social worker—for one thing he cannot take action under the Mental Health Act, 1959—but psychiatric nurses are experienced in managing the behaviour of psychotic patients and are able to give injections. Where community nursing has been well developed, many families are already looking to the community psychiatric nurse as a primary source of help. However, in Surrey one nurse was found to be solely responsible for a district with 138 000 people (Priestley, 1979).

An examination of the use of hospital services by chronic schizophrenics in Salford (Freeman et al, 1979a) showed that only 8 out of 102 had made heavy demands during a year, mainly through hospital admission. Medium use of services was by prolonged day care (14) while the great majority were light users (63) receiving depot injections and outpatient supervision. Use of social services followed the same trend as hospital services rather than making up for them.

Medical treatment

The details of medical treatment in schizophrenia are not covered here but are dealt with by Johnson (1977) and Freeman (1978). Neuroleptics represent the foundation of current treatment and are generally effective in controlling abnormal experiences and disturbed behaviour but not negative symptoms or chronic handicaps. Given prophylactically they can also prevent many relapses and the problems of noncompliance have been overcome by the development of depot injections. Hirsch et al (1973) proved the superiority of depot administration of neuroleptics over placebo injections. Also, a series of mirror-image studies, for example those of Johnson and Freeman (1972), agreed in finding a marked superiority of depot over oral treatment in reducing hospitalization; only Falloon et al (1978) came to a different conclusion.

Since neuroleptics were first introduced there has been dispute as to how long treatment should be continued. The idea that schizophrenia becomes "burnt out" over time is now largely discredited, certainly in respect of patients outside an unstimulating hospital milieu. Medication is still important by the fourth year, particularly for those who have remained in a steady mental state until then, although the rate of relapse is up to 40 per cent even on uninterrupted treatment (Johnson, 1979). Stopping drugs after 2 years' remission was followed in the next year by relapse in 68 per cent of one group; in this study the superiority of maintenance treatment over no treatment increased with time and the view that patients with good prognostic signs do not need prophylaxis was not supported (Hogarty, 1979). This author has also shown that a combination of social therapy and medication is more effective than either alone. As a result of side effects (sometimes irreversible) prescribing must be kept to the minimum that will prevent relapse, a level that can be found only by trial and error.

Although medication may be needed, getting it to the large number of people involved outside hospitals over long periods of time causes great problems of management and information. During the process patients are easily lost and so there is a need for some form of continually updated register to prevent this from happening, such as the one that has been developed in Salford (Freeman et al, 1979b). However, conventional medical treatment is not universally accepted and success has been claimed for psychological interpersonal methods (Berke, 1977; Mosher and Menn, 1978); so far these alternatives have not been evaluated in samples of undoubted schizophrenics.

Neuroleptics appear to reduce the physiological responsiveness of schizophrenics to environmental stimuli, including emotional interactions with relatives. If this is so, pharmacological effects may differ according to the social environment and the need for long-term treatment might be determined by physiological measures of arousal (Leff, 1979). However, this is not yet clinically possible.

Rehabilitation and home life

In a condition causing such widespread impairment rehabilitation is crucial but should be seen as "a continuous process of accommodation" rather than steady progress towards a role in the community (Bennett, 1978). The pursuit of unrealistic goals of "success" in terms of work and social functioning is likely to be disastrous because of the frequent cognitive defects that make patients abnormally distractible and unable to process information, including language. These problems call for a simplified environment and for freedom from the need for complex decision-making. A series of limited objectives must be defined with a programme of specific action to reach them, proceeding by trial and error until an optimum level is obtained; the aims then are to prevent relapse and develop any personal assets (Wing, 1978b).

This often means treading a knife-edge between the dangers of social withdrawal and understimulation on the one hand and those of excessive arousal on the other—a process that also has to continue in the home. It is made more difficult by the fact that many patients have fluctuating insight and are periodically affected by delusions and hallucinations, although careful attention to medication may reduce such changes. Behaviour therapy would seem to provide a possibility of improving the quality of life, but so far remains at an experimental stage (Gwynne Jones, 1978). The response of schizophrenics to rehabilitative efforts is often disappointing and it is said that "what they want to do they can't, and what they can do they don't want to". Although many will never return to open employment, a properly organized system of industrial rehabilitation can make the most of their residual capacity. However, the pioneering Bristol scheme (Early, 1978) has been little emulated elsewhere.

An understanding of these problems has been greatly increased by the research on family environment by the Institute of Psychiatry. The original finding was that a patient discharged to lodgings had a lower relapse rate than one returning to his family (Brown et al, 1958), and subsequently it was noted that the quality of family relationships influenced the course of illness independently of the individual's past history and his condition on discharge (Brown et al, 1962). The critical factor was shown to be expressed emotion (EE) on the part of relatives, its intensity being directly related to the risk of relapse (Brown et al, 1972). Relapse was also found to be related to the frequency of life events, which Schwartz and Myers (1977) have shown to occur more often in schizophrenics than in normals. Whereas regular medication appears to protect patients to a large extent from the risk of relapse due to a high degree of EE, it often fails to do so with life events (Leff et al, 1973). It was also found that 35 hours of contact per week was the critical point beyond which the influence of high EE was likely to have a harmful effect (Vaughn and Leff, 1976).

These findings show that schizophrenics, even when outwardly impassive, are abnormally sensitive to the effects of the social environment. There are many cases where contact with a key relative (showing high EE) should be minimized, for example by day care of even by moving to a hostel. It would be valuable to have a measurement of EE available as a clinical tool, but this is not yet possible. However, some patients have separated themselves from family contacts, perhaps as a self-protective mechanism.

Our knowledge of schizophrenia is therefore considerable although incomplete along any one dimension. The task ahead is to make full use of this knowledge in the services that are actually available to patients and their families.

References

Bennett, D H (1978) in Schizophrenia: Towards a New Synthesis (edited by Wing, J K). Academic Press, London

Berke, J H (1977) Butterfly Man. Hutchinson, London

Brown, G W, Carstairs, G M, Topping, G G (1958) *Lancet*, ii, 685

—, Monck, E M, Carstairs, G M, Wing, J K (1962) *British Journal of Preventive and Social Medicine*, **16**, 55

—, Bone, M, Dalison, D, Wing, J K (1966) Schizophrenia and Social Care, Maudsley Monograph No. 17. Oxford University Press, London

—, Birley, J L T, Wing, J K (1972) *British Journal of Psychiatry*, **121**, 241

Cheadle, A J, Freeman, H L, Korer, J R (1978) *British Journal of Psychiatry*, **132**, 221

Cooper, B (1961) *British Journal of Preventive and Social Medicine*, **15**, 17

— (1978) *in* Schizophrenia: Towards a New Synthesis (edited by Wing, J K). Academic Press, London

Creer, C (1978) ibid.

—, Wing, J K (1974) Schizophrenia at Home. National Schizophrenia Fellowship, Surbiton

Cunningham Owens, D G, Johnstone, E C (1980) *British Journal of Psychiatry*, **136**, 384

DHSS (1975) Better Services for the Mentally Ill. HMSO, London

Early, D F (1978) *International Journal of Mental Health*, **6**, 80

Falloon, I, Watt, D C, Shepherd, M (1978) *Psychological Medicine*, **8**, 59

Freeman, H I(1968) *British Medical Journal*, iv, 371

—(1978) *in* Schizophrenia: Towards a New Synthesis (edited by Wing, J K). Academic Press, London

—, Cheadle, A J, Korer, J R(1979a) *British Journal of Psychiatry*, **134**, 417

—, Cheadle, A J, Korer, J R(1979b) *ibid*. **134**, 412

Gwynne Jones, H (1978) *in* Schizophrenia: Towards a New Synthesis (edited by Wing, J K). Academic Press, London

Hewett, S, Ryan, P (1975) *British Journal of Hospital Medicine*, **14**, 65

Hirsch, S R, Gaind, R, Rohde, P D, Stevens, B C, Wing, J K (1973) *British Medical Journal*, i, 633

Hogarty, G E (1979) *in* Management of Schizophrenia (edited by van Praag, H M). Van Gorcum, Assen

Johnson, D A W (1977) *British Journal of Hospital Medicine*, **17**, 546

— (1979) *in* Management of Schizophrenia (edited by van Praag, H M). Van Gorcum, Assen

—, Freeman, H L (1972) *Practitioner*, **206**, 395

Korer, J R, Freeman, H L, Cheadle, A J (1978) *International Journal of Mental Health*, **6**, 45

Leff, J P (1979) *in* Management of Schizophrenia (edited by van Praag, H M). Van Gorcum, Assen

—, Hirsch, S R, Gaind, R, Rohde, P D, Stevens, B C (1973) *British Journal of Psychiatry*, **123**, 659

Levy, L, Rowitz, L (1973) Ecology of Mental Disorder. Behavioural Publications, New York

Mann, S, Cree, W (1975) *British Journal of Hospital Medicine*, **14**, 56

Mills, E (1962) Living with Mental Illness. Routledge and Kegan Paul, London

Mosher, L R, Menn, A Z (1978) *in* Alternatives to Mental Hospital Treatment (edited by Stein, L I, Test, M A). Plenum Press, New York

National Schizophrenia Fellowship (1979) Home Sweet Nothing. National Schizophrenia Fellowship, Surbiton

Office of Health Economics (1979) Schizophrenia. Office of Health Economics, London

Parkes, C M, Brown, G W, Monck, E M (1962) *British Medical Journal*, i, 972

Priestley, D (1979) Tied Together with String. National Schizophrenia Fellowship, Surbiton

Schwartz, C C, Myers, J K (1977) *Archives of General Psychiatry*, **34**, 1238

Soni, S, Soni, S D, Freeman, H L (1978) *International Journal of Mental Health*, **6**, 66

Turner, J (1978) Mimeographed Reports. National Institute of Mental Health, Washington DC

Vaughn, C F, Leff, J P (1976) *British Journal of Psychiatry*, **129**, 125

WHO (1979) Schizophrenia: An International Follow-up Study. Wiley, Chichester

Wing, J K (1978a) Schizophrenia and its Management in the Community. National Schizophrenia Fellowship, Surbiton

— (1978b) *in* Schizophrenia: Towards a New Synthesis (edited by Wing, J K). Academic Press, London

Chapter 18

The causes of alcoholism

Anthony W Clare, Medical College of St Bartholomew's Hospital, London

Considering that the definition of alcoholism is itself a subject of some controversy (WHO, 1952; Keller, 1960; Edwards et al, 1976) it is not surprising that theories about what actually causes the condition are numerous, diverse, and sometimes contradictory. Alcohol is widely available in most cultures and so any explanation has to account for the differences between the minority who become alcoholics and the majority who do not. Many attempts to provide such an explanation have been made but to date no single theory has proved adequate. Indeed, partly as a consequence of this failure many experts subscribe to the view that there is no single cause and alcoholism is best envisaged as a condition in which several factors operate to produce the final clinical picture (Chafetz, 1966; Criteria Committee of the National Council on Alcoholism, 1972). The major explanatory models are discussed in detail below. However, it is important to bear in mind that while many of these theories contain useful insights concerning the nature of alcoholism at present, none can be considered in isolation from the others.

Any explanation of alcoholism needs to take into account the particular properties of the drug (alcohol), the constitution and personality of the individual consuming it and the social and cultural milieu in which alcohol use and abuse occur. Each of the following three major categories of aetiological theories places special emphasis on one of these factors.

Biological models of alcoholism primarily focus on the pharmacological properties of alcohol and its effects on the CNS. The alcoholic tends to be portrayed as a person who, by virtue of some previously unexplained disturbance in his ability to metabolize alcohol normally or some particular sensitivity to alcohol or one of more of its breakdown products, is constitutionally predisposed to develop physiological dependence on the substance.

Psychological theories tend to rest on the assumption that alcoholics share certain personality traits or tendencies believed to be of crucial importance in the development of the disorder. In the past such a view has led to attempts to describe the so-called alcoholic personality, that is a constellation of traits, attitudes, and aptitudes thought to constitute a specific psychological vulnerability to develop alcoholism. More recently, psychological theorists have turned their attention to the manner in which individuals learn to use and misuse alcohol and the view of alcoholism as a learned piece of maladaptive behaviour has consequently gained ground.

170

The last category of explanatory theories goes outside the drug and the individual and explores the strong empirical relationship that exists between sociocultural variables and the incidence of alcohol use, abuse, and dependence. In the view of those who advance this sociocultural model of alcoholism the reasons why a person drinks and hence the reasons why he abuses drink are primarily sociological and anthropological rather than physiological or medical.

Biological causes

The earliest biological models of alcohol dependence tended to suggest that the circumstances of intoxication were themselves a necessary and a sufficient reason to explain the remorseless spiral towards ever-increasing drinking, craving, tolerance, dependence, and harm (Emerson, 1934). Within the framework of such explanations the potent addictive properties of alcohol were emphasized, in particular the tissue tolerance, withdrawal symptoms, subjective craving, apparent loss of control over consumption, and the steady physical and mental deterioration.

Much research has been directed at detecting biochemical, physiological and neurophysiological abnormalities to explain the mechanisms of alcohol addiction. However, the great bulk of such research has tended to be concerned with individuals *already* heavily dependent on alcohol. Thus, while a number of possible disturbances in physical functioning have been reported in alcoholics, there is much uncertainty about the actual causal status of such abnormalities since they may be as much the consequences of alcohol abuse as its antecedents.

Metabolic causes

The search for some metabolic defect in individuals physiologically dependent on alcohol is constant but to date has not been particularly fruitful. Alcoholics have been reported to metabolize alcohol at a faster rate than nonalcoholics. Other physiological and biochemical measures that have been claimed to differentiate alcoholic from nonalcoholic populations include sleep patterns (Johnson, 1971), salivary flow, glucose metabolism, and the excretion of certain metabolic products in the urine (Kissin et al, 1973). In all of these studies the alcoholic populations showed abnormalities that were altered in the direction of normality following the ingestion of alcohol (Kissin, 1974).

This has led to a suggestion that alcohol exercises a normalizing effect in alcoholics; that is in a dry state the alcoholic's physical condition is thought to differ significantly from that of nonalcoholic controls, but when drinking it moves back to normality. If such physiological or biochemical differences between alcoholics and nonalcoholics could be shown to antedate the onset of alcohol dependence than this would indeed be powerful evidence in favour of the view that alcohol has a unique functional value to the incipient alcoholic. However, once again it has to be acknowledged that such differences may well be the result rather than the cause of excessive alcohol ingestion and until there is conclusive evidence to demonstrate the proper causal sequence this normalizing theory will remain speculative.

Neurotransmitter alterations

Recently there has been increased interest in the roles of certain specific neurotransmitter systems in the genesis and presentation of psychiatric disorders including alcohol dependence. The monoamine neurotransmitters suspected to be involved in mood disturbances, anxiety and tension have been particularly studied (Israel et al, 1972; Griffiths et al, 1973; Post and Sun, 1973). Experiments on ethanol-dependent animals have shown an increase in catecholaminergic activity in the brain when compared with controls. Catecholamine turnover in the CNS continues at a high rate during the early period of withdrawal but probably falls thereafter (Littleton, 1977). Urinary catecholamine secretion in man has been shown to increase in alcoholics during a drinking bout and at the time of the subsequent physical withdrawal syndrome; the results are similar to those reported in animals (Feldstein, 1971).

The role of brain amino acids that are thought to have neurotransmitter functions, for instance gamma-aminobutyric acid, proline and aspartic acid, has been recently studied (Griffiths and Littleton, 1977) and it is interesting that many of the changes in concentrations may well be the precursors of the monoamine transmitter alterations mentioned above. It has also been suggested that during chronic alcohol ingestion derivatives of neurotransmitters and of alcohol may act on centres in the brain, rather like the way metabolic products of morphine and other opiates are believed to act on specific opiate receptors in the brains of seriously drug-dependent individuals. The discovery of naturally occurring morphine-like substances (enkephalins) that act on morphine receptors in the brain and exert powerful analgesic effects (Hughes et al, 1975) has provoked a new enthusiasm among researchers anxious to clarify the physiological basis of drug and alcohol dependence (Littleton, 1977).

Genetic factors

Given that the rates of alcoholism are much increased among the relatives of alcoholics compared with the general population, the question arises as to whether genetic mechanisms are involved in the condition. There have been reports of associations between alcoholism and known inherited characteristics or genetic markers such as colour blindness, of preference for alcohol in genetic strains of mice, and of an increased incidence of alcoholism among adopted individuals with a known alcoholic biological parent from whom they were separately reared (Goodwin et al, 1973, 1974).

Human populations have been found to differ in their responses to alcohol for reasons that are clearly not entirely cultural. For example Koreans, Chinese, and Japanese become flushed more often than caucasians after small doses of alcohol (Wolff, 1973). Furthermore, there are differences between populations in the relative frequencies of various types of the enzyme alcohol dehydrogenase which is crucially involved in the metabolic breakdown of alcohol in the body (Shields, 1977). There are also reported differences in the rates at which ethnic groups eliminate ethanol from the blood (Fenna et al, 1971).

To date, explanations other than the genetic ones for such phenomena have not been disproved. There are also those, for example Pattison (1974), who argue that on intuitive grounds alcoholism seems too complex a behaviour pattern to be explained solely by genetic determinants or biological defects. However, in a recent detailed review of the subject Shields (1977) concluded that despite many uncertainties and inconsistencies there is growing evidence "that genetic factors, some general, others perhaps relatively specific, are probably involved (along with others) in the development of alcoholism in man".

Psychological causes

An influential explanatory model is the one that derives its theoretical framework from classic psychoanalytical theory. This theory locates the source of problem drinking within the individual's psychological make-up. From such a position has developed the idea of the alcoholic personality, a personality-type vulnerable to alcohol and prone to develop alcohol dependence. An alternative psychological view is that derived from behavioural theory: this considers alcoholism, like any other deviant behaviour or symptom, to be the result of maladaptive learning which must be corrected by a process of retraining. A strikingly different conception derived from the principles of transactional analyses explains alcoholism as a game, a consciously adopted stratagem that enables the alcoholic (and those around him) to cope with his and their personalities, difficulties, and interactions.

Psychoanalytical theories of causation

Psychoanalysts define addiction in terms of a dependence on a substance, an activity, or a person which is believed to provide pleasure on the one hand and relief from psychic pain or anxiety on the other. Such a dependence is thought to result from a failure of personality development on the part of the addict. Addiction is seen as a protective defence against the graver consequences of such a failure, for instance suicide, psychosis, or asocial or criminal behaviour. This double function of the addictions led some analysts to place them midway between the neuroses (conceptualized as attempts to avoid psychic pain) and the perversions (attempts to obtain pleasure). From the psychoanalytical viewpoint alcoholism can be considered as a substitute for emotionally mature adaptation, a means of coping with conflicts, or the result of a variety of specific failures in emotional growth (Blum, 1966).

Some analysts stress the aspects of general dependency exhibited by many alcoholics and relate them to unresolved conflicts over parental relationships in early childhood. Others emphasize the element of modelling in child–parent relationships. The adult alcoholic's pathological behaviour is seen to reflect actual pathological recollections of what his parents were like as well as false recollections based on childhood fantasies and impressions.

The so-called ego-defence methods employed by the alcoholic, namely the denial of unpleasant reality and the projection of blame, are viewed as relating to the inability to delay the gratification of impulses and drives. The alcoholic is seen as an economically and emotionally dependent person, passive and lacking in perseverance and devoid of interest in achieving anything other than immediate pleasure or relief. His love relationships are characterized by a self-centredness and a clinging to mothering persons, with depressive moods when such support is not forthcoming.

The major problem with such an explanatory theory is that it is too all-embracing. While it is true that alcoholism is a pathological condition characterized by immature functioning, regression and denial are also associated with a number of other forms of psychiatric illness and deviant behaviour. Why does alcoholism develop in some and not in others? Moreover, the disinhibiting effects of alcohol that facilitate the overt expression of repressed feelings and regressed behaviour are commonly observed among drinkers who have not progressed to alcohol abuse and dependence. Similarly, while the disruptive experiences of early childhood may increase vulnerability to the development of alcoholism, they are far from specific to alcoholism and are reported in a wide variety of psychopathological conditions.

Finally, there is a very serious shortcoming of such theories which has been remarked on by critics of psychoanalysis, namely that they are difficult to disprove. It is impossible to disprove the immaturity of the alcoholic personality since his alcoholism is evidence of it and all the explanations of the genesis of that personality are retrospectively based.

Personality theories

For many years attempts have been made to delineate a consistent set of personality attributes that correlate with the development of alcoholism. However, despite a wealth of studies no specific personality traits have been linked to alcoholics. In so far as unusual or abnormal traits have been found, they have been attributed to the effect of alcohol abuse with as much ease as they have been blamed for its cause.

The best evidence for the causal status of trait variables in the development of alcoholism is to be found in longitudinal studies of personality but these are relatively rare. In one celebrated study Jones (1968) described the personality characteristics of 66 boys studied during childhood. Six of them subsequently manifested problem drinking and were reported to have been uncontrolled, impulsive, and rebellious during childhood. However, the small numbers in the study suggest that the results should be interpreted with caution. McCord et al (1962) followed-up 255 boys after 18 years and found 29 who exhibited alcohol problems. When their childhood records were matched with a control group of nonalcoholic boys early personality traits of unrestrained aggression, hyperactivity, denial of childhood fears, and inferiority feelings (hypermasculinity) were identified to a significantly greater extent in the alcoholic subjects' childhood assessments.

A related explanation involves the fact that alcohol acts as a potent tranquillizer for highly anxious individuals. There is some support for the view that some alcoholics manifest high levels of anxiety and that alcohol has depressant and sedative pharmacological properties (Vogel-Sprott, 1972; Barry, 1974). In addition, there is evidence that the precipitating occasion for the onset of drinking episodes in alcoholics is often the occurrence of heightened anxiety (Belfer et al, 1971). There appears to be a number of reasons why people drink and it has been suggested that those who drink merely for alcohol's psychotropic effects are especially prone to encounter alcohol-related problems (Edwards et al, 1972). However, there is still insufficient evidence for the notion that anxiety is more prevalent among alcoholics than among other groups of disturbed individuals for whom alcohol has not become an important method of coping. Nevertheless, many alcoholics spontaneously list as one of their main motivations for drinking the fact that alcohol does provide a tranquillizing effect.

It has also been suggested that alcoholics are individuals who suffer from pervasive feelings of inferiority that result in an enhanced need for power in the face of inadequate personality resources for achieving it. Confronted with frustrated ambitions the alcoholic resorts to drinking in order to have a sense of self-satisfaction and achievement as well as a release from tension (McClelland et al, 1972). At present this striving for power formulation remains an interesting but unsupported hypothesis.

Behavioural theories

A relatively simple psychological theory of alcoholism is that based on behavioural principles. Alcoholic behaviour is understood to be caused and maintained by the simple association of drinking with a positive and rewarding experience. Alcoholism is regarded as a conditioned behavioural response that can be unlearned through the appropriate modification of environmental stimuli and reinforcement situations. More complex theories acknowledge that alcohol abuse is a highly complicated form of behaviour. However, the major assumption remains the same, namely that alcoholics begin and continue drinking because alcohol ingestion is followed by a fall in anxiety, stress, or tension.

A two-stage model to explain the genesis of excessive drinking has been suggested by Bandura (1969). According to this the positive value of alcohol initially derives from the central depressant and anaesthetic properties of the substance. Thus, individuals who are subjected to stressful situations may obtain relief through drinking alcohol due to its pharmacological effects. The behaviour of drinking is reinforced by the reduction in unpleasant experience that follows it. Repeated experiences in which the drinking of alcohol leads to a lessening of anxiety, stress, or other aversive stimuli result in a progressive strengthening of the alcohol habits. Once established the excessive use of alcohol begins to have aversive effects on the individual that in turn set up renewed stimulus conditions for continued drinking. With prolonged heavy drinking physiological alterations eventually occur in the body resulting in physiological dependence. As a consequence the distressing withdrawal symptoms themselves become the stimulus conditions for alcohol consumption. In second-stage conditioning drinking is reinforced automatically and continually through the alleviation and termination of withdrawal symptoms which alcohol provides.

Support for such a tension-reducing hypothesis has been obtained from animal studies. However, to consider tension and its reduction as the sole causal factor is not warranted by the facts (Cappell and Herman, 1972). Nevertheless, other behavioural factors may have aetiological significance. Social reinforcement (such as peer approval) or imitative behaviour (for example of parental drinking attitudes and habits) may serve to initiate and/or maintain excessive drinking (Orford, 1977). More recent behavioural approaches to alcoholism have tended to see the specific antecedents and reinforcers of excessive drinking as highly variable from one individual to another. Such theories indicate that a careful analysis of the precise stimulus–response–reinforcement relationships in each case is essential for an understanding of aetiology (Sobell and Sobell, 1972).

Alcoholism as a game

Some theorists, drawing on the concepts employed in transactional analysis, have argued that alcoholism (like other forms of deviant behaviour) is best understood as a game, that is a complicated series of transactions engaged in for the purpose of obtaining an interpersonal advantage. By this it is implied that alcoholism should be understood as a sequence of interpersonal moves with an ulterior motive or pay-off rather than as an addiction, illness, or psychological defect. Steiner (1969) has even gone so far as to identify three distinct games.

There is the aggressive game in which the alcoholic puts himself in a position of being obviously disapproved of and allows those who disapprove to appear virtuous and blameless. The specific thesis of the game is "you're good, I'm bad, try to stop me". It is suggested that the alcoholic player is basically interested in making persecuting parental figures so angry that they show their impotence and foolishness.

There is also the self-damaging game usually played with a partner who is unable or finds it very difficult to provide emotional or sexual support. As a consequence the alcoholic's continued drinking is to the partner's advantage since as long as the drinking continues the partner's own emotional deficiency and his part in the game will not be exposed.

The third game, based on tissue self-destruction, is characterized by the alcoholic obtaining satisfactions (or strokes as transactional analysts term them) by making himself physically ill. By sacrificing his bodily integrity he forces others to take care of him. The pay-off in this game is the provision of medical care and treatment, nursing attention, and accommodation.

The attractiveness of such conceptualizations of alcoholism is that they provide some useful insights into the phenomena of alcoholism. However, caution needs to be exercised in handling them. Once again it is the behaviour of the alcoholic and those close to him *after* he has developed his alcoholism which forms the foundation of the explanatory theory. Many of the interactions observed by behavioural analysts result from the alcohol misuse and cannot logically be identified as causes of the condition. The other problem with such approaches is that they embody a strong moralistic and punitive flavour hardly warranted by the evidence.

Sociocultural causes

The facilitating effect of certain cultural factors on the development of alcoholism is well recognized. Mortality rates from cirrhosis of the liver vary greatly from country to country. Schmidt (1977) points out that rate differences among general populations of such magnitude usually indicate a priori the importance of environmental influences in the aetiology of the disease. Since the mortality rate from cirrhosis of the liver due to factors other than alcohol use has varied very little over the last 20 years in most Western countries, alterations in the rate can be attributed to changes in the number of chronic heavy users of alcoholic beverages.

Over the past two decades mortality from cirrhosis of the liver has increased at a steady and often rapid rate in many parts of the world (Massé et al, 1976). During this same period the idea that the rate of an alcohol-related problem in a population is associated with the per capita level of alcohol consumption has gained ground. Such a view shifts the search for *causes* of alcoholism away from the individual's psychopathology and biochemistry and towards those factors (potentially within society's grasp) that may influence overall consumption rates.

Occupational factors

Occupation appears to play an important role in alcoholism (Plant, 1977). Working in the drink trade as a barman, publican, wine merchant, or brewer places the individual at a high risk but others including seamen, printers, salesmen and businessmen also show high rates of alcoholism (Registrar General, 1971). Murray (1978) has drawn attention to the fact that doctors too exhibit high rates of alcoholism. Predisposing effects of occupation include the availability of cheap or free alcohol, strong peer pressure to drink, lack of supervision at work, and separation from normal social and sexual relationships.

Ethnic factors

Ethnic and subcultural differences in the use and abuse of alcohol suggest that prealcoholic learning factors are important in the development of alcoholism. That is to say, the proper and controlled use of alcoholic beverages may depend on underlying attitudes towards alcohol and mores regulating drinking practices. Children are socialized into culturally established attitudes, beliefs, and practices regarding alcohol consumption.

   Thus the extremely low rates of alcoholism reported among for example Jews, Moslems and Mormons might be accounted for by the cultural prohibitions against the use or abuse of the drug formulated by these groups. Certain countries including Scotland, Ireland and the USA have been characterized as ambivalent cultures, that is they have contradictory attitudes towards the use of alcohol and oscillate between a permissive tolerance of drunkenness and heavy drinking and a moral denunciation of physiological dependence (O'Connor, 1978). Permissive cultures where attitudes towards the use of alcohol are favourable but where there are strong and consistent social sanctions against intoxication, drunkenness, or other forms of deviant drinking have also been noted, examples being found in Spain and Portugal. An overpermissive culture in which the attitudes towards drinking and deviant behaviour while drinking are favourable is that of France.

   In general those ethnic groups with a permissive yet moderate attitude towards alcohol and a system of firm, consistent, and acknowledged social sanctions against its misuse have low rates of alcoholism and alcohol-related problems. However, the hazards of generalizing from inadequate or largely anecdotal evidence concerning ethnic and rational patterns of drinking are exemplified by the discussion of Italian drinking. It has been customary to assert that in countries such as Italy where drinking is largely confined to meals the rates of alcoholism and alcohol-related problems are low (Plaut, 1967). Now it appears that this conclusion needs drastic modification (Schmidt, 1977). Alcohol use in Italy is not restricted to mealtimes but is an incidental part of many occasions including work and recreation. As a consequence of such a pattern there are high levels of overall consumption and problems related to chronic heavy use. Not only is the death rate from cirrhosis high in Italy but so are the rates of alcoholism and acute problems including alcohol-related industrial and traffic accidents (Bonfiglio, 1963; Ledemann, 1964).

Familial factors

Sociocultural factors may also operate through familial mechanisms. Family studies from Sweden, Switzerland and the USA all agree in finding very much higher rates of alcoholism in the parents and siblings of alcoholics than those thought most appropriate for the general population (O'Connor, 1978; Stacy and Davies, 1970; Zucker, 1976). As discussed above a genetic factor may be operating, but one reason for doubting that this is the only explanation is the high rate often reported for relatives genetically one degree less close than parents or siblings and on average sharing only 25 per cent and not 50 per cent of their genes with the affected individual. Genetic theories, in contrast, predict much lower risks for second-degree than first-degree relatives.

A number of familial behaviour patterns have been implicated in the transmission of alcoholism. Parental conflict about drinking, parental disagreement and ambiguity concerning drinking practices, and parental abuse of alcohol have all been noted by observers. Paternal punitiveness and paternal escapist reactions to crisis were identified by McCord et al (1962) in their study of the family backgrounds of male alcoholics. It has even been claimed (Cahalan and Room, 1974) that problem drinking among males can be predicted quite effectively using only the traditional variables of age, socioeconomic status, urbanization, ethnic origin, and religious affiliation. The detailed study by O'Connor (1978) of drinking practices in two ethnic groups, English and Irish young drinkers, lends considerable substance to the view that it is parental attitudes towards alcohol as perceived by the young and the effect of peer pressures that constitute the important ethnic factors concerned with alcohol intake. This reduces still further the claims for the more traditional view that it is constitutional factors of a metabolic or psychological variety that are crucially important.

Stress

Social, cultural, and familial factors may also operate by increasing or aggravating conditions of environmental stress that provoke or precipitate episodes of alcohol abuse (Bales, 1946). Alcoholism has been reported to develop during periods of crisis or following significant life events that have led to serious instability, confusion, and role stress (Coleman, 1972). For example, women who have commenced excessive drinking in their late 30s or early 40s have attributed the onset of their drinking problems to alterations in their roles as wife and mother; these may include the menopause, loss of husband, and children leaving home (Curlee, 1969). Other instances of stress include marital disharmony, unemployment, and death of a relative. It is suggested that during such periods of heightened stress an individual's normal coping mechanisms are overwhelmed and he or she resorts to more extreme means of easing the stress including in some cases heavy consumption of alcohol.

High rates of separation and divorce have been reported among alcoholics and some commentators have interpreted this as evidence of disabling psychological factors in the personality structure of the alcoholic. It has been argued that their social behaviour alternates between cycles of sociability and alienation, a pattern that makes the maintenance of normal marital relationships difficult (Barry, 1974). Others have blamed the high marital failure rate on the alcoholic's poor choice of a spouse which arises out of strong dependency needs or fantasies of acquiring power. However, such explanations apart, it seems reasonable to hold that the presence of alcoholism in a marital partner might by itself constitute a sufficient incentive to divorce or separation. Once again we are confronted with the problem that it is as easy and as reasonable to consider a possible cause, in this case crisis or stress, as being an effect of alcoholism.

Availability of alcohol

The idea that it is alcohol that causes alcoholism needs both attention and qualification. Until recently such a view tended to be somewhat neglected in favour of the notion that the alcohol consumption of heavy drinkers and alcoholics is symptomatic of a distinct disorder and that the problems are drunkenness (not drinking) and alcoholism (not alcohol).

This position has always been favoured by the alcohol industry and was tersely formulated in a submission to the Canadian Government by the Association of Canadian Distillers (1973): "Alcohol and alcoholism are two entirely different subjects—while alcoholism is a major health problem, alcohol is not. Just as sugar is not the cause of diabetes, alcohol is not the cause of alcoholism." Such a view is now being contested by those who argue that there is a direct relationship between per capita consumption in a population and the extent of excessive and problem-related consumption (Schmidt and de Lint, 1972). The factors known to have a bearing on per capita consumption include the real price of the alcoholic beverages in question, the cost of related commodities that serve as substitutes or complements, changes in taste as reflected in trends in beverage preferences, and the value of what economists have termed personal disposable income (that is the income left to the individual when taxes, basic food, and other requirements have been taken care of).

There is mounting evidence that international and regional differences in rates of death from liver cirrhosis are very closely associated with differences in the apparent per capita consumption of alcoholic beverages. When the availability of alcohol has been curtailed, as happened in France during the Second World War, there has been a dramatic fall in cirrhosis mortality. Between 1954 and 1973 alcohol consumption and cirrhosis mortality rates in the UK rose in parallel. A relatively high level of general consumption of alcohol does not necessarily imply a high prevalence of heavy users and abusers and conversely a lower per capita consumption does not preclude the existence of higher rates of alcoholism. However, the relationship between consumption levels and the proportion of problem drinkers in a given population is such as to suggest to a number of researchers that one significant response to the growing problem of alcoholism may well lie in the adoption of stricter controls over the licensing, retailing, taxing, and advertising of alcoholic beverages.

Conclusion

The majority of contemporary researchers in the area of alcoholism (Seeley, 1960; Makela, 1970; Robinson, 1977; Schmidt, 1977) espouse a multifaceted approach to the study of causes of alcohol abuse and dependence. Such an approach incorporates elements from the broad areas of psychology, physiology, and sociology. One such model has been summarized by Plaut (1967) and is quoted in the survey of current theories of causation contained in the Rand Report on alcoholism and treatment (Armor et al, 1976):

A tentative model may be developed for understanding the causes of problem drinking, even though the precise roles of the various factors have not yet been determined. An individual who, (1) responds to beverage alcohol in a certain way, perhaps physiologically determined, by experiencing intense relief and relaxation and who, (2) has certain personality characteristics, such as difficulty in dealing with overcoming depression, frustration, and anxiety, and who (3) is a member of a culture in which there is both pressure to drink and culturally induced guilt and confusion regarding what kinds of drinking behaviour are appropriate, is more likely to develop trouble than will most other persons. An intermingling of certain factors may be necessary for the development of problem drinking, and the relative importance of the differential causal factors no doubt varies from one individual to another.

The implications of such a view for the understanding and treatment of alcoholism are obvious. With a simple disease model of alcoholism that envisages the cause as an organically based defect rendering the alcoholic vulnerable to alcohol, the therapeutic solution is a strict adherence to an abstinence regimen pending some medical breakthrough aimed at remedying the defect. A view of alcoholism as learned maladaptive behaviour, on the other hand, holds out the possibility of retraining some alcoholics to drink socially and responsibly. An emphasis on sociocultural causation directs attention to such factors as the availability of alcohol in society, its advertising, marketing and retailing, the societal value placed on its consumption, the manner in which alcohol use is initiated and maintained, the relative cost of the substance, and the legal controls on its use and abuse. It seems clear that a proper and comprehensive approach to the treatment of alcoholism needs to reflect the multifactorial approach that is now implicit in current theories of causation.

References

Armor, D J, Polich, J M, Stambul, H B (1976) Alcoholism and Treatment. National Institute of Alcohol Abuse and Alcoholism. The Rand Corporation, Santa Monica, California

Association of Canadian Distillers (1973) Submission to the Government of Ontario

Bales, R F (1946) *Quarterly Journal of Studies on Alcohol*, **6**, 480

Bandura, A (1969) Principles of Behavior Modification. Holt, Rinehart and Winston, New York

Barry, H (1974) *in* The Biology of Alcoholism, Vol. 3 (edited by Kissin, B, Begleiter, H). New York, Plenum Press. p. 53

Belfer, M L, Shader, R I, Carroll, M, Harmatz, J S (1971) *Archives of General Psychiatry*, **25**, 540

Blum, E M (1966) *Quarterly Journal of Studies on Alcohol*, **27**, 259

Bonfiglio, G (1963) *British Journal of Addiction*, **59**, 3

Cahalan, D, Room, R (1974) Problem Drinking Among American Men. Rutgers Center of Alcohol Studies, New Jersey

Cappell, H, Herman, C P (1972) *Quarterly Journal of Studies on Alcohol*, **33**, 33

Chafetz, M E (1966) *Annals of the New York Academy of Sciences*, **133**, 808

Coleman, J (1972) Abnormal Psychology and Modern Life, 4th edn. Scott, Foresman and Co., Glenview, Illinois

Criteria Committee of the National Council on Alcoholism (1972) *Annals of Internal Medicine*, **77**, 249

Curlee, J (1969) *Bulletin of the Menninger Clinic*, **33**, (3), 165

Edwards, G, Hensman, C, Chandler, J, Peto, J (1972) *Psychological Medicine*, **2**, (3), 260

—, Gross, M M, Keller, M, Moser, J (1976) *Journal of Studies on Alcohol*, **37**, 1360

Emerson, H (1934) Alcohol: Its Effect on Man. Appleton-Century-Crofts, New York

Feldstein, A (1971) *in* The Biology of Alcoholism, Vol.1 (edited by Kissin, B, Begleiter, H). Plenum Press, New York, p.127

Fenna, D, Mix, L, Schaefer, O, Gilbert, J A L (1971) *Canadian Medical Association Journal*, **105**, 472

Goodwin, D W, Schulsinger, F, Hermansen, L, Guze, S B, Winokur, G (1973) *Archives of General Psychiatry*, **28**, 238

—,—, Møller, N, Hermansen, L, Winokur, G, Guze, S B (1974) *ibid*. **31**, 164

Griffiths, P J, Littleton, J M (1977) *British Journal of Experimental Pathology*, **58**, 19

—,—, Ortiz, A (1973) *British Journal of Pharmacology*, **48**, 354

Hughes, J, Smith, T W, Kosterlitz, H W, Fithergill, L A, Morgan, B A, Morris, H R (1975) *Nature*, **358**, 577

Israel, M A, Kimura, H, Kiriyama, K (1972) *Experientia*, **28**, 1322

Johnson, L C (1971) *in* Recent Advances in Studies of Alcoholism (edited by Mello, N K, Mendelson, J H). NIMH, Washington. p.288

Jones, M C (1968) *Journal of Consulting and Clinical Psychology*, **32**, (1), 2

Keller, M (1960) *Quarterly Journal of Studies on Alcohol*, **21**, 125

Kissin, B (1974) *in* The Biology of Alcoholism, Vol. 3 (edited by Kissin, B, Begleiter, H). Plenum Press, New York. p.1

Kissin, B, Gross, M M, Schutz, I (1973) *in* Experimental Studies of Alcohol Intoxication and Withdrawal (edited by Gross, M M). Plenum Press, New York

Ledemann, S (1964) Alcool, Alcoolisme, Alcolisation, Mortalité, Morbidité, Accidents de Travail. Institut National d'Etudes Démographique, Travaux et Documents, Cahier No 41. Presses Universitaires de France, Paris

Littleton, J M (1977) *in* Alcoholism: New Knowledge and New Perspectives (edited by Edwards, G, Grant, M). Croom Helm, London. p.112

McClelland, D C, Davis, W N, Kalin, R, Wanner, E (1972) The Drinking Man. The Free Press, New York

McCord, J, McCord, W, Thurber, E (1962) *Journal of Abnormal and Social Psychology*, **64**, 361

McCord, W, McCord, J, Gudeman, J (1960) Origins of Alcoholism. Stanford University Press, California

Makela, K (1970) *Alkoholpolitukka*, **35**, 246

Massé, L, Juillan, J M, Chisloup, A (1976) *World Health Statistical Report*, **29**, (1), 40

Murray, R M (1978) *Journal of the Royal College of Physicians of London*, **12**, 403

O'Connor, J (1978) The Young Drinkers, Tavistock Publications, London

Orford, J (1977) *in* Alcoholism: New Knowledge and New Responses (edited by Edwards, G, Grant, M). Croom Helm, London. p.88

Pattison, E M (1974) *in* The Biology of Alcoholism, Vol. 3 (edited by Kissin, B, Begleiter, H). Plenum Press, New York. p.587

Plant, M (1977) *in* Alcoholism and Industry (edited by Grant, M, Kenyon, W H). Alcohol Education Centre/Merseyside, Lancashire and Cheshire Council on Alcoholism, Liverpool. p.28

Plaut, T F A (1967) Alcohol Problems: A Report to the Nation by the Cooperative Commission on the Study of Alcoholism. Oxford University Press, New York

Post, M E, Sun, A Y (1973) *Research Communications in Chemical Pathology and Pharmacology*, **6**, 887

Registrar General (1971) Decennial Supplement for England and Wales, 1961: Occupational Mortality. HMSO, London

Robinson, D (1977) *in* Alcoholism: New Knowledge and New Perspectives (edited by Edwards, G, Grant, M). Croom Helm, London. p.60

Schmidt W (1977) *ibid.* p.15

—, de Lint, J E(1972) *Quarterly Journal of Studies on Alcohol*, **33**, (1), 171

Seeley, J R(1960) *Canadian Medical Association Journal*, **83**, 1361

Shields, J (1977) *in* Alcoholism: New Knowledge and New Perspectives (edited by Edwards, G, Grant, M). Croom Helm, London. p.117

Sobell, M B, Sobell, L C (1972) California Mental Health Research Monograph, No 13. Department of Mental Hygiene, Sacramento, California

Stacy, B, Davies, J (1970) *British Journal of Addiction*, **65**, 203

Steiner, C M (1969) *Quarterly Journal of Studies on Alcohol*, **30**, 920

Vogel-Sprott, M (1972) *in* The Biology of Alcoholism (edited by Kissin, B, Begleiter, H). Plenum Press, New York. p.48

WHO (1952) Expert Committee on Mental Health Alcoholism Subcommittee, 2nd Report. WHO Technical Report Series, No 48. WHO, Geneva

Wolff, P H (1973) *American Journal of Human Genetics*, **25**, 193

Zucker, R (1976) *in* Alcoholism Problems in Women and Children (edited by Greenblatt, M, Schuckit, M A). Grune and Stratton, New York. p.211

Chapter 19

The alcoholic doctor

Robin M Murray, Institute of Psychiatry, London

Most doctors are interested in the health, particularly the mental health, of members of their own profession. Normally sceptical individuals, they frequently accept statements about the health of other doctors that are based on reasoning so false that they would immediately reject it for anyone else. The few established facts regarding the occurrence of disease in doctors are outnumbered by a profusion of explanatory theories usually based on little more than the personal experience of their originators. Such views often gain widespread acceptance when they accord with popular prejudices.

It is, for instance, a common belief that doctors, perhaps because of their life-style, long hours of work, or close contact with illness, have a shorter life-expectancy than the general population. The evidence does not support this conclusion. The latest report on occupational mortality (Office of Population Censuses and Surveys, 1971) shows that English doctors have an overall death rate 11 per cent less than that of the rest of the population. Two American studies (Williams et al, 1971; Everson and Fraumeni, 1975) have reported similar deficits in the expected death rates among doctors.

The frequency of alcoholism

While it seems that on average doctors are physically healthier than the general population, the opposite appears to be true of their mental health (Vaillant et al, 1972; Murray, 1974; Waring, 1974). The results of five major retrospective studies of doctors treated for psychiatric illness are summarized in *Table 1*, and confirm that drug dependence and alcoholism are disturbingly common. Glatt (1974) has also reported that over a 25-year period the proportion of doctors among alcoholic patients admitted to two English alcoholic units was 2–4 per cent. All these studies, however, can be criticized on the grounds that they were carried out in prestigious hospitals or clinics to which sick doctors would be preferentially attracted; where controls were used, neither they nor the doctor patients were drawn from populations of known size.

To obtain a more representative sample Murray (1976a) studied the admissions to and discharges from all Scottish hospitals of male doctors aged 25 years and over, and compared them with the figures for all nonmedical social class I males. Over the period 1963–72 alcoholism was the primary diagnosis of 39.8 per cent of all male doctors and of 32.5 per cent of all other social class I males discharged from Scottish

TABLE 20.1. Diagnostic breakdown in different studies of mentally ill disorders

Diagnosis	Duffy and Litin (1964) 93 American inpatients	a'Brook et al (1967) 192 British inpatients and outpatients	Vincent et al (1969) 93 Canadian inpatients	Pond (1969) 83 British inpatients and outpatients	Small et al (1969) 40 American inpatients
	(%)	(%)	(%)	(%)	(%)
Alcoholism		12	27	20	18
Drug dependence	} 51*	17	30	?	15
Affective psychosis	21	28	14	28	15
Schizophrenia	7	9	5	12	52†
Organic psychosis	9	5	5	7	?
Neurosis	20	16	14	21	?
Personality disorder	7	13	4	?	?

* Includes secondary diagnosis
† Broad category of schizophrenic reactions

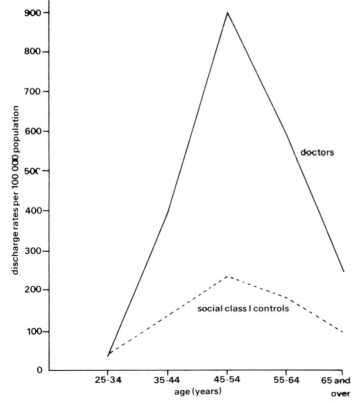

Figure 20.1 Discharge rates of alcoholic doctors from Scottish psychiatric inpatient beds. Reproduced by kind permission of the editor and publisher of the *Lancet*.

psychiatric inpatient beds. When population rates were calculated the differences were even more striking (*Figure 20.1*). The rates for both groups were highest between 45 and 54 years, but the peak was very much higher for doctors.

   This study confirms the suspicions of those who have maintained that doctors are a high risk group for alcoholism (DHSS, 1973; Glatt, 1974). Independent evidence of this comes from an examination of the death rates for cirrhosis of the liver in England and Wales, which for doctors is 350 per cent of that for the general population (Office of Population Censuses and Surveys, 1971).

The characteristics of alcoholic doctors

Two studies published in 1976 dealt specifically with alcoholic doctors. Bissell and Jones (1976) interviewed 98 American doctors who were members of Alcoholics

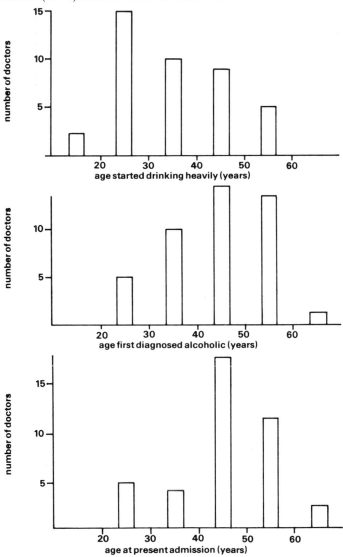

Figure 20.2   Drinking habits in 41 alcoholic doctors.

Anonymous (AA) and had been abstinent for a minimum of one year, while Murray (1976b) followed-up 41 alcoholic doctors who had been treated at a London postgraduate hospital. From these two studies it appears that only a minority of alcoholic doctors have a family history of alcoholism or psychiatric disorder. Their prealcoholic careers range from repeated failure to spectacular success. Among British alcoholic doctors a surprisingly high proportion have graduated from Scottish or Irish medical schools, and such graduates are similarly overrepresented among doctors appearing before the disciplinary committee of the General Medical Council on charges arising out of alcohol abuse (Cargill, 1976).

There has been continuing controversy over whether psychiatrists are generally more prone to mental illness than their medical colleagues, and this argument also applies to alcoholism. Bissell and Jones (1976) noted that "a striking proportion of the alcoholic physicians identified themselves as psychiatrists". In contrast, Murray (1976b) found that only 6 per cent of the psychiatrists referred to the Maudsley Hospital were diagnosed as alcoholic compared with 33 per cent of the surgeons, although he concluded that "this might have reflected not more alcoholism among surgeons but a higher incidence of other psychiatric disorders among psychiatrists". Such disparities are most likely a reflection of the unrepresentative nature of the samples studied.

Murray (1976b) found that alcoholic doctors had most often begun to drink heavily in their 20s and 30s (*Figure 20.2*), and the length of time from the start of heavy drinking to the diagnosis of alcoholism ranged from 6 months to 25 years. Many alcoholic doctors also abuse drugs; a minority begin drinking in the wake of well established drug dependence, but more commonly the hung-over doctor begins to experiment with other drugs and becomes dependent on them too.

The alcoholism may occasionally arise in the context of a psychiatric illness such as anxiety neurosis, depression, or personality disorder. However all too frequently those whom the drinking doctor eventually consults refuse to deal with the alcoholism itself and regard it merely as a symptom of an underlying disorder. Bissell and Jones (1976) found that 34 of their 98 alcoholic doctors had discussed the question of alcoholism with a therapist only to have the latter dismiss the possibility.

Consequences of alcoholism

Alcoholic doctors accumulate many of the same sequelae of their addiction as alcoholics without medical qualifications. Upper alimentary disorder, delirium tremens, marital breakdown, and drunken-driving offences are especially common. Although police are reluctant to apprehend a doctor, Bissell and Jones (1976) reported that their 98 physicians had accumulated a total of 219 arrests and 170 jailings. A doctor's physical symptoms and outrageous social behaviour are particularly often wrongly attributed to organic disease with resultant unnecessary investigation.

There are further hazards for the alcoholic doctor. Forging prescriptions can insidiously become a habit, careers are damaged, and patient care is invariably affected. Inevitably a minority come before their professional disciplinary board. Of 97 doctors whose cases were considered by the Penal Cases Committee of the General Medical Council in 1974 but not referred further, 39 resulted from the abuse of alcohol; 14 of the 46 more serious cases considered by the Disciplinary Committee of the same body also arose from alcohol abuse (General Medical Council, 1974).

Referral and treatment

Edwards (1975) has written perceptively of the way in which doctors only too often fail to help their alcoholic colleagues:

For the doctor alcoholic, the familiar history is therefore of a period of very dangerous drinking during which his colleagues have turned a blind eye, with the story developing to a crisis which is met with misunderstanding and rejection. This biphasic course is predictable.

Illustrations of connivance are many. A surgeon has obviously unsteady hands, but no one likes to do anything too positive. He is persuaded on bad days to let his registrar take the list. A consultant physician is drunk on teaching rounds and is simply regarded as a well known figure of fun.

Alcoholic doctors only rarely seek help entirely of their own accord, and even then they are concerned not so much about their alcohol consumption but about the adverse consequences of that consumption. It is therefore imperative that family, friends and colleagues make it clear to a doctor drinking excessively that they are worried about him. Refraining from expressing private concern only hastens the day when one will have to act, perhaps dramatically, because of the obvious danger to patients.

Once the alcoholic doctor is referred to a psychiatrist his care is essentially that of any alcoholic. This is more difficult than it sounds since, as Edwards (1975) states, "the temptation at this stage is for each actor to be telephoning all other parties at dead of night, giving information which is on no account to be passed on, and trying to set up a series of secret contacts". Furthermore, some doctors find it difficult to adopt the patient's role, and their psychiatrists frequently find it impossible to adhere to the consistent therapeutic policies that they apply to other patients.

In most instances the alcoholic doctor should be admitted to a specialized inpatient alcoholic unit. This may involve hospitalization some distance from home, but this is not necessarily a disadvantage since it may prevent the precise nature of the illness becoming public knowledge among the doctor's colleagues and patients. All alcoholic doctors should at least be introduced to AA. Not all will find it useful, but for those who do there is a British section of international doctors in AA with over 80 members.

Following hospitalization, which may last for anything from a few weeks to several months, therapy should be continued on a long-term supportive basis. The question will inevitably arise as to whether or not the patient-doctor should return to clinical practice. Any doctor who is drinking should be very strongly advised against working with patients since he runs the risk of destroying both his patients' health and his own career. Some experienced psychiatrists insist on their doctor alcoholics avoiding patient care until they have been sober for at least 6 months.

Outcome

Murray (1976b) followed-up 36 alcoholic doctors for a mean period of 63 months. Four killed themselves, one died from cirrhosis, and two died of causes unconnected with their alcoholism. Of the total 36 only seven completely overcame their drinking problem, and 10 had less than one relapse per year. But 10 suffered more than one relapse per year and nine continued almost constant dependent drinking. Of the 29 doctors alive at follow-up, only eight were practising satisfactorily and a further six with varying degrees of incompetence.

The high risk of suicide is hardly surprising since the suicide rate of all hospitalized alcoholics is about 25 times that of the general population (Nicholls et al, 1974). Indeed, alcoholism may be a major contributory factor to the high suicide rate generally recorded for doctors (Office of Population Censuses and Surveys, 1971; Rose and Rosow, 1973). Blachly et al (1968) studied 80 doctors who killed themselves and found that 39 per cent were described as alcoholic, while Simon and Lumry (1969) reported that 25 of their 36 suicidal physicians were alcoholic.

In my study (Murray, 1976b) it was disappointing that so many potentially able doctors were unable to overcome their addiction and return to practising good medicine. But the study may have been biased towards such a finding by the fact that two thirds of the subjects had previously undergone psychiatric treatment and had failed to achieve a lasting recovery. Both Glatt (1974) and Bissell (1977) believe that the prognosis is much less bleak. Certainly, the fact that Bissell and Jones (1976) were able to collect 98 abstinent doctors attests the existence of many who do overcome alcoholism.

Conclusion

Occupation is an important aetiological factor in alcoholism (Murray, 1975; Plant, 1977), but as yet the causes of the medical profession's increased liability to the disorder are poorly understood. Medicine may preferentially attract a minority of students who are especially vulnerable to later breakdown (Vaillant et al, 1972), and there is some partially convincing evidence that the practice of clinical medicine may be particularly anxiety-provoking (Cramond, 1969). These factors go some way towards explaining the increased rates for admission to psychiatric hospitals found among doctors (Murray, 1977), but do not account for the particularly high rates for alcoholism.

An ability to hold one's liquor is said to be almost mandatory for medical students. The majority of them enjoy trying to measure up to this caricature, but for an unfortunate few heavy drinking as undergraduates or housemen may be the prelude to later alcoholism. Furthermore, ready access to drugs may predispose doctors not only to drug dependence but also to switch to alcohol abuse if suspected of overprescribing for themselves. Once heavy drinking patterns are established, they may be reinforced by the relatively affluent social and economic milieu in which doctors live and work.

References

a'Brook, M F, Hailstone, J D, McLaughlin, I E J (1967) *British Journal of Psychiatry*, **113**, 1013
American Medical Association Council on Mental Health (1973) *Journal of the American Medical Association*, **223**, 684
Bissell, L (1977) personal communication
—, Jones, R W (1976) *American Journal of Psychiatry*, **133**, 1142
Blachly, P H, Disher, W, Roduner, G (1968) *Bulletin of Suicidology*, December 1
Cargill, D (1976) *World Medicine*, **11**, 22
Cramond, W A (1969) *Australian and New Zealand Medical Journal*, **3**, 324
DHSS (1973) Report of the Standing Medical Advisory Committee on Alcoholism. HMSO, London
Duffy, J C, Litin, E M (1964) *Journal of the American Medical Association*, **189**, 989
Edwards, G (1975) *Lancet*, ii, 1297

Everson, R B, Fraumeni, J F (1975) *Journal of Medical Education*, **50**, 809
General Medical Council (1973) Memorandum on the Registration of Doctors Suffering from Psychiatric Illness. General Medical Council, London
—(1974) Annual Report. General Medical Council, London
Glatt, M M (1974) *Lancet*, ii, 342
Merrison, A W (1975) Report of the Committee of Inquiry into the Regulation of the Medical Profession. HMSO, London
Murray, R M (1974) *Lancet*, i, 1211
—(1975) *Journal of Alcoholism*, **10**, 23
—(1976a) *Lancet*, ii, 729
—(1976b) *British Medical Journal*, ii, 1537
—(1977) *British Journal of Psychiatry*, **131**, 1
Nicholls, P., Edwards, G, Kyle, E (1974) *Quarterly Journal of Studies on Alcohol*, **35**, 841
Office of Population Censuses and Surveys (1971) Registrar General's Decennial Supplement on Occupational Mortality 1959–1963. HMSO, London
Physicians Committee Special Report (1975) *New York State Journal of Medicine*, **75**, 420
Plant, M (1977) *British Journal of Addiction*, **72**, (4), 309
Pond, D A (1969) *New Zealand Medical Journal*, **69**, 131
Rose, K D, Rosow, I. (1973) *Archives of General Psychiatry*, **29**, 800
Simon, W, Lumry, G K (1969) *Drug Dependence*, July 11
Small, I F, Small, J G, Assue, C M, Moore, D F (1969) *American Journal of Psychiatry*, **125**, 1333
Vaillant, G E, Sobowale, N C, McArthur, C (1972) *New England Journal of Medicine*, **287**, 372
Vincent, M O, Robinson, E A, Latt, L (1969) *Canadian Medical Association Journal*, **100**, 403
Waring, E M (1974) *Comprehensive Psychiatry*, **15**, 519
Williams, S V, Munford, R S, Colton, T, Murphy, D A, Poskanzer, D C (1971) *Journal of Chronic Diseases*, **24**, 393

Chapter 20

The sexual problems of diabetic men

Christopher Fairburn, Warneford Hospital, Oxford

Over the two centuries since Rollo (1798) reported an association between diabetes and erectile failure, the raised prevalence of impotence among diabetic men has been repeatedly recognized. Naunyn (1906) regarded impotence as one of the commonest symptoms of the disease, reporting its occurrence both in patients debilitated by loss of sugar and in healthy patients little troubled by the illness. The dramatic improvement in the treatment of diabetes that followed the introduction of insulin led many clinicians to expect that the association between diabetes and impotence would disappear. Unfortunately, their optimism was misplaced since one third to a half of diabetic men continue to develop erectile failure and a smaller number experience other disturbances of sexual function.

Clinical features of diabetic impotence

Difficulty in obtaining or maintaining a full erection is the best recognized of the sexual problems of diabetic men. It exists in two forms (Naunyn, 1906; Rubin, 1958; Cooper, 1972; Kolodny et al, 1979). In the first, failure of erection occurs in the context of poor diabetic control. Erectile failure and loss of libido accompany the general malaise and all three reverse once the patient's physical condition improves. This type of impotence is not specific to diabetes but is also found in other debilitating conditions. The second and more common form is said to be characteristic of diabetes. This "diabetic impotence" occurs independently of the quality of diabetic control. Indeed, it may precede the onset of diabetes by months or years and under these circumstances it is often regarded in retrospect as having been the first sign of the disease. It is not known whether there is a relationship between these types of diabetes-related impotence.

Although there have been many clinical descriptions of the erectile problems of diabetic men (for example Rubin and Babbott, 1958; Cooper, 1972; Kolodny et al, 1974, 1979; Schiavi and Hogan, 1979; Ellenberg, 1980) there has been no controlled descriptive study. The onset of erectile failure is said to be gradual with the individual experiencing increasing difficulty in obtaining and maintaining an erection. At first the erection is less firm and its duration is diminished but gradually the erectile failure becomes profound, often culminating in a permanent loss of erection. All erections are said to be affected: the individual loses his ability to obtain erections on waking, on masturbating, and spontaneously through the

189

day. Interest in sex is intact although two recent studies have found reduced libido in a quarter of their sample (Jensen et al, 1979; McCulloch et al, 1980). Ejaculation generally remains undisturbed with the result that the individual may ejaculate and experience orgasm while having a flaccid or partially erect penis.

This clinical picture is frequently contrasted with that of nondiabetics (for example Cooper, 1972; Kolodny et al, 1974). Largely on the basis of clinical reports and Kinsey's findings of over 30 years ago (Kinsey et al, 1948) the impotence of nondiabetics is usually characterized as being abrupt in onset and often related in time to an identifiable environmental stress. The erectile failure varies in severity and is selective: morning, masturbatory and spontaneous erections are not affected. Interest in sex is frequently reduced.

TABLE 21.1. Clinical stereotypes of impotence among diabetic and nondiabetic men

	Impotent diabetic men (diabetic impotence)	Impotent nondiabetic men
Onset of erectile failure	Gradual	Rapid
Integrity of morning, masturbatory and spontaneous erections	Impaired	Unimpaired
Interest in sex	Intact	Reduced
Presumed aetiology	Physical	Psychological

The differences between these clinical pcitures (*Table 21.1*) are widely used in the assessment of diabetic men with erectile failure. Patients showing the symptomatic picture of diabetic impotence tend to be viewed as having erectile problems of physical origin, whereas patients presenting with clinical features resembling those of nondiabetics are often regarded as having a psychogenic form of impotence which may respond to sex therapy (Ellenberg, 1980).

Prevalence of impotence in diabetes

Although impotence has long been known to be associated with diabetes there have only recently been studies of its prevalence. These studies have varied in their case-finding techniques and definitions of impotence. However, despite their differences they have without exception noted a markedly raised prevalence of impotence compared with the estimates of Kinsey et al (1948) for the general population. *Table 21.2* summarizes the findings of the larger studies.

A relationship between age and the frequency of impotence has been found in most studies with the prevalence rising with age and being consistently higher than in the general population. It was thought that like most diabetic complications the frequency of impotence was directly related to the duration of the disorder (Schoffling et al, 1963), but recent studies have either failed to confirm this (Ellenberg, 1971; Kolodny et al, 1974) or attributed the relationship to the associated increase in other factors of likely aetiological significance such as diabetic microangiopathy and neuropathy (McCulloch et al, 1980).

Most studies have failed to find a relationship between impotence and antidiabetic medication although the large study of McCulloch et al (1980) noted a significant

TABLE 21.2. Prevalence studies of diabetic impotence

Authors	Number in sample	Percentage impotent
Rubin and Babbott (1958)	198	55
Montenero and Donatone (1962)	436	37
Schoffling et al (1963)	314	51
Ellenberg (1971)	200	59
Kolodny et al (1974)	175	49
Faerman et al (1974)	299	40
McCulloch et al (1980)	541	35

association with the use of an oral agent or insulin compared with treatment by diet alone. This study also differs from others in its finding of a strong correlation with the presence and severity of retinopathy. However, there is unanimity over the association between impotence and evidence of an autonomic neuropathy.

While these studies suggest that there is a raised prevalence of impotence among diabetic men, the strength of this conclusion is eroded by the absence of satisfactory comparison figures for both the general population and patients with other conditions. The recent study of Lester et al (1980) has highlighted this deficiency. Using an unvalidated questionnaire and a small patient sample they found the frequency of impotence to be similar among diabetics and nondiabetics. Obviously further research along similar lines is required.

Ejaculatory disturbances in diabetes

Disturbances of ejaculation are also found in diabetes, the best described disorder being so called retrograde ejaculation (Greene et al, 1963; Ellenberg and Weber, 1966; Greene and Kelalis, 1968). This is thought to be an uncommon problem; for example in the series of Kolodny et al (1974) only two patients out of 175 diabetic men had retrograde ejaculation whereas 85 were impotent. It is characterized by a progressive diminution in the volume of ejaculate ending with its eventual absence. This reduction is attributed to semen passing in a retrograde direction into the bladder rather than outwards along the anterior urethra. In support of this mechanism there is in some patients cloudy postorgasmic urine which on microscopic examination contains numerous spermatozoa.

The same clinical phenomenon is a recognized complication of bladder neck surgery, bilateral lumbar sympathectomy, and the taking of certain drugs. In these instances the competence of the internal sphincter of the bladder is thought to be compromised whether surgically or pharmacologically, with the result that it fails to close at the moment of ejaculation when semen is propelled into the urethra. A similar mechanism may occur in diabetes with a sympathetic neuropathy interfering with the function of the sphincter. However, this mechanism may not be the sole explanation for the phenomenon since some diabetics who complain of a reduced or absent ejaculate have no spermatozoa in their postorgasmic urine (Klebanow and MacLeod, 1960). In these cases there may be a genuine decline in a semen production or alternatively interference with its passage into the urethra.

Diabetics may develop other forms of ejaculatory disturbance. For example, diabetes is said to be a cause of retarded ejaculation (Munjack and Kanno, 1979) and partial ejaculatory incompetence (Kaplan, 1974). In the former there is a difficulty or an inability to ejaculate; orgasm occurs if ejaculation takes place. In the latter the expulsion phase of the ejaculatory reflex is inhibited while the emission phase remains intact. The result is that semen trickles out of the penis and orgasm is altered in quality. The relationship between these ejaculatory disorders and erectile failure is uncertain. They can occur independently of one another.

These disturbances may be more common than hitherto recognized. Fairburn et al (1982b) found partial ejaculatory incompetence in one third of their sample of impotent diabetic men. It is probable that many cases fail to come to attention and it is doubtful whether they are amenable to treatment. However, occasionally the result is infertility and when this is the case, should adequate numbers of spermatozoa be present in postorgasmic urine specimens, it may be possible to overcome the problem by artificial insemination (Bourne et al, 1971).

Aetiology of impotence in diabetes

The understanding of the aetiology of erectile impotence is hampered by ignorance over the mechanism by which erections are obtained and maintained. Endocrine, vascular, neurological and psychological disorders may produce erectile failure as may excessive alcohol consumption and the taking of certain drugs. In the majority of cases it is likely that erectile failure results from a combination of these factors.

Endocrine factors

Endocrine studies of nondiabetic impotent men have yielded conflicting results and the place of hormonal treatments is uncertain (Bancroft, 1977).

For some years it was thought that a specific endocrine abnormality might be relevant to the impotence of diabetics. In support of this idea were the observations of Schoffling et al (1963) who not only found abnormalities in the hypothalamic–pituitary–gonadal axis of impotent diabetics but also reported successful treatment with chorionic gonadotrophin and testosterone. Recent studies have failed to confirm these findings. Normal gonadotrophin levels (Faerman et al, 1972), total testosterone levels (Ellenberg, 1971; Faerman et al, 1972; Kolodny et al, 1974), gonadotrophin responses to LH–RH stimulation (Rastogi et al, 1974; Wright et al, 1976), and prolactin levels (Jensen et al, 1979) have been found and attempts at replacement therapy have proved fruitless (Ellenberg, 1971; Kolodny et al, 1974). However, Geisthovel et al (1975) observed lowered levels of free testosterone, the physiologically active form. This finding requires confirmation.

On balance, it seems unlikely that endocrine abnormalities play a major role in the genesis of diabetic impotence. It is possible that there may be subgroups of patients in whom endocrine factors are relevant; in addition a two-way interaction between hormones and sexual behaviour may operate such that the sexual inactivity that often follows erectile failure results in a secondary endocrine disturbance.

Vascular factors

There is no doubt that an adequate arterial blood supply to the penis is necessary for the development and maintenance of a normal erection. Large-vessel disease may result in erectile failure as seen in Leriche's syndrome, but it is possible that in some cases small-vessel disease may be responsible (Ginestie and Romieu, 1978). This suggestion is supported by the work of Herman et al (1978) who found significantly greater stenosis in the internal pudendal arteries of impotent patients than in those of potent controls. Whether more subtle disturbances of vascular dynamics may result in impotence is uncertain.

It is not clear whether vascular abnormalities contribute to the impotence of diabetics. The fact that cardiovascular disease is associated with diabetes might appear to be of relevance. However, prevalence studies have failed to demonstrate a significant association between indices of cardiovascular disease and the presence of impotence (Rubin and Babbott, 1958; McCulloch et al, 1980). One angiographic study found an absence of blood supply to the corpora cavernosa in diabetics (Fournier and Huguet, 1968), but this important observation remains unconfirmed. Measurement of penile blood pressure has also suggested that the blood supply to the penis may be impaired in some diabetics (Gaskell, 1971; Abelson, 1975; Engel et al, 1978; Karacan et al, 1978a; Karacan, 1980), but this finding must be interpreted with caution in view of the paucity of normative data and the poor correlation between penile blood pressure and the findings of angiography (Engel et al, 1978).

Diabetics are also subject to diabetic microangiopathy. It is possible that this disorder might interfere with the microvascular blood supply to the penis. Again indirect evidence is not conclusive. The studies of Rubin and Babbott (1958), Kolodny et al (1974), and Jensen et al (1979) found no relationship between impotence and diabetic retinopathy. whereas the much larger study of McCulloch et al (1980) found a strong relationship not only with the presence of diabetic retinopathy but also with its severity.

Overall, it is not possible to conclude whether vascular abnormalities are of importance in the aetiology of diabetic impotence. Psychophysiological studies of erectile function may well clarify this issue as may the relatively new radioisotope techniques for studying penile blood flow (Shirai et al, 1973; Shirai and Nakamura, 1975). From the findings of the angiographic and penile blood pressure studies it seems that a proportion of diabetic and nondiabetic men with erectile failure have an impaired vascular supply to their penis, but the relevance of this abnormality to their erectile problems is unclear. It is equally uncertain whether impotent diabetics are any more likely to show these abnormalities than their potent diabetic counterparts.

Neurological factors

For over 30 years it has been recognized that diabetic impotence is frequently associated with evidence of an autonomic neuropathy (Rundles, 1945; Ellenberg, 1971; Faerman et al, 1974; Kolodny et al, 1974; Jensen et al, 1979; McCulloch et al, 1980). However, the absence of satisfactory tests of erectile function has prevented any direct connection being drawn between autonomic nerve dysfunction and erectile failure. Strong indirect evidence has come from investigations into the relationship between bladder dysfunction and impotence, the bladder and the penis sharing the same peripheral autonomic pathways (Learmouth, 1931). In the best known study of this type, Ellenberg (1971) found abnormal cystometrograms in 37 out of 45 impotent diabetic patients compared with three out of 30 potent diabetic controls. Buck et al (1976) have since reported similar findings. Further evidence comes from the observation that the bulbocavernosus reflex response latency is prolonged in impotent diabetic men compared with potent, nondiabetic controls (Karacan, 1980); no data on potent diabetic men were provided.

More direct support for the role of autonomic damage in diabetic impotence comes from the research of Faerman et al (1974). They performed histochemical studies on the corpora cavernosa of five impotent diabetics and five potent nondiabetic controls. Four out of five impotent patients had evidence of autonomic nerve abnormalities whereas no abnormalities were present in the control group. In a similar study Melman and Henry (1979) found lower noradrenaline concentrations in the spongy erectile tissue of impotent diabetic men compared with a mixed group of nondiabetic controls; again there were no comparison figures for potent diabetic men.

In summary, there is strong evidence for an association between pelvic autonomic neuropathy and impotence. It is likely that the neuropathy affects the nerves involved in the formation and maintenance of erections, but this has yet to be confirmed.

Psychological factors

It is generally accepted that psychological factors are of prime importance in the aetiology of most cases of erectile impotence. Particular emphasis has been placed on those factors in the individual or couple that may directly result in erectile dysfunction and these factors are the focus of modern sex therapy (Masters and Johnson, 1970; Kaplan, 1974). However, with regard to diabetic impotence, psychological factors have received scant attention. This neglect may stem from the widespread assumption that diabetic impotence is physical in origin. There are, nevertheless, a number of ways in which psychological factors might contribute to the problem (Fairburn et al, 1982a).

First, since both diabetes and erectile dysfunction are relatively common (Kinsey et al, 1948; Frank et al, 1978), it is to be expected that a proportion of cases arises from the chance association of the two conditions and that the origin of the impotence in these cases is similar to that in nondiabetics.

Secondly, diabetic men may be peculiarly vulnerable to psychogenic impotence since, although the concept of a diabetes-prone personality is discredited (Menninger, 1935; Dunbar, 1954; Kubany et al, 1956), there is no doubt that being diabetic causes a variety of psychosocial problems (Entmacher and Marks, 1971; Kravitz et al, 1971) and that many of these affect not only the individual but also his marriage (Campbell and McCulloch, 1979). Furthermore, episodes of impotence at times of poor diabetic control may erode the sexual self-confidence of some patients with the result that their susceptibility to psychogenic impotence is increased. These possibilities await investigation.

Lastly, the psychological reaction to developing erectile failure may itself worsen the sexual problem since performance anxiety is currently regarded as one of the prime causes of sexual difficulty (Masters and Johnson, 1970; Kaplan, 1974). Moreover the reaction of the sexual partner may complicate matters, particularly if the quality of the relationship is poor, sexual adjustment is precarious, and communication is limited.

Other factors

Erectile function is sensitive to many influences in addition to the endocrine, vascular, neurological and psychological factors discussed above. These influences include certain other physical diseases (Cooper, 1969), acute alcohol intoxication and chronic alcoholism (Lemere and Smith, 1973; Wilson, 1977), and the ingestion of a wide variety of drugs (Bell, 1972; Taylor Seagraves, 1977). None of these factors has been systematically assessed in studies of diabetic impotence, yet they may be of considerable importance since diabetics not only are subject to a wide range of physical disabilities but also are prescribed many different drugs.

Objective measures of erectile function

Over the last 10 years it has been claimed that the measurement of sleep erections might provide an objective means of assessing erectile function. Since Karacan (1970) first suggested this application of sleep research a number of studies have been reported in which the sleep erection of differing groups of patients have been measured (for example Fisher et al, 1975; Karacan et al, 1977, 1978b; Hosking et al, 1979; Karacan, 1980). These studies have shown that in comparison with control subjects some diabetic men spend less time having sleep erections and have less nocturnal penile circumference change. These observations have been taken to indicate that abnormal sleep erections are indicative of organogenic impotence. In contrast, one recent British study (Hosking et al, 1979) found that two thirds of the patients had sleep erections of circumference and duration similar to those of healthy controls. On this basis it was concluded that in most impotent diabetic patients the problem is psychological rather than organic.

Not surprisingly, concern has been expressed over the interpretation of these studies (Fisher et al, 1979; Schiavi, 1979; Bancroft and Wu, 1980). There are no firm grounds for concluding that normal sleep erections indicate that impotence is psychogenic, and abnormal sleep erections that impotence is organogenic. Furthermore it is well recognized that certain diabetic men have occasional full sleep erections despite having total erectile failure at other times. Lastly, it is easily forgotten that sleep erections, as assessed by penile circumference measures, are not necessarily full erections adequate for sexual intercourse since penile circumference may increase without a rigid erection being present.

It is likely that direct measures of erectile function will prove to be an invaluable aid in the assessment of patients with erectile failure. However, at present they are research procedures and their findings are open to a variety of differing and sometimes contradictory interpretations.

Assessment of diabetic impotence

Relatively little has been written about the assessment and treatment of this problem. In addition to a careful history being taken, most authorities recommend the evaluation of the patient's endocrine, cardiovascular and neurological status (for example Mills, 1976). However, it is largely on the basis of the symptomatic picture that patients are subdivided into organogenic and psychogenic groups; the physical investigations indirectly facilitate this process by revealing abnormalities that have an association with impotence.

This mode of assessment may be criticized on several grounds. First, in view of the absence of descriptive studies of erectile impotence, the validity of the clinical stereotypes is open to doubt. Schiavi and Hogan (1979) reported that many patients showed intermediate features and one recent study found that the clinical picture was both varied and variable (Fairburn et al, 1982b). Secondly, our understanding of sexual dysfunction is not sufficiently sound to legitimize assumptions regarding aetiology based largely on the symptomatic profile. Finally, it is most improbable that erectile problems are either organic or psychological in origin (Schiavi, 1980); instead, there is likely to be an interaction between physical and psychological factors.

Assessment should therefore encompass both physical and psychological influences (Fairburn et al, 1982a). Physical assessment should place particular emphasis on the identification of potentially reversible disorders. Poor diabetic control, impaired exercise tolerance, excessive alcohol consumption, and the taking of drugs that interfere with sexual function are all factors of importance in the evaluation of the patient's physical state. Psychological assessment should involve both partners with the emphasis being on past and present sexual adjustment, the quality of the relationship, and the nature of the reaction to the sexual problem.

Management of diabetic impotence

Psychological methods

The place of psychological treatment methods in the management of diabetic impotence has yet to be evaluated. There have been a number of reports of the successful use of these methods (Renshaw 1976, 1978, 1979; Waxberg, 1978) and several authors have made general recommendations on the best approach to adopt. What might be termed the traditional stance has been outlined by Campbell and Clark (1975): "Psychological counselling. This involves explaining to the diabetic and his spouse the nature of the impotence—that it is not due to lack of virility, but it is caused in some way by the diabetic disorder. The physician should be frank with the patient from the outset and explain that once good diabetic control is achieved then treatment is expectant."

This style of approach has been criticized by Renshaw (1976, 1978) who argues that attributing the sexual problem to the diabetes is not only unjustifiable in the majority of cases but is also liable to produce "iatrogenic psychogenic impotence", imposing on the patient a fatalistic attitude to the problem.

Schiavi (1980) and Fairburn et al (1982a) suggest that most patients would benefit from a modified form of sex therapy in which special emphasis is placed on enhancing the couple's enjoyment of nongenital sexual activities. In this way the inhibiting influence of performance anxiety would be lessened while adjustment to the limitations posed by physical factors might be facilitated. Obvously this mode of treatment would also incorporate an educative component in which the relationship between diabetes and sexual dysfunction is discussed with the couple. The dangers of inducing iatrogenic impotence are likely to be minimal so long as the couple are encouraged to adopt a positive attitude to the problem.

Surgical methods

The place of penile prosthetic surgery in the treatment of impotence is controversial. It has been argued that this is the only means of treating organogenic impotence and that recipients are generally satisfied with the outcome of surgery (Scott et al, 1980). However, for some patients the results are less than satisfactory. Kramarsky-Binkhorst (1978), for example, on interviewing the wives of recipients of a Small Carrion prosthesis found that several men had not used their implant and some wives were not aware that the operation had taken place. Sotile (1979) has argued that the stability of the patient's relationship with his sexual partner should be assessed preoperatively and that care should be taken to ensure that both have realistic expectations regarding the effect of implantation.

It is possible that such surgery is the appropriate treatment for certain diabetic men with erectile failure. However, before referral to a surgeon is contemplated it would seem judicious to explore the potential benefits of sexual therapy. It is all too easy for patients and clinicians alike to equate genital performance with sexual satisfaction.

Summary

Diabetic men are prone to develop sexual problems, the most common being erectile failure. In the past this diabetic impotence has been regarded as a discrete clinical entity, providing one of the best examples of a physically induced failure of erection. It now appears likely that the clinical picture and aetiology are more involved than had been suspected, there being a complex interaction between physical and psychological influences. Assessment and treatment need to take account of this interaction by concentrating not only on the form of the sexual disturbance but also on its context.

References

Abelson, D (1975) *Journal of Urology*, **113**, 636
Bancroft, J H J (1977) *Psychological Medicine*, **7**, 553
—, Wu, F C W (1980) *British Medical Journal*, **280**, 483
Bell, C (1972) *Pharmacological Review*, **24**, 657
Bourne, R B, Kretzschmar, W A, Esser, J H (1971) *Fertility and Sterility*, **22**, 275
Buck, A C, Reed, P I, Siddiq, Y K, Chisholm, G D, Fraser, T R (1976) *Diabetologia*, **12**, 251
Campbell, I, Clark, B (1975) *Medical Aspects of Human Sexuality*, **5**, 157
—, McCulloch, D K (1979) *Practitioner*, **223**, 343
Cooper, A I (1969) *Journal of Nervous and Mental Disease*, **149**, 337
—(1972) *British Medical Journal*, ii, 34
Dunbar, F (1954) Emotions and Bodily Changes. Columbia University Press, New York
Ellenberg, M (1971) *Annals of Internal Medicine*, **75**, 213
—(1980) *ibid*. **92**, 331
—. Weber, H (1966) *ibid*. **65**, 1237
Engel, G, Burnham. S J, Carter, M F (1978) *Fertility and Sterility*, **30**, 687
Entmacher, P S, Marks, H H (1971) in Joslin's Diabetes Mellitus (edited by Marble, A, White, P, Bradley, R F, Krall, L P). Lea and Febiger, Philadelphia. p. 783
Faerman, I et al (1972) *Diabetes*, **21**, 23
—, Glocer, I, Fox, D, Jadzinsky, M N, Rapaport, M (1974) *ibid*. **23**, 971
Fairburn, C G, McCulloch, D K, Wu, F C W (1982a) *Clinics in Endocrinology and Metabolism*, **11**, 741
Fairburn, C G, Wu, F C W, McCulloch, D K, Borsey, D Q, Ewing, D J, Clarke, B F, Bancroft, J H J (1982b) *British Journal of Psychiatry*, **140**, 447
Fisher, C, Schiavi, R, Lear, H, Edwards, A, Davis, D M, Witkin, A P (1975) *Journal of Sex and Marital Therapy*, **1**, 277
—, —, Edwards, A, Davis, D M, Reitman, M, Finn, J (1979) *Archives of General Psychiatry*, **36**, 431
Fournier, A M, Huguet, J F (1968) *Journal de radiologie, d'electrologie et de medicine nucleaire*, **49**, 515
Frank, E, Anderson, C, Rubenstein, D (1978) *New England Journal of Medicine*, **299**, 111
Gaskell, P (1971) *Canadian Medical Association Journal*, **105**, 1047
Geisthovel, W, Niedergerke, U, Morgner, K D, Willms, B, Mitzkat, H J (1975) *Medizinische Klinik*, **70**, 1417
Ginestie, J-F, Romieu, A (1978) Radiologic Exploration of Impotence. Martinus Nijkoff Medical Division. London

Greene, L F, Kelalis, P P (1968) *Journal of Urology*, **98**, 693

—,—, Weeks, R E (1963) *Fertility and Sterility*, **14**, 617

Herman, A, Adar, R, Rubinstein, Z (1978) *Diabetes*, **27**, 975

Hosking, D J, Bennet, T, Hampton, J R, Evans, D F, Clark, A J, Robertson, G (1979) *British Medical Journal*, ii, 1394

Jensen, S B, Hagen, C, Frøland, A, Petersen, P B (1979) *Acta medica Scandinavica supplementum*, **624**, 65

Kaplan, H S (1974) The New Sex Therapy. Brunner Mazel, New York

Karacan, I (1970) *Medical Aspects of Human Sexuality*, **4**, 27

—(1980) *Annals of Internal Medicine*, **92**, 334

—et al (1977) *Biological Psychiatry*, **12**, 373

— et al (1978a) *Sleep*, **1**, 125

— et al (1978b) *American Journal of Psychiatry*, **135**, 191

Kinsey, A C, Pomeroy, W B, Martin, C E (1948) Sexual Behaviour in the Human Male. Saunders, Philadelphia

Klebanow, D, MacLeod, J (1960) *Fertility and Sterility*, **11**, 255

Kolodny, R C, Kahm, C B, Goldstein, H H, Barnett, D M (1974) *Diabetes*, **23**, 306

—, Masters, W H, Johnson, V E (1979) Textbook of Sexual Medicine. Little, Brown and Company, Boston

Kramarsky-Binkhorst, S (1978) *Urology*, **12**, 545

Kravitz, A R, Isenberg, P L, Shore, M F, Barnett, I M (1971) in Joslin's Diabetes Mellitus (edited by Marble, A, White, P, Bradley, R F, Krall, L P). Lea and Febiger, Philadelphia. p. 767

Kubany, A J, Danowski, T S, Moses, C (1956) *Diabetes*. **5**, 462

Learmouth, J R (1931) *Brain*, **54**, 147

Lemere, F, Smith, J W (1973) *American Journal of Psychiatry*, **130**, 212

Lester, E, Grant, A, Woodroffe, F (1980) *British Medical Journal*, **281**, 354

McCulloch, D K, Campbell, I W, Wu, F C, Prescott, R J, Clarke, B F (1980) *Diabetologia*, **18**, 279

Masters, W H, Johnson, V E (1970) Human Sexual Inadequacy. Little, Brown and Company, Boston

Melman, A, Henry, D (1979) *Journal of Urology*, **121**, 419

Menninger, W C (1935) *Journal of Mental Science*, **81**, 332

Mills, L C (1976) in Sex and the Life Cycle (edited by Oaks, W W. Meldiode, G A, Ficker, I). Grune and Stratton, New York. p. 163

Montenero, P, Donatone, E (1962) *Diabète*, **10**, 327

Munjack, D J, Kanno, P H (1979) *Archives of Sexual Behaviour*, **8**, 139

Naunyn, B (1906) Der Diabetes Mellitus. Alfred Holder, Vienna

Rastogi, G K, Chakraborti, J, Sinha, M K (1974) *Hormone and Metabolic Research*, **6**, 335

Renshaw, D C (1976) *Comprehensive Therapy*, **2**, 47

— (1978) in Handbook of Sex Therapy (edited by Lo Piccolo, J, Lo Piccolo, L). Plenum Press, New York. p. 433

—(1979) *British Journal of Sexual Medicine*, **6**, 48

Rollo, J (1798) John Rollo's Book. Dilly, London

Rubin, A (1958) *American Journal of Obstetrics and Gynecology*, **76**, 25

—, Babbott, D (1958) *Journal of the American Medical Association*, **168**, 498

Rundles, R W (1945) *Medicine*, **24**, 111

Schiavi, R C (1979) *Sexuality and Disability*, **2**, 66

— (1980) *Annals of Internal Medicine*, **92**, 337

—, Hogan B (1979) *Diabetes Care*, **2**, 9

Schoffling, K, Federlin, K, Ditschunheit, H (1963) *Diabetes*, **12**, 519

Scott, F, Fishman, I, Light, J (1980) *Annals of Internal Medicine*, **92**, 340

Shirai, M, Nakamura, M (1975) *Tohoku Journal of Experimental Medicine*, **116**, 9

—, —, Matsuda, S (1973) *ibid*. **111**, 187

Sotile, W M (1979) *Diabetes Care*, **2**, 26

Taylor Seagraves, T (1977) *Journal of Sex and Marital Therapy*, **3**, 157

Waxberg, J D (1978) *Connecticut Medicine*, **42**, 555

Wilson, G T (1977) *Behaviour Research and Therapy*, **15**, 239

Wright, A D, London, D R, Holder, G, Williams, J W, Rudd, B T (1976) *Diabetes*, **25**, 975

Chapter 21

Exhibitionism: an eclectic approach to its management

Graham Rooth, Barrow Hospital, Bristol

About 10 years ago I read extensively in the world literature in an attempt to find an adequate explanation for the puzzling phenomenon of exhibitionism. This term refers to intentional genital display under inappropriate circumstances, almost invariably by a man to adults or children of the opposite sex. I discovered that exhibitionism is widely recognized throughout the world as abnormal behaviour although it appears to be comparatively rare in Eastern and African countries. Its relatively common occurrence in this country seems to be a recent phenomenon (Rooth, 1970, 1973).

As far as explanations are concerned there seems to be general agreement that a symptomatic exhibitionism can occur. The behaviour may present as part of a general deterioration caused by a major psychosis such as schizophrenia or by organic brain damage. There is also an association with subnormality.

However, most men who develop exhibitionism are not psychotic or brain-damaged. They are ordinary people, unremarkable until their deviation manifests itself and sets them apart. For the majority the exhibitionistic phase is short-lived, a temporary aberration. But there are a few, a small proportion of the total, in whom the desire to expose is tenacious and persistent and often part of a wider disturbance of the personality. They are responsible for a disproportionate number of sexual offences every year and seem to be unresponsive to both psychiatric treatment and legal sanctions.

Troubled family relationships, immature personality traits, and adult under-achievement are themes that emerge consistently from studies of exhibitionists but they do not point to a group of features that are specific to exhibitionism. The case for regarding exhibitionism as a syndrome rather than a symptom is weakened by work showing an overlap between exhibitionism, paedophilia, and some kinds of indecent assault. As a guide to treatment the label exhibitionist also proves unhelpful—the literature describes a wide range of approaches to treatment and there is little to suggest that the diagnostic label has much bearing on results or carries any specific implications for treatment. Social factors and personality traits are more important.

Indeed it will be apparent that the section on treatment below could be applied with little alteration to the management of any socially stigmatized impulsive behaviour.

Treatment

General considerations

After 10 years of treating exhibitionists I now see them as members of a much larger group of men who have difficulty in establishing adult sexual behaviour and who fail to develop a comfortable adult male role and identity for themselves. The specific deviation represents an idiosyncratic extra rather than the essential syndrome, and for lack of a better explanation I assume that the choice of deviation is ultimately dictated by an innate predisposition. Most members of this vulnerable group do not develop manifest deviations but show a range of difficulties in relating emotionally and physically to the opposite sex. In those who do act out the deviant behaviour it shows differing degrees of penetration as shown by the age of its first manifestation, its frequency of expression, and the part played by stress in its release.

The majority of exhibitionists do not warrant treatment. Their behaviour can be seen as a public demonstration of the fact that sexual development in men is often not straightforward. Difficulties in sexual development are so widespread in our culture that their minor manifestations must be regarded as a common hazard of growing up, although this perhaps raises questions about the ways in which we prepare our children for adulthood.

The suggestions that follow concern men in whom the difficulties are not transient but persist so that repeated exposing or recurring urges to expose are the leading complaint. The approach and techniques described below have not been validated as a "package" by research although most of the individual measures recommended here have a respectable research background to which a few references allude. However, the main reason for including these methods is personal experience in their use over a number of years during which many ideas have been discarded while a few have retained a modest credibility.

Issues of general psychiatric management are largely ignored, but it should be remembered that in many cases the exhibitionism proves to be a minor concern and the treatment is directed to depression or to marital difficulties or very rarely to an underlying psychosis or dementia.

During the initial assessment the psychiatrist decides whether his patient's exhibitionism needs to be treated as a target symptom. Having made this decision he then has a number of options open to him. His choice of which to exercise is influenced by his estimate of the likely return in terms of benefit to the patient compared with the deployment of scarce resources and restricted specialist time.

Interventions can be grouped according to their focus: education, symptom control, personal growth; and grouped according to their arena: the individual, his family or his marriage, or his wider social nexus.

Education

This aspect should never be omitted; it involves representing the individual's behaviour to him, to his wife or family, and if necessary to the courts in a way that makes it understandable and relates it to ordinary experience and development. The purpose of this crucial intervention is to oppose at all levels—intrapsychic, interpersonal and social—the splitting-off that turns anomalous sexual behaviour into something alien and therefore monstrous, inexplicable, frightening, and something to be denied.

To aid this kind of understanding the psychiatrist stresses the common occurr- ence of exhibitionism and other sexual anomalies and relates them to the difficulties experienced by many men in establishing adult sexuality. He portrays exhibitionism as the persistence into adulthood (or adolescence) of a behaviour pattern that was once a normal part of childhood but is now inappropriate. He explains that this behaviour derives some of its compulsiveness from its links with the sex drive but also appeals to a persisting area of immaturity within the subject's personality. It is usually possible to lend force to the idea of areas of immaturity by pointing to other aspects of the individual's life in which he also appears to be a late developer. Finally, where appropriate, connections are drawn between the emerg- ence of this regressive behaviour and failure to cope adequately with life's stresses. Such a failure may have produced other symptoms of distress, for example depression and anxiety, or disturbances in vital functions with a consequent impairment of sleep, appetite, and sexual interest.

It can be seen that the whole aim of this part of the treatment is to demystify the symptom and depict it to the individual and his family in a way that allows them to think about it and talk about it in everyday language. This keeps it connected to ordinary experience and resists the process whereby the behaviour becomes almost impossible to acknowledge or discuss. I also believe that family or conjoint interviews contribute powerfully to healing the split within the individual by building connections between the real world and the compartmentalized exhibi- tionist frame of mind. So long as the exhibitionistic urges are compartmentalized, that is dissociated from more age-appropriate and realistic areas of functioning, the patient runs the risk of relapse.

Symptom control techniques

We now move into a more labour-intensive area, but one that offers good opportunities for involving less experienced colleagues. Symptom control should only become a focus for treatment if the subject complains that he cannot control his behaviour and wants to do something about it. Without his cooperation none of the methods described below has anything to offer. The behavioural techniques in particular are weak and may involve a lot of work for relatively small returns. This is acceptable providing it is clear from the outset that it is the work done by the patient that matters.

There are two groups of exposer whose rather different needs must be borne in mind at this point. First, there are men who experience very persistent exhibitionis- tic urges and tend to belong to type 2 in my classification, often showing lack of control and moderately sociopathic behaviour in other areas of their life. Secondly, there is a larger episodic group who may go for long periods without wishing to expose or even think about it. They function better on the whole and the overcontrolled type 1 exposer is more often found in this group than among the persistent exposers (Rooth, 1971).

Self-monitoring

Both categories require instruction in self-monitoring. The purpose of this is to build up their understanding of the situations in which they are most at risk and to enhance their vigilance against further episodes. This concept includes an aware- ness of the obvious external triggers such as a tempting situation and a suitable witness. But more important the subject learns to recognize the subtle shifts in mood and ideation that indicate the imminence of a take-over by the exhibitionistic complex with the consequent exclusion or impairment of the maturer aspects of the psyche. The process can be very rapid or may develop gradually over days, weeks, or even longer.

Self-monitoring is aided by detailed discussion with the therapist who can direct his patient's attention to less obvious sources of the shift such as hurts and injuries to his self-esteem, particularly those collected during the course of his relationships with the opposite sex. Where possible a diary should be kept at this stage.

Drugs and self-discipline

As patterns begin to emerge two main strategies can be considered—first, approaches that discourage the build-up of those tensions (both sexual and affective) that apparently predispose to exposing and, secondly, approaches that make the behaviour itself less attractive and more "costly".

Pharmacology   The reduction in sex drive through the use of cyproterone acetate can be very useful, particularly as a first-aid measure during a crisis. It usually takes about 10 days to produce its maximum effect with a dosage of 50 mg twice daily, although higher dosages may be required at first. Used in this way it can sometimes help the individual through a vulnerable phase or make his task easier while he tries to bring his behaviour under control. With lower dosages some men report that they can maintain normal sexual activity without feeling the same need for the different kind of release provided by exposing.

If the individual fails to control his exposing on regimens of this kind (that is short-term, intermittent, or low dose) it may be worth trying a longer course. Side effects such as breast tenderness and hair loss may become more of a problem and the patient must be warned of the uncertain long-term effects on fertility. Loss of energy may be troublesome during the early weeks of treatment. As a useful bonus some men report a decline in irritability.

Unfortunately the persistent exposer may be unsuitable for this treatment. If exposing has come to play a very important part in his life then reducing his sex drive may have little effect on the urgency of the behaviour, or if it does and thus begins to make his exposing significantly less satisfying and effective he may become depressed and miserable or, more usually, he stops taking the tablets.

Drugs affecting mood   Cyproterone acetate is proposed as the drug of first choice during crises when extreme measures are justified in order to anticipate a prison sentence, loss of employment, or marital breakdown. However, the situation is usually less urgent and one is able to avoid introducing medication whose long-term effects are uncertain and whose short-term effects may be very unwelcome both to the patient and his partner. In such cases it is worth considering anxiolytic medication, not on a regular basis but to be taken at times when the individual becomes aware of a growing restlessness and tension that he cannot deal with in other ways.

The benzodiazepines should be used with caution for this purpose because of their known liability to disinhibit. Flupenthixol 0.5—1 mg, trifluoperazine 1—2 mg, or antidepressants with relatively rapid sedative effects such as dothiepin and mianserin could be considered. It must be stressed that the correct use of anxiolytics by the subject requires him to have made some progress in self-monitoring.

Behavioural and psychological methods

Relaxation techniques   A well learned relaxation technique can contribute to a reduction in background and acute tension states. It can also provide a behavioural alternative to the exposing response and can open the way to the use of autohypnosis and autosuggestion techniques. (Details of a comprehensive relaxation technique are available from the author.)

Planned avoidance of trigger situations   This method is self-explanatory. It is an example of something that may seem too obvious to be stated: that the more tempting and ideal the situation the stronger is the urge to expose and the greater the effort needed to resist it. (See Bergin's (1969) discussion of the impulse chain.)

Masturbation   This often plays a large part in the exhibitionist's life. It can be turned to good use as another means of reducing sexual tension but it is important that he does not masturbate to fantasies of exposing. If exhibitionistic fantasies have been prominent they should be replaced by fantasies of more appropriate sexual behaviour. The content of the normal fantasies should be discussed in some detail in order to establish a safe nonexhibitionistic scenario that the subject finds arousing. If none can be found he has to continue with his previous fantasies but shape them by gradually altering them in the desired direction.

Methods that make the behaviour itself less attractive and increase its cost

The court report   Society, in the shape of the local magistrate and the Vagrancy Act, 1824, offers a number of approaches to the problem. It must be admitted that the majority of convicted exposers apparently stop after their first court appearance thus arguing that deterrence has a part to play. Psychiatrists preparing court reports are aware of the need to find some recommendation for the individual that encourages the magistrate to strike the most useful balance between deterrence and sympathy. For instance, the type 1 exhibitionist may have already suffered so much from his arrest and appearance in court that further punishment adds little. The more sociopathic individual may interpret magisterial leniency as an invitation to continue his practices unchecked whereas overpunishment and apparent vindictiveness on the part of the Bench may leave him resentful and rebellious and therefore more difficult for others to help.

   The psychiatrist must also bear in mind that the subject of his report will probably have access to it at some stage. He can therefore usefully discuss his conclusions and recommendations when he explains to the patient his proposals for treatment.

Behavioural techniques   Cautela (1967) described a technique called covert sensitization in which the subject is trained to associate the deviant behaviour with some undesired outcome. For instance, he might fantasize about being arrested at the moment of exposure or imagine exposing to a group of women who make jeering unflattering remarks.

In aversion therapy either the therapist or the subject himself delivers electric shocks to the forearm. Portable shock boxes make it possible for the patient to use this approach in real situations. The details of aversion therapy have been extensively researched and variations in timing and procedure seem to make little significant difference. (See Rooth and Marks (1974) for further discussion and references.)

Although early hopes for the usefulness of aversion therapy have not been met, it does seem to have a part to play in the treatment of some patients, particularly those less able to use techniques requiring ability in introspection and imagination. Aversion produces a reliable short-term reduction in the compulsiveness and attractiveness of the target behaviour. My impression is that this effect does not last and is not of much practical importance but that favourable results in the long term are more plausibly explained in terms of the decompartmentalization referred to above and the effect of the repeated intentional rehearsal of the fantasy or act of exposing on the subject's future ability to self-monitor. I suspect that there is also an investment effect of the kind conceptualized in Festinger's cognitive dissonance theory. (See Jensen (1979) for a recent discussion of the clinical applications of dissonance theory.) The possibility of being offered this unpleasant treatment again at a future date must also act as a deterrent.

A milder aversive experience (without electric shocks or other obvious punishment) seems to occur when patients hear themselves giving a tape-recorded account of their exposing.

For completeness I should mention here a new Australian initiative which I have not tried. The aversive element involved is shame accompanied by high levels of anxiety: the subject is required to undress in the presence of a mixed audience of hospital staff. As he does so he describes his exposing and his ideas about it. The audience questions him and discusses the subject objectively; videotape is also used (Jones and Frei, 1977). Very good results have been reported for most of the 15 persistent exhibitionists treated in this way.

The approaches described in this section contain some common ingredients: they spoil the fantasy by sharing it with other people who are not excited by it and they invade it with unpleasant or dissonant associations that make the fantasy less effective in engendering the particular frame of mind in which exposure can be used as a source of excitement and satisfaction.

Well motivated subjects may also use a gentler self-fining and self-rewarding approach based on criteria such as time spent on deviant fantasies in excess of an agreed limit. This approach has some of the features of symptom-prescription (Newton, 1968).

General comments

Rehearsal and training in the use of complex coping strategies

In the last two decades clinical psychologists have taken a welcome interest in mental processes. This has resulted in a more disciplined approach to the question of how people develop self-control and also emphasis has been placed on the importance of cognitive training and rehearsal in the acquisition of new coping skills.

Meichenbaum's (1977) review of the cognitive therapies contains a full discussion of these issues. In it he describes a procedure called stress-inoculation which is of particular interest. It has been used to improve control over pain, anger, and fear but the ideas have a wider relevance. Very briefly, this procedure has three stages. The first is an educational phase in which the subject is taught how to think about his problem and he is given various behavioural and mental techniques for approaching it; these techniques are rehearsed in the second phase. The third phase provides opportunities for applying the new skills to a variety of stressful situations. Meichenbaum has been particularly interested in the things people say to themselves and an important part of the training involves the selection and use of key self-statements designed to facilitate and organize the new responses and discourage the old.

Apart from the attention given to modifying mental processes by introducing selected self-statements the main interest of this approach lies in its insistence on a detailed and carefully structured training programme with both behavioural and mental aspects taken into consideration.

Motivational issues in symptom control

One of the advantages of incorporating behavioural tasks (whether they be pill swallowing, keeping a diary, or practising relaxation) is that they provide early and frequent opportunities for the therapist to test the working relationship and to clarify mutual expectations within the agreement to treat and be treated.

Many of the approaches suggested are difficult and require a degree of self-discipline that has to be acquired slowly. The therapist's enthusiasm and patience must be matched by a willingness to confront and explore his patient's failure to maintain his contribution to the treatment programme. The therapist's morale and credibility are helped if he has a good range of techniques at his disposal so that he can offer convincing alternatives when a particular approach has resulted in failure and mutual frustration.

The therapist's qualities are not within the scope of this article, but it should be stressed in passing that the therapist's willingness to confront and to use controlling techniques must be complemented by an ability to offer sensitive support and understanding. To increase his understanding of these patients and his capacity to empathize with them the therapist may find it helpful to turn to some of the more recent psychoanalytic writings on the narcissistic personality. Kohut's (1977) work in particular is recommended for its contribution to our understanding of personality structure and symptoms in deviant behaviour.

Help with personality problems

A proportion of patients is considerably disadvantaged in other aspects of personality function. This may make it impractical to adopt a symptom-focused approach on its own without more extensive support or treatment being directed towards other areas of their lives.

Poor impulse control in other situations, narcissistic preoccupations and vulnerability, and social incompetence are common themes. They may incapacitate an individual to a point where he scarcely seems able to look after himself in the adult world let alone sustain a commitment to the kinds of treatment outlined above.

For such people by far the best option is membership of a long-term group for sex offenders. This approach was described by English and American psychiatrists in the 1960s (for example Mathis and Collins, 1970) and has now been taken up by the probation service in a number of centres in this country of which Bristol is fortunate in being one. Groups of this kind can offer support over months and years while their members assimilate ideas and techniques outlined above. They also provide opportunities for developing social skills and confidence through discussion, role play, and the group experience itself.

There are advantages in restricting membership of these groups to people in whose lives exposing (or similar antisocial deviant sexual acts) is playing a significant part. To facilitate acceptance and identification there must be some clearly perceived common ground between these vulnerable and often isolated men. Those whose deviant behaviour is better controlled and is less of an issue in their lives do not wish to identify with a group catering for more persistent offenders with a poor social image. In any case such men could be considered for membership of an ordinary psychotherapy group if their personality difficulties warrant this.

A further advantage of the probation service group for persistent exposers is that attendance can be made compulsory and supervised under the terms of a probation order. This can sometimes be the only means of keeping these often poorly organized and easily discouraged men in one of the few situations where they can be helped.

References

Bergin, A E (1969) *Psychotherapy: Theory, Research and Practice*, **6**, 113
Cautela, J A (1967) *Psychological Reports*, **20**, 459
Jensen, R E (1979) *American Journal of Psychotherapy*, **33**, 303
Jones, I H, Frei, D (1977) *British Journal of Psychiatry*, **131**, 295
Kohut, H (1977) The Restoration of the Self. International Universities Press, New York
Mathis, J L, Collins, M (1970) *International Journal of Group Psychotherapy*, **20**, 163
Meichenbaum, D L (1977) Cognitive Behaviour Modification. Plenum Press, New York
Newton, J R (1968) *Psychotherapy: Theory, Research and Practice*, **5**, 95
Rooth, F G (1970) *Medico-Legal Journal*, **38**, 135
—(1971) *British Journal of Hospital Medicine*, **5**, 521
—(1973) *Archives of Sexual Behaviour*, **2**, 351
—, Marks, I M (1974) *ibid.* **3**, 227

Chapter 22

Homosexuality and sexually transmitted diseases

J L Fluker, Charing Cross and Hammersmith Hospitals, London

Homosexuality is as old as the human race. Although it has long been known that infection in man can be caused by homosexual practices (Harkness, 1948) it is only within the last 25 years that it has become important. Jefferiss (1956), Nicol (1960), Mascall (1961), and King (1962) showed varying rates at their respective hospitals. At St Mary's Hospital 8.4 per cent of 1000 cases of both syphilis and gonorrhoea in 1956 were homosexually acquired, and at St Thomas' 32 per cent of syphilis cases, St Paul's 79 per cent, and The London 14 per cent. The last would have fewer homosexuals attending in any case since it is in the East End. Jefferiss (1966), 10 years after his former paper, found that "out of a total of 1997 new male cases of all diagnoses, 281 (14 per cent) admitted homosexual contact; 31 (62 per cent) of 50 cases of early syphilis and 89 (14.7 per cent) of 604 cases of gonorrhoea".

Over the years 1968–71 at the West London Hospital (Charing Cross Hospital) the proportion of known male homosexuals ranged from 15.0 to 16.9 per cent and in 1971 there were 1773 homosexuals out of 11 174 men. From the same 4 years the syphilis rate in homosexuals ranged from 78.1 to 85.5 per cent and the gonorrhoea rate from 26.0 to 31.0 per cent, both of which have been maintained ever since (Fluker, 1976).

These high rates are atypical of the UK as a whole. The British Cooperative Clinical Group (Wright and Ginger, 1973) found the homosexual transmission rate for early (infectious) syphilis to be 73 per cent in the west of London as opposed to 37 per cent in the rest of the capital with corresponding rates for gonorrhoea of 28 per cent and 8 per cent. This pattern exists in most large cities of the Western developed countries. However, in the smaller towns and rural areas the pattern is quite different. The author had only one known case in over 7 years at the Chester Royal Infirmary.

Mode of infection

A myth was once held that venereal disease was not transmissible homosexually. Certainly mutual masturbation is relatively safe, except perhaps in secondary syphilis. Prolonged, especially lingual, kissing carries a similar slight risk but a social kiss does not. Orogenital contact in both sexes carries some risk but the danger is with penile–anal contact, especially intromission although less than half of all male homosexuals practise sodomy (Schofield, 1964). Anal–oral or penile–anal and then penile–oral with the same or another partner carries considerable risk of infection.

Almost all clinic patients indulge in anal sex. Most are versatile being both active and passive. A few are exclusively one or the other. In history taking the patient should be asked if he was active or passive on a particular occasion and not "Are you active or passive?". In practice, infections tend to be classified as active (genital) or passive (rectal) although some patients have both at once. In the Charing Cross Hospital series (Fluker, 1976) the ratio of active to passive was about 45.55 throughout.

Social characteristics

Although society has rightly become more tolerant, many homosexuals have difficulty in settling down with a single partner since family or social pressures discourage this. Some admit to having had at least 100 different partners and a few to many more. This explains the high repeater rate, some patients having had 40–50 new infections over the years in the same clinic—possibly an indication of satisfaction with their treatment. Regular attendance and checkups every 3 months should be encouraged. Waugh (1972) has shown that the exclusive homosexual is exemplary both in this and in producing his sexual contacts while the bisexual is often difficult, furtive, and untruthful, particularly as to the likely source of his infection. Married patients, especially if there is conjugal involvement, present the physician with a great challenge in trying to treat the couple and yet preserve the family intact.

Tables 23.1 and 23.2 show the categories and distribution of clinic patients (Fluker, 1976).

TABLE 23.1. Categories of homosexuals treated from 1962 to 1971 (Fluker, 1976)

	Number	%
Exclusively homosexual	6520	83.5
Bisexual	1128	14.5
Married	156	2.0
Total	7804	100.0
(Coloured)	(314)	(4.0)

TABLE 23.2. Ethnic distribution of homosexuals treated from 1972 to 1974 (Fluker, 1976)

	Number	%
White	4832	93.8
Coloured	324	6.2
Total	5156	100.0

Even an expert cannot always detect a male homosexual; many are athletic and masculine types. Neither does the author believe the relative laxity or tightness of the anal sphincter to be a reliable guide. The funnel-shaped anus is mostly confined to young male prostitutes (few of whom attend Charing Cross Hospital) or to much older men.

Management

Many doctors are repelled by homosexuality while a few are orientated towards it themselves. In professional dealings this should not count; the good of the patient ranks above all else. A doctor who cannot so adjust is incompletely educated professionally. It is satisfactory to see medical students eventually accepting this after initial distaste. After all, this is a part of the art of medicine which in this specialty has to be very highly developed since a good doctor–patient relationship is crucial.

Syphilis

The potential course of this disease is the same in everyone, only anal chancres betraying any difference in homosexuals. Such sores may be perianal or within the anal canal and rectum and so visible only on proctoscopy. A classic sore is obvious but many here present as painful fissures. The fact that traumatic fissures often occur compounds the difficulty. With a chancre a proctoscope can usually be passed but with a true fissure it frequently cannot. In the former event, tests for rectal gonorrhoea are advised.

Clinical examination may reveal a suspicious inguinal adenitis, especially lateral-ly, or some of the many symptoms are signs of secondary syphilis. In suspicious cases a darkground test will clinch the diagnosis by revealing *Treponema pallidum* and if the test is negative in known homosexuals it should be repeated for 2–3 days if necessary. In the presence of local sepsis a sulphonamide is helpful (and will not mask syphilis) while normal saline is the only permissible local treatment. With darkground-negative lesions blood tests should be done weekly for a month, fortnightly during the second month, and finally after the third calendar month. It takes from 10 to 90 days after the appearance of the primary sore for the blood tests to show positively, the same as the incubation period. The time-lag occurs because it is a delayed antibody response that is being tested for.

The usual order in which the tests become positive is fluorescent treponemal antibody test, VDRL slide test, and *T. pallidum* haemagglutination test, but this is frequently not adhered to. A rising titre in the VDRL test is virtually diagnostic and may herald a new infection in a patient previously treated and cured but left with positive treponemal tests (fluorescent treponemal antibody test and *T. pallidum* immobilization test) and negative reagin (VDRL test). The *T. pallidum* immobi-lization test remains negative at this stage of the disease. Finally, specialist help may well be desirable.

Gonorrhoea

Urethral gonorrhoea is the same in all men. Nevertheless, it should be remembered that it may be both symptomless and signless and therefore unrecognizable on simple clinical examination. Intraurethral smears and cultures and similar tests on any urinary threads are necessary with contacts of known cases, and if all these prove negative similar examinations of the prostatic fluid are required before the patient can be discharged.

Rectal gonorrhoea is often symptomless. *Table 23.3* shows the symptoms of 1867 patients including a proportion of repeaters.

TABLE 23.3. Symptoms shown by 1867 patients with rectal
gonorrhoea

	Number	*%*
None	988	53.0
Slight itching	839	45.0
Mucoid discharge — wetness	762	40.8
Greenish-yellow discharge	150	8.0
Bloodstained discharge	27	1.4
Passage of blood	8	0.4
Acute tenesmus	4	0.2
Retention of urine (only)	3	0.15

Repeaters tend to be more sensitive to slight symptoms but the disease seems to be becoming milder so the number of symptomless cases may well increase.

Proctoscopy is essential as an aid to diagnosis, for tests of cure, and as above to exclude associated conditions such as primary syphilis (14 cases in the series in *Table 23.3*), condylomata acuminata (35), herpes genitalis (2), and chlamydial infection—tests for *Chlamydia trachomatis A* (types D–K) could not then be done.

The proctoscopic appearances range from normal in most cases to an excess of mucus, strips or ribbons of mucopus adherent to the rectal wall, or (uncommonly) thick greenish-yellow pus on an intensely red background. Such pus must be swabbed away lest it conceal another lesion. Smears and cultures are essential, particularly the latter on which at least half the diagnoses depend.

All homosexuals and heterosexuals who have orogenital sex require pharyngeal smears and cultures. Verification of the latter by fluorescent antibody methods and sugar fermentation is essential to distinguish between the various *Neisseria* species in the throat. These may also appear in genital sites and the rectum (Beck et al, 1974).

In London and other areas with a high proportion of insensitive but not fully resistant strains (Lynn et al, 1970) treatment is best given by the single large dose method. A suitable treatment is ampicillin 3 g plus probenecid 1 g orally. This is better than giving multiple small doses. Penicillin is contraindicated in those with known hypersensitivity to it or with an associated possible syphilitic lesion as yet undiagnosed, or after exposure to known beta-lactamase infection. Alternative but more costly methods are a single intramuscular injection of spectinomycin 2 g (Gerken et al, 1980), a similar dosage of kanamycin 2 g although its potential ototoxicity (cochlea) tends to disqualify it (Fluker and Hewitt, 1970), and in a beta-lactamase infections only, cefuroxime 0.75 g with probenecid 1 g orally (Price and Fluker, 1977). Lastly co-trimoxazole three or four tablets twice daily (each containing trimethoprim 80 mg and sulphamethoxazole 400 mg) may be given orally for 4–5 days (Waugh, 1971). Tetracycline and erythromycin give poorer results and are not recommended for the initial treatment of gonorrhoea.

Nonspecific genital infection

This may be transmitted by penile–anal intercourse. Those few clinics able to grow *C. trachomatis* are finding it in the rectums of patients who have been in contact with urethral cases (Goldmeier and Darougar, 1977). The treatment of choice is either a tetracycline (oxytetracycline 500 mg twice daily) or, as a second string to the bow, erythromycin in a similar dosage for 14 days.

Genital warts

The wart viruses flourish in the anorectal mucosae. The genital wart, spread through sexual activity, is generally softer than the tough cutaneous wart which may also get implanted here. Thus anal warts are not conclusive proof of homosexual activity. As these lesions are often treated by other than genitourinary physicians, their frequent association with other conditions—mainly syphilis and gonorrhoea—means that these should always be excluded before starting treatment.

Soft pedunculated or cauliflower warts usually respond better to treatment than the flat sessile ones which often infiltrate the entire thickness of the skin and mucosa. Self-treatment should not be allowed. Podophyllum resin 25 per cent may be tried first, but despite occasional success it tends only to produce excessive soreness. Trichloroacetic acid acts similarly on hard warts and also tends towards subsequent scarring. Single large warts may respond to cryosurgery, but the author finds electrocautery using a local anaesthetic very satisfactory. Surgery may be needed for extensive warts and in such cases and in those of poor morale a general anaesthetic may be necessary. At Charing Cross Hospital it is customary for patients to be referred to genitourinary medicine for follow-up since rapid and extensive recurrence is all too common.

Herpes genitalis

The incidence of anal herpesvirus infections is increasing. The eruption is often preceded by intense pain for up to 2 days before its appearance. The diagnosis may be confirmed by virus isolation and associated infections appropriately excluded (Goldmeier, 1980).

Conditions such as chancroid, lymphogranuloma venereum, and granuloma inguinale may be transmitted homosexually but call for no further comment here.

Hepatitis B

This is spread by sexual contact—mainly homosexual. Coleman et al (1977) at Charing Cross Hospital found that 31 (5.2 per cent) of 600 patients were positive for hepatitis B antigen, and of 85 tested for antibody by radioimmunoassay 30 (35 per cent) were positive. In a larger study at Charing Cross and St Thomas' Hospitals, Murray-Lyon et al (1979) found that 129 (5 per cent) of 2612 homosexual males harboured the hepatitis B surface antigen. Liver biopsy in 25 patients with no clinical symptoms or signs but with abnormal liver function tests showed 14 (56 per cent) with chronic active hepatitis or cirrhosis. Of 118 with hepatitis B surface antigen, 38 per cent were positive for the electrophoresis antigen (hepatitis B e antigen) and therefore likely to infect their nonimmune sexual partners.

In short, homosexual males should all be investigated for hepatitis B, ideally at 3-monthly intervals. A word of warning: do not start telling jaundiced patients that they may have venereal disease!

Bowel infections

The homosexual practices already considered may be a means of spreading enteric diseases. More attention has been paid to this in the USA so far (Felman, 1980). In the UK, infestations with threadworms and *Giardia lamblia* have been met with in the clinics. Examination of stools is now becoming almost routine to exclude such parasitic infestations (Macmillan, 1980).

Other conditions

As the author has pointed out elsewhere (Fluker, 1966, 1976) few homosexuals wish for sexual reorientation—out of 700 personally interviewed only 15 desired it and of these eight attempted treatment. They seem no more prone to major psychiatric disorders than anyone else although Wells and Schofield (1972) concluded that their Glasgow patients were significantly more neurotic than the general population.

Trauma of the rectum and anus is common resulting in tears, fissures, fistula in ano, and even ischiorectal abscess (in 10 years the author found 15 cases in homosexuals and none in heterosexuals). Spasm of the anal sphincter occasionally requiring dilatation is seen but, curiously enough, no cases of anal incontinence. Nor do there seem to have been any cases of proctalgia fugax although this has sometimes occurred in heterosexual patients.

Mucus in excess is doubtless a response to unnatural trauma and to what is surely a physiological outrage, but in introspective patients irritable bowel syndrome and even ulcerative colitis may occur.

Proctoscopy has sometimes revealed foreign bodies, knowledge of which may have prompted the patient's attendance. The use of vibrators has led to occasional rupture of the bowel and peritonitis. One such patient (who recovered after operation) collapsed after walking 3 miles to our department. He said that he had come to us because he knew that whatever he had done we would always be kind to him.

References

Beck, A, Fluker, J L, Platt, D J (1974) *British Journal of Venereal Diseases*, **50**, 367
Coleman, J C, Waugh, M A, Dayton, R (1977) *ibid.* **53**, 132
Felman, Y M (1980) *Practitioner*, **224**, 1151
Fluker, J L (1966) *British Journal of Venereal Diseases*, **42**, 48
—(1976) *ibid.* **52**, 155
—, Hewitt, A B (1970) *ibid.* **46**, 455
Gerken, A, Platt, D J, Fluker, J L, Deheragoda, P (1980) *ibid.* **56**, 397

Goldmeier, D (1980) *ibid.* **56**, 111
—, Darougar, S (1977) *ibid.* **53**, 184
Harkness, A H (1948) *Proceedings of the Royal Society of Medicine*, **41**, 476
Jefferiss, F J G (1956) *British Journal of Venereal Diseases*, **32**, 17
— (1966) *ibid.* **42**, 46
King, A J (1962) *Proceedings of the Royal Society of Medicine*, **55**, 869
Lynn, R, Nicol, C S, Ridley, M, Rimmer, D, Symonds, M A E, Warren, C (1970) *British Journal of Venereal Diseases*, **46**, 404
Macmillan, A (1980) *Scottish Medical Journal*, **25**, 33
Mascall, N (1961) *British Medical Journal*, i, 899
Murray-Lyon, I M et al (1979) *Lancet*, i, 903
Nicol, C S (1960) *Practitioner*, **184**, 345
Price, J D, Fluker, J L (1977) *Proceedings of the Royal Society of Medicine*, **70**, Suppl. 9, p.125
Schofield, M (1964) *British Journal of Venereal Diseases*, **40**, 129
Waugh, M A (1971) *ibid.* **47**, 34
— (1972) *ibid.* **48**, 534
Wells, B W P, Schofield, C B S (1972) *ibid.* **48**, 75
Wright, D J M, Ginger, C D (1973) *ibid.* **49**, 329

Chapter 23

The assessment and management of transsexual problems

Kurt Schapira/Kenneth Davison, University of Newcastle upon Tyne
Harry Brierley, Newcastle Area Health Authority

Until the early 1950s transsexual phenomena were included with other gender-identity problems under the heading of transvestism (transvestitism). Havelock Ellis (1928) described a group of cases that he called aesthetic inversion or eonism after the Chevalier d'Eon de Beaumont, an 18th century French diplomat/spy who for many years masqueraded as a female. Eventually a distinct syndrome was delineated to which the term transsexualism was applied (Cauldwell, 1949).

Nowadays the term transsexual is used for persons of either sex who display the following characteristics (Wålinder, 1968):

1. A sense of belonging to the opposite sex, having been born into the wrong sex, and being one of nature's extant errors
2. A sense of estrangement from one's own body; all manifestations of sex differentiation are regarded as repugnant
3. A strong desire to resemble physically the opposite sex and seek treatment, including surgery, towards this end
4. A wish to be accepted in the community as belonging to the opposite sex.

The condition is to be distinguished from transvestism in which individuals (usually males) dress in the clothes of the opposite sex but do not regard themselves as belonging to that sex. This cross-dressing may be either a symptom of some other sexual deviation (occasionally homosexuality) or employed as a means of fetishistic sexual excitement.

Benjamin (1966), a pioneer in this difficult field, sees transsexualism and transvestism as parts of a continuum, some transitional cases having features of both. Thus some males become dissatisfied with cross-dressing and in an effort to approximate more closely to the feminine role begin to demand hormone therapy to induce breast enlargement, but they usually stop short of requesting surgical remodelling of their external genitalia. This contrasts with the full-blown transsexual to whom all external manifestations of his/her physical sex are sources of disgust and regarded as alien to his/her true inner being.

Transsexuals should be distinguished from pseudohermaphrodites who are wrongly assigned to a sex because of equivocal genital anatomy. They usually regard themselves as belonging to the assigned sex (Armstrong, 1966).

Prevalence

Using Wålinder's criteria the prevalence of transsexualism in Sweden has been estimated as 1 in 54 000: 1 in 37 000 for men and 1 in 103 000 for women (Wålinder, 1968). Hoenig and Kenna (1974) calculated that there are some 537 male and 180 female transsexuals in England and Wales, and Pauly (1969) estimated about 2000 cases in the USA. Such figures are likely to repesent the tip of the iceberg.

Sexual identification

The seven criteria for establishing sexual identity (Money, 1963) are:

1. Chromosomal sex (normal male 46/XY and normal female 46/XX)
2. Gonadal sex (the histological structure of the ovary or testis)
3. Hormonal function
4. Internal genital morphology
5. External genital morphology and body image
6. Assigned sex
7. Psychosexual differentiation.

In transsexualism there is no evidence of abnormality in the first five of these variables and assigned sex conforms to biological sex. There is, however, a severe disturbance in psychosexual differentiation, particularly in the sphere of gender identity.

Gender identity

This term refers to an individual's sense of masculinity or femininity as distinct from sex which is the sum of the biological attributes that contribute to the making of a male or a female (Stoller, 1976). Stoller considers gender identity as arising from the interaction of three forces: biological, biopsychic and intrapsychic.

The biological components derive from prenatal endocrine influences. In mammals the basic state of resting tissue is female and male organs are produced only under the influence of androgens (Jost, 1972) which must be available at a critical (species-specific) time if the brain is to be organized towards maleness (Money and Erhardt, 1972).

As we ascend the evolutionary scale the influence of environmental factors becomes increasingly important and the organism's repertoire of behaviour exhibits greater flexibility. Thus the general rule that maleness and masculinity or femaleness and femininity inevitably go together is most frequently broken in humans (Stoller, 1969).

The biopsychic factors include imprinting and conditioning, and the intrapsychic ones the resolution of oedipal conflicts. The gender identity of transsexuals is incongruous in that it is contrary to biological and anatomical sex, in contrast to homosexuals in whom it may be uncommitted but not incongruous.

Aetiology

There are two schools of thought about this. One theory considers that the condition is caused by pathogenic, social and psychological factors in child rearing (Money et al, 1957). For example, Ball (1967) consistently found in the history of male transsexuals an absent or unsatisfactory paternal figure and a corresponding excessive dependence on, and preference for, the mother.

Other workers believe that transsexualism is due to a subtle organic dysfunction, possibly related to prenatal endocrine influences on the developing thalamus (Baker and Stoller, 1968). Certainly a female pattern of behaviour has been observed in anatomically male animals after prenatal or early postnatal hormonal administration (Harris and Michael, 1964). However, in man, although boys born to mothers given large dosages of oestrogen during pregnancy were subsequently shown to be less masculine in activity and interests than a control group, none showed any transsexual features (Yalom et al, 1973).

Other conditions that have been reported to be associated with transsexual behaviour include Klinefelter's syndrome (Money and Pollitt, 1964), both functional psychosis (Lukianowicz, 1959) and amphetamine-induced psychosis (Roth and Ball, 1964), and temporal lobe epilepsy (Davies and Morgenstern, 1960; Hunter et al, 1963). Wålinder (1965) found a high prevalence of EEG abnormalities in a group of transvestites.

Levine (1971) combined the two theories into a hypothesis involving the sequential actions of chromosomes, hormones, and learning mechanisms at critical stages in development.

Assessment procedure

From the above observations it is clear that the proper assessment of a patient presenting with transsexual features demands the most detailed and careful collection and analysis of data relating to the person and his environment from the moment of conception onwards. Whenever possible, information should be sought from independent sources as well as the patient. Such areas of information may conveniently be classified as follows.

Physical development

The possibilities of unusual prenatal or perinatal conditions, illnesses or operations in childhood, and exposure to male or female hormones should be considered. The patient's birth weight and age at milestones in development should also be assessed.

Psychological and psychosexual development

Information should be sought concerning the patient's position in sibship, ages of first cross-dressing and wish for reassignment, menarche and breast development in females, spontaneous erections and emissions in males, homosexual and/or heterosexual activities. masturbatory fantasies, sadomasochistic tendencies, sociability, hobbies and interests, marriage and parenthood, and nonsexual behavioural problems.

Environmental influences

Consideration should be given to the parental attitudes to the birth and the sex of the patient and the presence of a dominant parent, an absent or ineffectual parent, and psychosexual problems in the parents.

Current psychosocial situation

This should be examined with particular reference to the patient's sexual orientation, cross-dressing behaviour, attitude to his own and the opposite sex, and employment record.

Physical examination

Observations should be made of the patient's height and weight, ratio of shoulder to hip width (androgyny score; Tanner, 1951), facial and body hair distribution, body fat, breasts, and external genitalia.

Psychological and psychiatric examinations

These should include an assessment of the patient's posture and mannerisms that indicate gender role, the extent of mental distress, psychopathic traits, and evidence of psychosis. Some objective assessments of intelligence, personality, sexual attitudes, and interests by means of recognized psychometric tests (for example the Wechsler Adult Intelligence Scale, the Cattell 16 personality factor questionnaire, and the Terman–Miles attitude-interest test) are useful for future reference. More sophisticated techniques such as the repertory grid and the semantic differential are useful in quantifying and investigating the individual's concept of himself and his world (Brierley, 1979).

Special investigations

These should include skull and chest X-rays, EEGs, and karyotypes. Hormonal abnormalities are rarely found except when the patient has been ingesting androgens or oestrogens, but it is usual to measure the serum levels of FSH and LH and the plasma concentrations of testosterone in males and 17-beta-oestradiol in females.

Photography and videotapes of the patient in the appropriate and the cross-dressing conditions, alone and interacting with both men and women, are useful for future comparison.

Management of the male transsexual

Before embarking on a scheme of management it is important to assess the individual's commitment to his proposed new identity. Is the problem really lifelong and fundamental or may it possibly be transient? Is the person fully aware of the extent of the readjustment he will have to make? Few can expect to receive the kind of tolerance and understanding accorded to Jan Morris (1974). Because of these factors it is advisable for reassignment attempts to proceed in stages with plenty of time allowed for the transsexual to change his mind before committing himself to any irrevocable procedure.

Stage one

The person is assisted in developing modes of behaviour and actions appropriate to his preferred gender role. This involves the learning of feminine deportment, speech, mannerisms, and many of the subtle aspects of behaviour that distinguish women from men. Transsexuals are often unaware of these aspects and although professing to be entirely feminine look grotesque in female clothes.

Yardley (1976) gives an excellent account of the training in feminine skills of a 20-year-old transsexual as part of a programme leading up to surgical remodelling of the external genitalia. Extensive use was made of videofilm of the cross-dressed patient interacting with both men and women. The film was reviewed by 20 student teachers, four clinicians and a behaviour therapist. From their comments certain target areas were selected for behaviour modification. These included body movements, body tonus, gestures, voice, control of interaction, content of conversation, manner of relating to others, appearance, and general impression. The procedure consisted of 20 weekly sessions each of 2 hours' duration. The individual's relationships with the female therapist and the male psychiatrist, who were both able to accept and relate to the patient as a woman, were regarded as important aspects of the treatment.

Advice from a beautician about make-up and from other female staff (such as nurses and occupational therapists) about mode of dress is an essential part of gender-role training. Many male transsexuals left to themselves choose clothing that highlights their femininity with an effect more appropriate to the theatre than to everyday life. They also tend to dress much younger than their actual ages. It may be these tendencies that lead many transsexuals to take up careers as models or actresses where the wearing of ultrafeminine garments is not only more acceptable but also positively advantageous.

Stage two

This involves medical management in the form of hormone therapy. It may be started during the period of training in social skills and gender role, but first the person must appreciate its effects, limitations, and potential hazards.

The ingestion of oestrogens cannot produce a female out of an anatomical male. Although the development of the glandular and fatty tissues causes some increase in the size of the breasts, in only a few cases do they assume a normal female contour. Oestrogens do not raise the pitch of the masculine voice—often a considerable problem—but vocal practice may help. Their effects on hair growth are also variable. In some the scalp hair grows more quickly and becomes softer in texture, but in others these changes are less striking. The beard is little affected and usually requires electrolytic depilation; this technique can produce satisfactory results, although it may be prolonged and is sometimes painful (Brierley, 1979).

Oestrogen therapy also induces a deposition of fat around the hips and thighs and often at other sites (especially the face) also, creating a more youthful and feminine appearance. However, the recipient should be warned that hormone therapy will not necessarily transform him into someone of perfect female proportions. He need only be reminded that there are many females who, although exposed to the influence of endogenous oestrogens from puberty, have failed to achieve this ideal!

Psychosexual changes are confined to reductions in sexual interests and drive. Some also claim a general decrease in assertiveness as well as describing themselves as more emotional, weeping more easily and expressing greater lability of mood. These features are usually welcomed by the recipient as representing feminine personality traits.

Side effects occasionally occur and include nausea, vomiting, and dizziness. More rarely thrombosis and malignant breast tumours have been reported (Symmers, 1968). Potential recipients of hormone therapy should be warned of the risks involved, but few are deterred from proceeding.

The feminizing drugs that are employed include stilboestrol 0.25–0.5 mg daily, ethinyloestradiol 0.02–0.05 mg daily, conjugated oestrogens (Premarin) 1.25–2.5 mg daily, and oestradiol valerate 5–20 mg twice weekly by injection (Money and Walker, 1977).

Stage three

The so-called sex-change operations have achieved an undesirable degree of notoriety in society and have aroused controversy within the medical profession. Their ethical justification has been questioned on the grounds that they are in effect mutilating since no anatomical anomaly is present and they are performed merely at the demand of the patient (Ostow, 1953). On the other hand, there is no doubt that some transsexuals suffer great anguish and misery which only in rare cases is alleviated by conventional psychiatric methods (Barlow et al, 1973). By definition transsexuals constantly importune for surgical correction of what they regard as their alien sexual anatomy; however, as Laub and Fisk (1974) point out, other types of individual with gender-identity problems also request sex-change surgery. These authors classify six distinct subgroups under the title of gender dysphoria syndrome which they define as "an emotional state characterized by anxiety, depression and restlessness" arising in individuals who are so dissatisfied with their sex that they seek surgical change. The syndrome includes classic transsexuals, some effeminate homosexuals, some transvestites, some psychotics with delusions regarding their sexual identity, some persons with neurotic thoughts of impulses towards their own genitalia, and some extreme sociopaths or psychopaths.

In the treatment programme at Stanford, California (Laub and Fisk, 1974) 74 out of 769 who requested surgery (9.6 per cent) were eventually operated on and they were only selected from the first three of the above subgroups. Of these 50 were male-to-female and 24 female-to-male operations. Surgery was only undertaken after a prolonged rehabilitation programme such as the one described above. The criteria employed in selection for surgery in this series are shown in *Table 24.1*.

TABLE 24.1. Criteria qualifying transsexuals for surgical intervention (from Laub and Fisk, 1974)

Age 21—58 years

Successful endocrine feminization

One to 3 years of total cross-living and working in the gender of choice

Success in social, psychological, employment and sexual spheres

Not married in the anatomical gender

Freedom from psychosis or significant sociopathy (jail or drugs)

No life-limiting medical diseases (for example diabetes and hypertension)

In her book *Conundrum* Jan Morris (1974) describes the criteria for operation that were applied in her case. These were her being nonpsychotic, having an ability to understand the procedure, being physically compatible with the new role, having already acquired the secondary female characteristics by prolonged hormone therapy, showing few if any masculine characteristics, and having lived for some years in the role of the preferred gender and proved that it was socially and economically possible.

Laub and Fisk (1974) described in detail the surgical techniques employed to reshape the genital anatomy in the required direction. In the male-to-female conversion a capacious vagina is constructed with skin grafts, the labia are constructed from scrotal and penile skin, the urethra is displaced posteriorly, and the meatus accurately directed. A dilating vaginal mould is used for 6 months postoperatively. It is claimed that sexual intercourse as a female can subsequently be achieved comfortably. The Stanford team performs other cosmetic procedures one week later. These include breast augmentation, rhinoplasty, thyroid cartilage reduction, and blepharoplasty.

In a review of postoperative follow-up for up to 6 years (mean 25.3 months) Laub and Fisk (1974) found that the significant factor leading to a satisfactory outcome (assessed in terms of economic, social, psychological, and sexual functions) was a successful preoperative adjustment to living in the gender of choice during a 1–3 year trial period. Physical complications such as infections and rectovaginal fistula occurred in 47 per cent of male-to-female operations and 25 per cent of female-to-male operations. Other problems have included a $2.5 million lawsuit, "excessive emotional attachment to surgeon", and a "desire to shoot the genitals of the surgeon with a shotgun". However, the authors concluded that overall the operations were beneficial, notably in improving social and sexual adjustments.

In this country Randell (1969), who directs the London Gender Identity Clinic at Charing Cross Hospital, reported that of 29 male transsexuals who underwent sex-reassignment surgery two thirds showed a marked amelioration in social and psychological adjustments.

Management of the female transsexual

The management of biological females wishing to adopt a male gender identity is similar in principle to that of male transsexuals. At the stage of the behavioural modifications (stage one) the emphasis is on body-building exercises and the encouragement of masculine behaviour patterns. Hormone therapy consists of androgens (for example monthly intramuscular injections of testosterone oenanthate 250 mg) which increase body weight and growth of facial hair, lower the pitch of the voice, and often suppress menstruation.

With regard to surgery, requests for mastectomy are most common followed by hysterectomy or possibly ovariectomy. Provision of a nonerectile phallus is also possible (Laub and Fisk, 1974). The criteria applied are the same as for males.

Legal and administrative issues

Without social and legal recognition of the new role the transsexual remains at a disadvantage no matter what medical or surgical measures have been undertaken. Legal attitudes to transsexual problems vary from country to country, Sweden being possibly the most liberal (Hoenig, 1977). The following comments apply to the situation in the UK.

There is no legal definition of sex and the precise meaning of man or woman has never been established. Society regards a person as either male or female according to the entry on his birth certificate which is based on the apparent anatomical sex of the infant. In the rare cases of intersex the assigned sex determines the subsequent rearing of the child and hence his/her gender identity (Money et al, 1957).

In the first judgement in this country to rule on the sex of an individual (Corbett v. Corbett, 1970) Sir Roger Ormrod held that the marriage of a surgically reassigned male-to-female transsexual (April Ashley) and a man was a nullity. In his opinion sex reassignment was no more than a doctor's decision on the gender in which a person can best be managed. In contractual relationships where sex is a relevant factor, such as life insurance, pension schemes, and other contracts involving personal documentation, there is nothing to prevent the parties from agreeing to treat an individual as either a man or a woman. However, in the context of marriage only biological criteria are relevant and these are the chromosomal constitution, the external genitalia at birth, and the nature of the internal gonads. If these three criteria are congruent, for the purpose of marriage they determine the sex of an individual and no operative intervention has any bearing on the matter (Corbett v. Corbett, 1970).

This important judgement acknowledges the differences between sex and gender and indicates those fields of human activity where the legal sex is entirely governed by the biological sex and other areas where gender assignment, even when contrary to the biological sex, might be legally recognized.

Returning to practical issues, a change of Christian name or forename is one of the matters requiring early legal consideration. It is not essential to apply for legal permission to change one's name since a person is entitled to assume a new name as long as this is not done for criminal purposes. Nevertheless, it is advisable to obtain a legal change of name with the support of medical evidence since this facilitates subsequent alterations in documents such as National Insurance card, driving licence, and passport as well as certificates of examinations and qualifications.

From an early stage of management the transsexual should carry a medical certificate to the effect that he/she is under medical care and in the process of gender reassignment. Although of no legal value, such a certificate gives the transsexual confidence and is useful evidence for the police or anyone else who may challenge the person's bona fides. Cross-dressing is in itself not a criminal offence, but it may be interpreted as conduct likely to provoke a breach of the peace.

Prevention

Since adult transsexualism is a serious condition that presents formidable therapeutic problems and because cross-gender behaviour may be evident in children under the age of 5 years (Green, 1968), follow-up of such children and therapeutic intervention at an early stage may achieve a more satisfactory end result by less drastic means as well as increasing understanding of the condition (Hampson, 1974).

A multidisciplinary approach

Transsexualism is a good example of a disorder in which a purely medical approach is inadequate. Also required are psychologists to help with behaviour modification, supported by beauticians, occupational therapists, and physiotherapists. Family incomprehension may necessitate the assistance of social workers, a lawyer is required for legal advice, and administrators are involved in providing the necessary documentation. The clergy may be helpful where religious or ethical conflicts arise.

Medical help is required for the physical assessment and the hormone therapy and a sympathetic plastic surgeon is needed for the surgical remodelling. However, the initial referral is usually to a psychiatrist and no matter how far along the road of gender reassignment the transsexual travels he/she will require nonjudgemental psychotherapeutic support. On rare occasions the patient may even need to be helped to achieve a reversal of his/her gender identity to one congruous with his/her biological sex (Barlow et al, 1973; Duffy and Davison, 1979).

Transsexuals suffer (Cowell, 1954; Morris, 1974). How best to alleviate their suffering is open to honest differences of opinion. At the very least they deserve not to be ignored.

References

Armstrong, C N (1966) *British Medical Journal*, ii, 1255
Baker, H J, Stoller, R J (1968) *American Journal of Psychiatry*, **124**, 1653
Ball, J R B (1967) *Australian and New Zealand Journal of Psychiatry*, **1**, 188
Barlow, D H, Reynolds, E J, Agras, W S (1973) *Archives of General Psychiatry*, **28**, 569
Benjamin, H (1966) The Transsexual Phenomenon. The Julian Press, New York
Brierley, H (1979) Transvestism. Pergamon Press, Oxford
Cauldwell, D O (1949) *Sexology*, **16**, 274
Corbett v. Corbett (1970) 2 All England Law Reports, 33. Probate, Divorce and Admiralty Division. Butterworths, London
Cowell, R E (1954) Roberta Cowell's Story. Heinemann, London
Davies, B M, Morgenstern, F S (1960) *Journal of Neurology, Neurosurgery and Psychiatry*, **23**, 247
Duffy, J P, Davison, K (1979) unpublished report
Ellis, H (1928) Studies in the Psychology of Sex, Vol. 7: Eonism and other Studies. F A Davis, London
Green, R (1968) *Journal of Nervous and Mental Disease*, **147**, 500
Hampson, J L (1974) *in* Proceedings of the Interdisciplinary Symposium on Gender Dysphoria Syndrome (edited by Gandy, P, Laub, D). Edwards Brothers, Ann Arbor
Harris, G W, Michael, R P (1964) *Journal of Physiology*, **171**, 275
Hoenig, J (1977) *Canadian Medical Association Journal*, **116**, 319
—, Kenna, J C (1974) *British Journal of Psychiatry*, **124**, 181
Hunter, R, Logue, V, McMenemy, W H (1963) *Epilepsia (Amsterdam)*, **4**, 60
Jost, A (1972) *Johns Hopkins Medical Journal*, **130**, 38
Laub, D R, Fisk, N (1974) *Plastic and Reconstructive Surgery and the Transplantation Bulletin*, **53**, 388
Levine, S (1971) *in* Personality and Science: An Interdisciplinary Discussion (edited by Ramsey, I T, Porter, R). Churchill Livingstone, Edinburgh and London. p.5
Lukianowicz, M (1959) *Psychiatria et neurologia*, **138**, 64
Money, J (1963) Determinants of Sexual Behaviour. Charles C Thomas, Illinois
—, Erhardt, A A (1972) Man and Woman, Boy and Girl. Johns Hopkins University Press, Baltimore
—, Pollitt, E (1964) *Archives of General Psychiatry*, **11**, 589
—, Walker P A (1977) *in* Handbook of Sexology (edited by Money, J, Musaph, H). Excerpta Medica, Amsterdam
—, Hampson, J G, Hampson, J L (1957) *Archives of Neurology and Psychiatry*, **77**, 333
Morris, J (1974) Conundrum. Faber and Faber, London
Ostow, M (1953) *Journal of the American Medical Association*, **152**, 1553
Pauly, I (1969) *in* Transsexualism and Sex Reassignment (edited by Green, R, Money, J). Johns Hopkins University Press, Baltimore. p.58
Randell, J B (1969) *ibid*. p.373
Roth, M, Ball, J R B (1964) *in* Intersexuality in Vertebrates including Man (edited by Armstrong, C N, Marshall, A J). Academic Press, London. p.395
Stoller, R J (1969) Sex and Gender: On the Development of Masculinity and Femininity. Hogarth Press and The Institute of Psychoanalysis, London
—, (1976) *in* The Sexual Experience (edited by Sadock, B J, Kaplan, H I, Freedman, A M). Williams and Wilkins, Baltimore

Symmers, W St C (1968) *British Medical Journal*, ii, 83
Tanner, J M (1951) *Lancet*, i, 574
Wålinder, J (1965) *International Journal of Neuropsychiatry*, **1**, 567
—, (1968) *Acta psychiatrica et neurologica Scandinavica*, Suppl. 203, p.255
Yalom, I D, Green, R, Fisk, N (1973) *Archives of General Psychiatry*, **28**, 554
Yardley, K M (1976) *British Journal of Medical Psychology*, **49**, 329

Chapter 24

Management of early childhood autism

Lorna Wing, MRC Social Psychiatry Unit, London

Childhood autism and related conditions almost always lead to lifelong handicaps, but the problems can, to some extent, be alleviated by appropriate management and education based on an understanding of the impairments underlying the abnormal pattern of behaviour. Good management also requires that the needs of the whole family, and not just those of the handicapped person, are considered.

The nature of childhood autism

Normal children are born "preprogrammed" to develop a wide range of skills over the course of time. Among these is the capacity to attribute meaning to experiences (Ricks, 1975; Ricks and Wing, 1975). In particular, the infant is able to recognize that human beings are of more interest and importance than other aspects of the environment and within the first few weeks he begins to initiate and respond to communication with other people (Schaffer, 1974; Trevarthen, 1974). The process of making sense of the world and communicating ideas speeds up and becomes much more efficient in the second year with the development of language and the ability to give symbolic labels to concepts. A further major step forward occurs when the child becomes able, around 18 months of age, to develop imaginative pretend play with toys, pets, and eventually other children. These interrelated skills are the basis on which the child builds his own private version of the rules governing the culture in which he lives. By the time he reaches adulthood his inner world is complex and stable enough to enable him to plan his own life and to become independent of his parents.

Autistic children appear to lack, or to be severely limited in, these in-built capacities (Ricks, 1975; Ricks and Wing, 1975). Many seem to be born without them and the rest lose them after a short period of apparently normal development. To the observer, the problem is shown in a triad of severe impairments affecting reciprocal social interaction, communication (nonverbal and verbal), and imaginative activities (Wing and Gould, 1979). The child or adult concerned fills his time with repetitive stereotyped routines; these vary from the simple (such as scratching on surfaces, gazing at lights, flicking objects, and even repetitive self-injury) to the elaborate (for example making complex but meaningless patterns with household objects or drawing pictures of trains over and over again).

224

The best known subgroup is that first described by Kanner (1943) who coined the term early infantile autism. This is characterized by marked social aloofness, especially to age peers (at least in the early years), and elaborate repetitive routines. However, there are other children with the triad of impairments described above who do not fit the classic autistic picture but who need the same kind of education and management (Wing and Gould, 1979). In nearly all cases the onset is before the age of 5 years. Such conditions are to be distinguished from the psychotic illnesses of adults, such as schizophrenia, which very rarely occur in childhood and virtually never before 7 years of age (Kolvin, 1971). In this paper the term childhood autism is used to cover all those with the triad of social and language impairments.

In addition to the features mentioned above, various other abnormalities are found (Wing, 1976a). There are likely to be odd responses to sensory stimuli, difficulty in imitating other people's actions, stereotyped movements of limbs and body, and odd posture and gait, disturbances of eating, drinking, and sleeping and of the vestibular system, and disturbed behaviour especially in response to any change in routine. Simple motor and visuospatial abilities and rote memory for verbal material are better than performance on tasks requiring understanding of symbolic ideas.

A variety of organic conditions affecting the CNS can be found in association with autism (Creak, 1963; Lotter, 1967; Rutter, 1970; Chess, 1971; Kolvin et al, 1971; Taft and Cohen, 1971; Folstein and Rutter, 1977; Wing and Gould, 1979).

Approximately 70–80 per cent of autistic children are mildly or severely mentally retarded (Carr, 1976; DeMyer, 1976; Lotter, 1967; Rutter and Lockyer, 1967; Wing and Gould, 1979) and even those of "normal" intelligence show evidence of subtle cognitive defects (Bartak et al, 1975).

Various physical disabilities, such as sensory impairments can occur in autistic children. In adolescents and adults, psychiatric conditions such as depression may complicate the clinical picture. It should also be remembered that autistic people vary in personality as much as the rest of humanity and this affects their reaction to their handicaps.

Medical aspects of management

Diagnosis

There is no evidence for or against the view that early intervention affects the basic impairments underlying autism, but early diagnosis is helpful for the parents. Naming the problem enables them to seek advice from experienced professionals and other parents and from reading and thus to find ways of coping with their child's strange behaviour.

When they consult a doctor they may find it difficult to put their fears into words. Faced with a vague history of an "odd" child, the doctor should never dismiss the parents as overanxious just because the child looks normal. Referral to an appropriate specialist centre should be arranged for a full examination and diagnostic assessment. If the parents make their own diagnosis from a book or from seeing another autistic child, this should be taken seriously since they are likely to be right. Even if the child is severely mentally retarded or has additional physical handicaps, it is worthwhile deciding whether or not he is also autistic because this affects his management and prognosis.

Telling the parents

Giving the parents full details of the diagnosis and explaining the possible causes and the likely prognosis are the basis of good management (Spain and Wigley, 1975). It is generally necessary to go over the same ground many times since most parents find it hard to take in the full implications at first. The experience is painful for them and for the doctor, but in the long term it is better to emphasize the severity of the problems and the likelihood of lifelong handicaps than to give false hopes. In the author's experience parents are happy if the child makes better progress than predicted, but find it hard to bear if their expectations are not fulfilled.

The prognosis is closely related to development of language, sociability, and visuospatial skills. The score, obtained in childhood, on standardized intelligence tests is a useful guide (Rutter, 1970). Only the small proportion with IQs in the normal or borderline normal range are likely to become independent as adults.

Medical treatment (see Corbett, 1976)

Autism is due to dysfunction of the brain produced by a variety of different aetiologies, but there is as yet no treatment for the underlying impairments. A few of the known causes (for example, maternal rubella and untreated phenylketonuria) are potentially preventable. Detection and correction of any associated physical conditions helps to reduce the degree of disability. This may be easier said than done since, for example, hearing and vision are difficult to assess in an uncooperative child. Previous experience with autistic children is particularly important in this situation.

Autistic adolescents with no previous history of epilepsy may have one or two fits and then no more, in which case it is unnecessary and undesirable to give any drug treatment. However, some autistic children or adults have recurrent seizures that do require medication. It is important to monitor the blood levels of the drug in order to control the fits adequately and to guard against overdosage. Both epilepsy and drug intoxication can precipitate or exacerbate behaviour problems (Corbett et al, 1975).

Unless there are visible signs, diagnosis of intercurrent illness can be extremely difficult. Most autistic children cannot describe their symptoms and many resist examination. They may give no indication of pain, even with conditions such as appendicitis or a broken bone. Parents usually become aware of some change in the child's pattern of behaviour which leads them to suspect illness. If the diagnosis cannot be made immediately, the child should be observed until the clinical picture becomes clearer or he reverts to his usual behaviour.

Medical management of behaviour problems

If possible, behaviour problems should be dealt with by appropriate organization of the child's environment and by techniques of behaviour management. These approaches are by no means always successful, either because the care givers do not apply the methods correctly or because the problems are not amenable to environmental manipulation of any kind. In this situation major tranquillizers are often tried. Sometimes the problems are alleviated, but in other cases the results are poor or the improvement is only temporary.

It is difficult to predict who will respond to drugs and which types of medication are likely to be successful (Corbett, 1972, 1976). Autistic people tend to be resistant to sedatives and hypnotics and may show paradoxical responses to barbiturates. If a drug proves ineffective or ceases to be helpful after a time, it should be stopped and another tried. There is a tendency to continue with medication, however useless, just because medical or nursing staff wish to feel that something is being done. This should be strongly resisted. If a drug does prove helpful, the opportunity to improve behaviour management techniques should be taken in the hope that eventually the latter alone will be sufficient.

There may be an exacerbation of behaviour problems in adolescence, which is sometimes related to a superimposed psychiatric illness. The diagnosis has to be made from the history and present behaviour as described by parents, teachers, and caring staff. Appropriate medication, for example antidepressive drugs, may alleviate the problem. A mildly handicapped autistic person with fairly good language development may become depressed as a reaction to his handicaps. Counselling given by someone experienced with autistic people could be helpful in such a case.

Other types of help

The behaviour of autistic children is particularly difficult in a strange place with people they do not know. It makes life much easier for parents and child if special appointments can be made to avoid long waiting times at clinics.

A doctor can use the authority conferred by his professional status to assure the parents that they did not cause their child's handicaps. Unhappily, despite the accumulation of evidence to the contrary (Cox et al, 1975; Wing, 1976b; DeMyer, 1979), it is still possible for parents to be told that their child's problems are due to their methods of child rearing, which does nothing to help but adds greatly to the family's distress (Eberhardy, 1967; Kysar, 1968).

Behaviour management and education

Since autistic people lack an inner world of ideas and rules for living, an external structure has to be provided for them. The techniques of behaviour modification, in which appropriate behaviour is encouraged and inappropriate behaviour is discouraged systematically and consistently, are helpful as long as they are regarded as one among a range of approaches and are applied with sensitivity to the needs of each individual. Some workers, faced with intractable behaviour problems, have used harsh "punishments". It is becoming clear that such methods, as well as being repugnant to most people, do not lead to improvement in the long term, except perhaps in cases where a single or a very few applications rapidly suppress the difficult behaviour. The practical and moral dilemmas posed by using or withholding aversion techniques are explored in a discussion edited by Sullivan (1978).

Considerable skill and experience are needed to devise programmes of behaviour management and teaching, but parents, teachers, and others can apply the methods under the supervision of a trained professional worker. Home-based programmes of management carried out by parents are described by Schopler and Reichler (1971) and Hemsley et al (1978).

Dealing with disturbed behaviour

The methods that have been developed for coping with behaviour problems are described in detail elsewhere (Howlin et al, 1973; Marchant et al, 1974; Hemsley and Howlin, 1976; Hemsley et al, 1978; DeMyer, 1979; Carr, 1980; Wing, 1980a, b). It is only possible to give a brief outline here.

Knowledge of the individual child may allow one to predict the situations that precipitate difficult behaviour, such as screaming or temper tantrums. A programme of carefully graded exposure may help the child eventually to accept such situations with equanimity. If difficult behaviour does occur, it should be ignored or the child should be removed from the scene with as little fuss as possible and not returned until he has calmed down. Buying temporary peace, by for example giving the child a sweet to keep him quiet, should be avoided since it leads to more problems than it solves.

Repetitive activities

Because of the impairment of development of imagination and social interests, autistic people always have some repetitive routines. The aim is to discourage those that are undesirable and to limit the more peculiar ones to the privacy of home rather than public places. Repetitive routines can become the cause of difficult behaviour, since any interference with the usual sequence of events or the loss of a special object may precipitate severe temper tantrums.

It may be possible to forestall the development of special routines (such as always following the same route for a daily walk or carrying some large object everywhere) by deliberately changing the daily activities or by removing unsuitable objects before they become an obsession. If the child has already developed an attachment to something of inconvenient size (for example a large blanket) this can be overcome by cutting a tiny piece off each day until it disappears, or by gradually limiting the time during which the child is allowed to hold it (Hemsley and Howlin, 1976).

Self-injury is rarely seen in more intelligent autistic children, but may occur in those who are severely retarded (Bartak and Rutter, 1976). It is particularly distressing and difficult to manage and is one of the problems for which harsh aversion methods have been used, although with little long-term success (Frankel and Simmons, 1976). If even carefully planned behaviour measures fail, then specially made protective clothing may be necessary. This should be used only during the times when the child cannot be prevented from harming himself by supervision and alternative occupation.

In some cases repetitive activities can be used constructively to help the child learn new skills, either by gradually extending his interests (say from drawing trains to other types of art) or by allowing indulgence in the activity for a brief period as a reward after some more constructive task has been accomplished.

Teaching new skills

Discouraging repetitive behaviour is more likely to be successful if some constructive activities are available to the child. Teaching self-care, practical tasks, language, school work, and leisure activities needs as much planning as does every other aspect of management (Everard, 1976; Jeffree and McConkey, 1976; Jeffree et al, 1977; Schopler et al, 1979; Carr, 1980). The skills to be taught should be appropriate to the child's level of development, so detailed assessment is necessary before teaching begins (Gould, 1976). Failure to generalize is a major problem in autism and therefore home and school should cooperate in the educational endeavour. Lovaas et al (1973) have shown that regression tends to occur unless the teaching and management programmes are consistently maintained.

Since imitation is often poor or absent, it is usually necessary to begin the teaching of practical skills by moving the child's limbs passively through the steps of the tasks so that he experiences the "feel" for himself.

Sometimes autistic children astonish everyone by suddenly acquiring a skill, such as riding a bicycle, apparently without any practice. Others appear to learn better if they overhear the teacher working with another child, rather than when they receive the attention directly. However, when there are major learning problems the tasks can be broken down into very small steps each of which can be mastered easily by the child, so that he is encouraged to progress by a series of successes. This is particularly helpful because many autistic children are highly sensitive to failure (Churchill, 1971).

"Backward chaining", that is teaching the last step in a task and then working in reverse order until the whole task can be completed, is useful for some skills such as dressing.

If the child's impairments prevent the acquisition of a skill, it may be possible to develop compensatory abilities. Approximately half of all autistic children do not learn to speak. In these cases it may be possible to teach an alternative system of expressing simple needs and comprehending instructions, such as manual signs or a set of picture cards, and thus reduce some of the frustration caused by inability to communicate (Deich and Hodges, 1977).

Lessons should, as far as possible, be enjoyed by the child and the atmosphere should be relaxed and peaceful. Some autistic children appear to learn more under pressure and a number of workers believe this to be justified. In the opinion of the author, learning under these conditions tends to be mechanical and meaningless and the strain may exacerbate behaviour problems outside the classroom.

It has to be remembered that even the least handicapped and most able autistic people have lifelong cognitive problems. Unless there is a good chance of achieving independence as an adult or unless the autistic person himself wants to learn, there seems little point in making him acquire more than is practically useful or interesting for him in the sheltered conditions in which he will always live.

Services

Part of the doctor's role is to help in obtaining services and appropriate placements for the child. An outline of the services needed throughout life is given by Wing and Wing (1976). They include advice on management and teaching in the home; nurseries for preschool children; education in specialized schools, schools for children with mixed handicaps, or even normal schools, depending on the needs and abilities of the individual child; sheltered or open employment for adults; provision for leisure activities (most difficult to organize); residential care when appropriate (usually in adult life) in a hostel, sheltered community, or hospital for the mentally handicapped, again depending on the individual concerned.

Some parents try hard to avoid any contact with the services for severe mental handicap. This is understandable since autistic people differ in many ways from those mentally retarded people who are sociable and communicative. However, many autistic people are also severely mentally retarded and are appropriately placed in the mental handicap services. The problem can be resolved only if the staff in these services are trained and have the facilities to help not only sociable retarded people in their care but also those, much harder to understand and manage, who are retarded and have autistic behaviour.

The needs of the family

The needs of the autistic child have to be seen in the context of those of the rest of the family. The medical adviser can encourage the parents to consider the effects of the handicapped child on his normal brothers and sisters and on themselves. Some families manage to cope without undue strain on the parents or children but in other cases there are many problems (see discussion edited by Sullivan, 1979). These may in some instances be alleviated by better methods of behaviour management, but sometimes the solution lies in frequent short-term or permanent long-term care for the autistic child. Residential places are difficult to find and parents need the support of the doctor when trying to make suitable arrangements.

Most parents find great help and comfort in meeting and talking to others who have similar problems. Some find special satisfaction in working to improve provision for their own and other children. The National Society for Autistic Children (1a Golders Green Road, London NW11 8EA) is an organization for parents and professional workers which can put members in touch with each other. It arranges meetings, provides practical advice, and publishes useful literature and a bibliography that includes books by parents describing the experience of bringing up an autistic child (for example, Park, 1968; Lovell, 1978).

References

Bartak, L, Rutter, M (1976) *Journal of Autism and Childhood Schizophrenia*, **6**, 109
—,—, Cox, A (1975) *British Journal of Psychiatry*, **126**, 127
Carr, J (1976) *in* Early Childhood Autism, 2nd edn (edited by Wing, L). Pergamon, Oxford. p.247
—(1980) Helping Your Handicapped Child. Penguin, London
Chess, S (1971) *Journal of Autism and Childhood Schizophrenia*, **1**, 33
Churchill, D W (1971) *Archives of General Psychiatry*, **25**, 208
Corbett, J A (1972) *British Journal of Hospital Medicine*, **8**, 141
—(1976) *in* Early Childhood Autism, 2nd edn (edited by Wing, L). Pergamon, Oxford. p.271
—, Harris, R, Robinson, R G (1975) *in* Mental Retardation and Developmental Disabilities, Vol. 7 (edited by Wortis, J). Brunner and Mazel, New York. p.79
Cox, A, Rutter, M, Newman, S, Bartak, L (1975) *British Journal of Psychiatry*, **126**, 146
Creak, E M (1963) *ibid.* **109**, 84
Deich, R, Hodges, P (1977) Language Without Speech. Souvenir Press, London
DeMyer, M (1976) *in* Early Childhood Autism, 2nd edn (edited by Wing, L). Pergamon, Oxford. p.169
— (1979) Parents and Children in Autism. Winston, Washington
Eberhardy, F (1967) *Journal of Child Psychology and Psychiatry*, **8**, 257
Everard, P (1976) Editor. An Approach to Teaching Autistic Children. Pergamon, Oxford
Folstein, S, Rutter, M (1977) *Journal of Child Psychology and Psychiatry*, **18**, 297
Frankel, F, Simmons, J Q (1976) *American Journal of Mental Deficiency*, **80**, 512
Gould, J (1976) *in* An Approach to Teaching Autistic Children (edited by Everard, P) Pergamon, Oxford. p.31
Hemsley, R, Howlin, P (1976) *in* An Approach to Teaching Autistic Children (edited by Everard, P). Pergamon, Oxford. p.53
—et al (1978) *in* Autism: Reappraisal of Concepts and Treatment (edited by Rutter, M, Schopler, E). Plenum, New York. p.379

Howlin, P, Marchant, R, Rutter, M, Berger, M, Hersov, L, Yule, W (1973) *Journal of Autism and Childhood Schizophrenia*, **4**, 308

Jeffree, D, McConkey, R (1976) Let Me Speak. Souvenir Press, London

—, —, Hewson, S (1977) Let Me Play. Souvenir Press, London

Kanner, L (1943) *Nervous Child*, **2**, 217

Kolvin, I (1971) *British Journal of Psychiatry*, **118**, 381

—, Ounsted, C, Roth, M (1971) *ibid*. **118**, 407

Kysar, J E (1968) *American Journal of Psychiatry*, **125**, 103

Lotter, V (1967) *Social Psychiatry*, **1**, 163

Lovaas, O L, Koegel, R, Simmons, J Q, Long, J S (1973) *Journal of Applied Behavioural Analysis*, **6**, 131

Lovell, A (1978) In a Summer Garment. Secker and Warburg, London

Marchant, R, Howlin, P, Yule, W, Rutter, M L (1974) *Journal of Child Psychology and Psychiatry*, **15**, 221

Park, C C (1968) The Siege. Colin Smythe, Gerrards Cross

Ricks, D M (1975) *in* Language, Cognitive Deficits and Retardation (edited by O'Connor, N) Butterworths, London

—, Wing, L (1975) *Journal of Autism and Childhood Schizophrenia*, **5**, 191

Rutter, M (1970) *Seminars in Psychiatry*, **2**, 435

—, Lockyer, L (1967) *British Journal of Psychiatry*, **113**, 1169

Schaffer, H R (1974) *Bulletin of the British Psychological Society*, **27**, 209

Schopler, E, Reichler, R J (1971) *Journal of Autism and Childhood Schizophrenia*, **1**, 87

—.—, Lansing, M (1979) Individualized Assessment and Treatment for Autistic and Developmentally Disabled Children, Vol. 2: Teaching Strategies for Parents and Professionals. University Park Press, Baltimore

Spain, B, Wigley, G (1975) Editors. Right From the Start. National Society for Mentally Handicapped Children, London

Sullivan, R C (1978) *Journal of Autism and Childhood Schizophrenia*, **8**, 99

—(1979) *Journal of Autism and Developmental Disorders*, **9**, 287

Taft, L T, Cohen, H J (1971) *Journal of Autism and Childhood Schizophrenia*, **1**, 327

Trevarthen, C (1974) *New Scientist*, **62**, 230

Wing, J K, Wing, L (1976) *in* Early Childhood Autism, 2nd edn (edited by Wing, L). Pergamon, Oxford, p.287

Wing, L (1976a) *ibid*. p 15

—(1976b) *ibid*. p.65

—(1980a) Autistic Children: a Guide for Parents, 3rd edn. Constable, London

—(1980b) Children Apart. National Society for Autistic Children, London

—, Gould, J (1979) *Journal of Autism and Developmental Disorders*, **9**, 11

Chapter 25

Stress, personality, and coronary artery disease

Martin H Davies, Midland Nerve Hospital, Birmingham

Arteriosclerotic heart disease is now one of the major causes of death and disability, especially in males of 45–64 years. In 1950 it represented about 20 per cent of the total male mortality rate. By 1973 this had risen to 30–40 per cent (Clayton et al, 1977). This is not only a relative change due to the decline of other causes of death, but also an absolute change in the majority of nations including the UK. But what is most striking is that the trend varies from country to country for reasons that are not yet fully apparent. The WHO Statistical Annual (1968–79) shows how the mortality rate from heart disease has changed, rising steeply in Finland and less steeply in other European countries, while falling in the USA from the highest level in the world in 1950 to one which in 1978 was approaching that of the UK. Japan has moved from a low level to an even lower one, although as we shall see below this is not true of Japanese living abroad.

The aetiology of cardiovascular disease is complex and those causative factors that appear to have been identified are not of proven relevance to these changes in mortality rate. It has been argued that the decline in coronary artery disease in the USA in recent years is a consequence of such changes in behaviour as altered diet, diminished cigarette smoking, increased physical activity, and earlier treatment of high blood pressure. Nevertheless, there is no clear-cut evidence that any of these factors has made a measurable contribution to this trend (*Lancet*, 1980).

The role of social or psychological factors is therefore one that deserves at least to be considered. The evidence generally indicates that such influences are important, but it is less clear how important and even less clear whether they can be ameliorated by the action of public health programmes or other medical measures. This evidence comes from several sources of enquiry and may be reviewed under the following headings:

Who? What kind of person might be predisposed to develop coronary artery disease?

When? Do life events and other environmental changes influence the onset of myocardial infarction?

Where? Do different social and cultural systems affect its incidence?

How? What are the postulated psychological and physiological mechanisms that might mediate these influences?

Why? Can we deduce a general theory of sociosomatic interaction based upon these mechanisms?

Personality and coronary artery disease

The concept of the "coronary personality" has been with us for many years. It was first propounded in the 1930s and 1940s by both Franz Alexander and Helen Flanders Dunbar. The influence of the psychoanalytical model of personality, especially the emphasis on repressed emotion, is evident in their approach. Each psychosomatic disease is seen to represent a particular style of behaviour in which unventilated affect takes its toll of the appropriate physiological system. These writers and their co-workers devised profiles of personality from the observation of large numbers of patients suffering from conditions such as asthma, peptic ulcer, and migraine.

In the case of coronary artery disease the following description (Dunbar, 1959) is fairly typical of their findings. The coronary personality exhibits a tendency towards considered consistent action and seizure of authority. This is to be contrasted with the accident-prone who act impulsively and avoid authority. The coronary personality plans his career, sticks to one job, works long hours, and attaches emotions to ideas and goals. Although he uses conversation as an instrument of domination he is extremely articulate about his feelings, establishes interpersonal relationships easily, and is rarely bored. He suppresses and restrains his inner feelings and imagination instead of acting them out. He has considerable trouble with his hostility but diverts it into a course of action that will ultimately place him in a position of dominance. He has an extremely positive self-picture.

In the last three decades this view has become less acceptable (Stonehill, 1980). More rigorous research conditions have indicated that the associations between personality types and physical disease are less clear when subjects are unselected and the methods of observation more objective. In other words biased selections and foreknowledge of the patient's personality status contributed to the kind of stereotype described above. Also, while stress may be important, the specificity of the organs affected seems to be due more to the inherited constitution of the individual than to the constellation of personality features that characterize him. The kind of frustrated emotional needs that may be associated with peptic ulceration in one person may be observed in another with migraine or asthma. Moreover the same characteristic of personality may be exhibited in varying degrees and observed in individuals who do not succumb to any of the diseases that are traditionally labelled as psychosomatic.

So it is of particular interest that coronary artery disease has been an exception to this debunking trend (Friedman and Rosenman, 1959). If we look at Dunbar's (1959) coronary personality we see that he is striving, ambitious, and authority seeking. Friedman and Rosenman recognized in their coronary patients competitiveness and an intense striving for achievement. Dunbar's coronary personality is said to be hard-working. Friedman and Rosenman described an overcommitment to work. They also found a profound sense of time urgency, impatience, and hostility. Dunbar's description does refer to these more aggressive social characteristics but sees them as being suppressed or diverted into a socially acceptable competition.

Friedman and Rosenman's (1959) initial findings were obtained retrospectively by structured interviewing but it was not long before a standardized 61-item questionnaire was developed (Jenkins et al, 1967) and both these methods of assessing the "type A behaviour pattern" as it is described have since been widely applied. The Jenkins activity survey has in fact made it possible to study very large numbers of patients. During the 1960s and early 1970s further work appeared to confirm Friedman and Rosenman's original observations. For example, 62 middle-aged male survivors of an initial myocardial infarction were compared with 109 male subjects without coronary artery disease (Theorell and Rahe, 1972). The myocardial infarction patients admitted that during the previous year they had worked more hours overtime, obtained less satisfaction from their jobs, and felt greater hostility when slowed down by others than did the control subjects. The controls registered not only more responsibilities and more supervision of others at work but also more time for physical and social activity outside work.

Other researchers have attempted to compare patients from different cultures, for example Finnish, Swedish and American patients suffering from myocardial infarction (Romo et al, 1974). It seemed that the postmyocardial infarction subjects in all groups tended to take more responsibility at work, do more overtime, have a greater sense of time urgency, exhibit more hostility when delayed, and feel more dissatisfaction with their educational level and achievement of life goals. However, there were differences between the patients from the three countries, the Finns scoring relatively low on work behaviour and time urgency but high on life dissatisfaction and the Americans scoring higher on work behaviour.

Prospective studies have also tended to confirm Friedman and Rosenman's (1959) findings, for example a prospective study of 10 years duration in which 65 patients who had suffered from myocardial infarction and 65 controls were interviewed and then followed up (Bruhn et al, 1974). These authors described what they called a Sisyphus pattern of behaviour—"striving without sense of satisfaction or fulfillment" like the legendary Greek giant who was forced by the gods whom he had offended to push a large stone up a hill, but the next day he always found that it had rolled back to where it had started. In fact there was an excess mortality rate from heart disease for those subjects in the myocardial group showing the Sisyphus pattern and extreme type A behaviour with which it appeared to be correlated. Depression was also correlated with the mortality rate although the two deaths by suicide in the group were not predicted.

Finally, the association of the type A behaviour pattern has also been confirmed in two large epidemiological studies of coronary artery disease: the Western Collaborative Group Study and the Framingham Heart Study, both in the USA.

The Western Collaborative Group Study began in 1960–61 when over 3000 men aged 29–59 years employed by 10 Californian companies were examined and subjected to an 8–9-year follow-up (Jenkins et al, 1971; Rosenman et al, 1975). During this period there were 257 cases of coronary artery disease, 140 deaths (31 of which were due to coronary artery disease), and 19 recurring coronary artery disease events. In the personality assessments obtained by the Jenkins activity survey, which were associated with a higher than expected incidence of coronary artery disease, the significant features were enhanced aggressiveness, ambitiousness, and competitive drive and a chronic sense of time urgency. Other relevant factors including parental history of coronary artery disease, reported history of diabetes, a lower level of education, cigarette smoking, high blood pressure, and high levels of serum lipids did not have any association with these personality features. In a subsequent analysis of these data (Jenkins et al, 1974) the type A behaviour score was found to be significantly greater in patients experiencing recurrent episodes of coronary artery disease than in those suffering a single episode.

The Framingham Heart Study was even more comprehensive including over 5000 subjects, both male and female, initially free of any manifestation of coronary artery disease who were followed-up biennially from 1949 onwards. The investigators designed an extensive life-history questionnaire of 300 items covering five areas of psychosocial stress and strain, and somatic stress (Haynes et al, 1978). This involved a 45-minute interview and answers were either dichotomous (yes or no) or Likert-type (four-point scale). The Framingham type A score correlated with other scales especially ambitiousness ($r=0.31$), emotional lability ($r=0.43$), tension ($r=0.42$), daily stress ($r=0.47$), anger symptoms ($r=0.34$), and marital dissatisfaction and disagreement ($r=0.44$).

The prevalence of coronary artery disease in 1822 subjects of 45–77 years in the eighth to ninth round of examination during 1965–67 appeared to correlate with psychosocial findings as follows: in men and women aged over 65 with marital dissatisfaction and disagreement; in women aged 45–64 with type A behaviour, emotional lability, ageing worries, tension, and anger; and in men aged 45–64 with type A behaviour, ageing worries, daily stress, and tension. (These findings were controlled for age, blood pressure, serum cholesterol, and smoking.)

So these two large-scale studies do seem to confirm the importance of certain psychosocial characteristics closely resembling those originally described by Dunbar (1959). It cannot be claimed for certain that the relationship is causal or that a differential mortality rate prior to the survey might not have been important. But there is no specific evidence in favour of these criticisms.

One other approach used to confirm the significance of type A personality has been to compare it directly with the degree of coronary artery narrowing measured by angiography. However, findings have not been consistent. In one study (Krantz et al, 1979) the investigation was repeated at an average interval of 17 months and showed a definite although not statistically significant deterioration positively related to the type A behaviour pattern. In another study (Blumenthal et al, 1978) the extent of coronary artery occlusion was assessed on a single occasion and found to be significantly correlated with type A personality independently evaluated by a structured interview in 156 consecutive referrals. However, a third study failed to confirm these results (Dimsdale et al, 1979).

Influence of life events

Do life events precipitate acute episodes of coronary vascular disease? There is a considerable research literature concerning the association of life events and physical illness. This suggests that life changes that deprive individuals of important sources of emotional security, self-esteem, or sense of identity are likely to be followed by a higher than normal risk of various kinds of disease. In the case of cardiovascular disease it has been found, for example, that widows suffer an above average mortality rate in the first 5 years after bereavement and much of this is accounted for by cardiovascular disease (Parkes et al, 1969). Fifty men of 40–60 years who had recently suffered a heart attack were compared with a matched control group and showed a significantly higher incidence of divorce and a tendency to report more frequent loss of close friends (Thiel et al, 1973). Other studies have suggested that heart disease is common in those who have emigrated, although this may be less in the first generation especially if they live among fellow countrymen and retain their cultural patterns (Medalie and Kahn, 1973).

Social and cultural factors

The question "Where does the disorder occur?" is probably inseparable from the question "When does it occur?". Stress is a complex interaction, often with a largely symbolic significance, between those factors that make the individual's social environemnt less secure and predictable and those that provide him with courses of action by which to maintain or regain his threatened sense of personal significance and capacity to control his destiny. The stressful event may itself act largely by removing a significant social support but if it is a fairly common occurrence, bereavement for example, the social network may respond to the sufferer's need by encouraging him to play out his grief and loss in such a way that he obtains a kind of meaning and even value from the situation which diminishes his previous sources of security and gratification.

In fact "When?" and "Where?" are also tied to "Who?" since the coronary-prone personality may indeed be a factor in determining what constitutes a stressful event. Students with a high type A score reported more life events than those with the opposite personality features (Suls et al, 1979). Moreover, on closer examination it appeared that type A students were particularly disturbed by events that they saw as undesirable, unexpected, or ambiguous in terms of their perceived control over them. Type B students became less distressed the more they perceived the events as out of their personal control. This implies that the type A individual's need to control makes it more difficult for him to fall back on external support even when this is clearly desirable and available.

But to return to the question "Where?" One of the more impressive reports of social influences is that of the Human Population Laboratory survey of a random sample of 7000 adults aged 20 years or over in a single county of California during a 9-year follow-up period beginning in 1965 (Berkman and Syme, 1979). Four sources of social contact were examined: marriage, contact with close friends, church membership, and informal and formal group associations. Mortality rate was clearly related to the total quantity of social support. Intimate contact had greater weight in this connection than less intimate (that is marriage partners and close friends more than church or group affiliations). For example, marriage plus a few friends was equivalent to many friends or to several relatives and several friends. Some of the excess mortality rate could be accounted for by emotionally mediated behaviour (for example suicide or accident) but there was also a contribution by heart disease and cancer.

An investigation invoking cultural factors sought to explain the gradient of incidence of coronary artery disease in Japanese males—lowest in Japan, highest in Japanese domiciled in California, and intermediate in those living in Hawaii (Marmot and Syme, 1976). Differences of diet, serum cholesterol level, blood pressure, and cigarette smoking apparently accounted for only part of the variation. Accordingly these authors classified a large sample of Japanese men living in California in terms of the degree to which they retained their traditional Japanese culture. Those most acculturated to the West had a three to five times higher prevalence of coronary artery disease than the least acculturated. This seemed to support the suggestion that in a stable society members enjoy the benefit of fellowship in a close-knit group and may be relatively protected against the forms of social strain that lead to coronary artery disease. The same kind of comparison has been suggested as between say Greece, Italy and Yugoslavia, with their cohesive family and village groups, and the countries of northwestern Europe where society is more unstable and individualistic.

This evidence strongly indicates that a combination of habitual patterns of social interaction, specific traumatic experiences, and a relative lack of social relationships of a supportive kind can trigger or contribute to physiological processes leading to heart disease. What are these processes? Or in terms of our original questions, "How does it come about?".

Mediating mechanisms

The trail begins in the 1930s with the physiologist Walter Cannon who pioneered the study of the adrenomedullary response to stress. More recently researchers have again become interested in the physiological changes occurring in real-life stress, for instance parachute jumping, motor racing, and public speaking (Carruthers, 1975). In tense competitive situations—not only motor racing but also ordinary traffic conditions—there are measurable rises in plasma noradrenaline level, blood pressure, and plasma lipid levels. There appears to be a linear relationship between the rapid rise of free fatty acids and the level of noradrenaline until a plateau of lipids is reached at a catecholamine level of about 2 µg/litre (Taggart and Carruthers, 1971).

Exercise appears to counteract these changes, which may affect the heart in two ways. First, the repeatedly raised levels of blood lipids may dispose to the development of atheroma and, secondly, the high level of sympathetic arousal may actually render the coronary circulation and cardiac metabolism less efficient, precipitating angina or even infarction. Animal studies support at least the first of these mechanisms. In one experiment the stress took the form of electric shocks applied to the animals' feet for 35 minutes every day (Bassett and Cairncross, 1977). At postmortem the experimental rats showed junctional gaps in the endothelium, large lipid-filled vacuoles in the arterial walls, and aggregation of platelets in the coronary system. Direct stimulation of the lateral hypothalamus leads to similar results (Gutstein et al, 1978).

Do type A patients respond with greater noradrenaline release to stress? The answer is probably "yes". In 15 men with high type A scores and 15 with opposite characteristics, plasma noradrenaline and adrenaline were assayed under resting conditions before, during and after a nonphysical competitive struggle (Friedman et al, 1975). The average catecholamine levels were similar in both groups under resting conditions but during competition the level rose much higher in the type A subjects.

Discussion

If these observations are confirmed, what conclusions can be drawn? The coronary profile behaviour pattern seems to be a valid phenomenon and may even be of greater significance in determining the incidence of heart disease than the other known risk factors. The behaviour is probably mediated by the sympathetic nervous system which may vary in its tendency to produce high levels of lipids and catecholamines even in individuals of similar temperament. The behaviour itself is, if not socially determined, at least socially modulated as the cross-cultural and other studies indicate.

Totman (1979) in his book *Social Causes of Illness* has argued that the important stressful quality of life events is best understood in terms of a model of behaviour of the following kind which he calls a "structural" theory. He suggests that individuals interpret the significance of their social environment by a set of rules which in turn prescribe their own behaviour. Their responses lead to social consequences which serve to validate the implicit rules that are used to determine what is expected of them in the given social setting. Consequently the disruptive impact of stressful change represents the failure of the affected person to continue to respond in roles that elicit validating and reassuring reaction from others. Totman calls this process the "testing of committed actions against rules". In short, purposeful activity demands a set of predictable responses.

The failure of such a system may occur in several ways. First, the rules themselves may be so severe and inflexible that they inhibit or restrict the satisfaction of biologically based needs or demand a performance beyond the biological limitations of the organism. This might well be another way of interpreting type A behaviour or the Sisyphus pattern. Secondly, there may be abrupt changes in the social environment in which familiar rules cease to operate and/or new rules are difficult to assimilate. Thirdly, the individual may be separated from a reference group (for example in bereavement, separation, or moving home) or the rules themselves may be undermined.

These ideas are not wholly new, and structural theory has some conceptual as well as verbal echoes in Kelly's personal construct theory. It does not explain why vegetative function is impaired, although Totman (1979) argues that if social involvement has important evolutionary survival value then the social isolate is of less biological use to the species and psychosomatic disease may be a kind of self-destructive mechanism. Before this hypothesis can be turned to practical use in a clinical setting there are certain crucial tests still to be performed. Further well designed large-scale studies are required as suggested by Jenkins (1976). However, intervention studies are already under way (Friedman, 1979). Studies of twins suggest that type A behaviour is learned rather than inherited (Rahe et al, 1978). Brief group therapy has already been attempted and initial results show reduced coronary morbidity and mortality rates after 4 years (Rahe et al, 1979). But the resistance of many such patients to therapy suggests that the behavioural character-istics may be deep-rooted (Friedman, 1979).

Can we identify type A individuals earlier in their lives and carry out a prophylactic trial? This would appear a difficult enterprise to organize because of a likely lack of motivation in young apparently healthy people. However, in California a group approach to teaching behaviour change to individuals already afflicted with coronary artery disease seems to be catching the enthusiasm of the public, especially as it offers support in the arduous task of altering long-standing habits (Friedman, 1980) and also provides practical advice about other risk factors in the precipitation of the coronary infarct. In Quebec a programme of behaviour modification for managers with type A features has been shown to lead to measurable changes which persist 6 months after completion of treatment. Moreover, as predicted, motivated subjects with clinical evidence of coronary artery disease showed significantly greater changes than those without such a history and all subjects exhibited a lowering of serum cholesterol levels (Roskies et al, 1979).

A prophylactic programme does seem to show promise and its long-term value should be more clearly determined in the next 10 years as more behaviour training becomes available and the effect on recurrence of myocardial infarction is assessed in larger numbers of subjects.

References

Bassett, J R, Cairncross, K D (1977) *Pharmacology, Biochemistry and Behaviour*, **6**, 311
Berkman, L F, Syme, S L (1979) *American Journal of Epidemiology*, **109**, 186

Blumenthal, J A, Williams, R B, Kong, Y, Schanberg, S M, Thompson, L W (1978) *Circulation*, **58**, 634

Bruhn, J G, Paredes, A, Absett, C A, Wolf, S (1974) *Journal of Psychosomatic Research*, **18**, 187

Carruthers, M (1975) *Proceedings of the Royal Society of Medicine*, **68**, 429

Clayton, D G, Taylor, D, Shaper, A G (1977) Health Treands, Vol. 9. DHSS Welsh Office, London. p.1

Dimsdale, J E, Hackett, T P, Catanzano, D M, White, P J (1979) *Journal of Psychosomatic Research*, **23**, 289

Dunbar, H F (1959) Psychiatry in the Medical Specialties. McGraw-Hill, New York

Friedman, M (1979) *American Heart Journal*, **97**, 551

—(1980) personal communication

—, Rosenman, R H (1959) *Journal of the American Medical Association*, **169**, 1286

—, Byers, S O, Diamant, J, Rosenman, R H (1975) *Metabolism*, **24**, 205

Gutstein, W H, Harrison, J, Parl, F, Kiu, G. Avitable, M (1978) *Science*, **199**, 449

Haynes, S G, Levine, S, Scotch, N, Feinleib, M, Kannel, W P. (1978) *American Journal of Epidemiology*, **107**, 362

Jenkins, C D (1976) *New England Journal of Medicine*, **294**, 987

—, Rosenman, R H, Friedman, M (1967) *Journal of Chronic Diseases*, **20**, 371

—, Zyzanski, S J, Rosenman, R H (1971) *Psychosomatic Medicine*, **33**, 193

—, Rosenman, R H, Zyzanski, S J (1974) *New England Journal of Medicine*, **290**, 1271

—, Zyzanski, S J, Rosenman, R H (1976) *Circulation*, **53**, 342

Krantz, D S, Sanmarco, M I, Selvester, R H, Matthews, K A (1979) *Psychosomatic Medicine*, **41**, 467

Lancet (1980) i, 183

Marmot, M G, Syme, S L (1976) *American Journal of Epidemiology*, **104**, 225

Medalie, J H, Kahn, H A (1973) *Journal of Chronic Diseases*, **26**, 63

Parkes, C M, Benjamin, B, Fitzgerald, R G (1969) *British Medical Journal*, i, 740

Rahe, R H, Hervig, L, Rosenman, R H (1978) *Psychosomatic Medicine*, **40**, 478

—, Ward, H W, Hayes, V (1979) *ibid.* **41**, 229

Romo, M, Siltanen, P, Theorell, T, Rahe, R H (1974) *Journal of Psychosomatic Research*, **18**, 1

Rosenman, R H, Brand, R J, Jenkins, C D, Friedman, M, Straus, R, Wurm, M (1975) *Journal of the American Medical Association*, **233**, 872

Roskies, E, Kearney, H, Spevack, M, Surkis, A, Cohen, C, Gilman, S (1979) *Journal of Behavioural Medicine*, **2**, 195

Stonehill, E (1980) *British Journal of Psychiatry*, **136**, 302

Suls, J. Gastorf, J W, Witenberg, S H (1979) *Journal of Psychosomatic Research*, **23**, 315

Taggart, P, Carruthers, M (1971) *Lancet*, i, 363

Theorell, T, Rahe, R H (1972) *Journal of Chronic Diseases*, **25**, 139

Thiel, H G, Parker, D, Bruce, T A (1973) *Journal of Psychosomatic Research*, **17**, 43

Totman, R (1979) Social Causes of Illness, Souvenir Press, London

WHO Statistical Annual (1968–79) World Health Organisation, Geneva

Chapter 26

Management of the acutely disturbed patient on the general ward

Jeremy M Pfeffer, The London Hospital

Patients are individuals with unique backgrounds, experiences and personalities who react differently to illnesses and hospitals (Chesser, 1975) and exhibit a wide range of behaviour on the ward. However, few are actually considered to be disturbed and this is related to variables in the patient himself, in the staff looking after him, and in the treatment setting. Disturbed behaviour can be defined as behaviour that is disturbing to others, particularly the patient's doctor and nurses (Meyer and Mendelson, 1961). It not only affects the treatment of the patient's underlying physical illness but also, by jeopardizing the smooth running of the ward, interferes with the care of the other patients. Management must therefore be rapid and effective, and involve the patient, the staff, and the treatment setting (Tonge, 1975).

Disturbed behaviour can take many forms including verbal and physical aggression aimed at others or self-directed, acting in a bizarre or confused manner, making excessive demands, and showing extreme levels of emotion particularly anxiety and unhappiness. This may be caused by a circumscribed psychiatric illness, a personality disorder, an understandable reaction to a severe stress, or a combination of these and it is further affected by the way in which staff and other patients cope with it.

The first stage in the treatment involves making an assessment of the underlying cause which necessitates taking a history from the patient, staff, and other relevant people including spouse, family, and GP and examining the patient's physical and mental state. Even if he is unwilling or unable to cooperate in this process or his behaviour demands urgent action to defuse a crisis it is rarely impossible to arrive at a hypothesis upon which you can act. A relatively short time spent with a disturbed patient usually gives enough information to enable you to carry out emergency treatment if it is still necessary after the interview. This is often, although not invariably, in the form of sedation which while relieving the acute behaviour disturbance need not preclude further assessment in order to arrive at an adequate formulation.

The following psychiatric conditions are most likely to underlie disturbed behaviour.

240

Toxic confusional and delirious states

Patients present with an acute onset of clouding of consciousness, with confusion, impairment of attention, grasp, memory and concentration, and disorientation particularly in time and place. They are often perplexed, frightened, and restless, with perceptual disturbances including illusions and hallucinations (commonly visual but also auditory and tactile), and paranoid ideas or delusions which may be centred around other patients or staff. The clinical picture characteristically shows a fluctuating pattern with periods of lucidity and deterioration at night-time due to tiredness and the absence of familiar cues as a result of darkness.

Such a condition is organic in origin, being due to disturbance of cerebral function either following a local insult or secondary to a systemic disorder. It may be caused by failure of any of the vital organ systems (cardiac, respiratory, renal, or hepatic), poisoning by or withdrawal of drugs, nutritional deficiency, endocrine and other metabolic disorders, and severe infections (Kiloh, 1977). It may occur postoperatively particularly following open-heart surgery (*British Medical Journal*, 1974) or may be the presenting feature of a silent myocardial infarct or broncho-pneumonia (Hore, 1972). It is especially likely to occur at ages when the brain is most vulnerable, namely in the very young or very old and in the latter it may be superimposed on an underlying dementia. One common and often preventable cause of a confusional state is delirium tremens following alcohol withdrawal which is discussed more fully below.

The diagnosis is not difficult given the characteristic clinical picture but where doubts arise an EEG is almost always abnormal with prominent slow activity (Roth and Meyers, 1969). Treatment is two-pronged, aimed first at resolving the underlying condition which must be exhaustively sought and secondly at relieving as far as possible the symptoms themselves by both general nursing and specific pharmacological measures.

The patient should be nursed in a side room with a night-light by the same nurse or nurses in order to limit the number of unfamiliar people he is faced by. To this end where necessary and feasible the aid of the family or close friends should be enlisted. He should be handled as gently as possible to avoid increasing any paranoid delusions he may have. During lucid moments when the patient is most approachable time should be spent talking to him to help relieve the considerable anxiety that confusional states engender.

Sedation

Whatever the cause of the disturbed behaviour, if pharmacological sedation is required the general principles remain the same. They are discussed in detail here and any differences to the following regimen mentioned where appropriate. Sedative drugs should only be given when necessary because they may mask important physical and mental signs. However, where they are needed doses must be adequate and tailored to the individual's clinical state with higher doses being given when he is most likely to be disturbed, for example at night. Drugs should be given orally where possible since injections not only are likely to be difficult to administer to an agitated paranoid patient but also may add to his delusions of persecution. Syrup may be more acceptable than tablets and makes it easier to ensure that he has actually taken his medication.

Where oral medicine is refused or where speed of action is essential parenteral drugs should be given. If the patient is likely to resist this then sufficient members of staff should be present to avoid any injury to patients or staff, although their mere presence may induce the patient to have his injection willingly and quietly. The drugs of choice are phenothiazine derivatives such as chlorpromazine and the butyrophenones such as haloperidol. Doses vary from patient to patient but chlorpromazine 100 mg orally or haloperidol 5–10 mg orally every 4–6 hours normally gives control within 24 hours. In the severely disturbed patient rapid control can be achieved within a few hours by the use of chlorpromazine 100–200 mg intramuscularly or 50 mg intravenously 4-hourly (Crammer et al, 1978) or haloperidol 2.5–10 mg intramuscularly at intervals of 30–60 minutes where patients usually settle on one to four injections (Donlon et al, 1979). As control is achieved oral drugs should be gradually substituted and the dose reduced when clinical improvement occurs as indicated by the patient's behaviour and examination of the mental state. In patients with acute confusional states this occurs after a shorter period of time than in those with the functional psychoses and it is usually possible to reduce the drug doses rapidly after 24 hours and to stop them within 2–3 days.

Alcohol-related confusional states

Many of the patients admitted to the general ward have drinking problems (Jarman and Kellett, 1979) but this is frequently missed partly due to failure to take an adequate drinking history (Barrison et al, 1980). Unfortunately, with such patients the first time that alcohol dependence is suspected is soon after admission to hospital when they develop delirium tremens, an illness that with adequate cover of alcohol withdrawal is largely preventable. It develops about 3–4 days after drinking stops and may be preceded by less serious withdrawal symptoms such as tremor, irritability and anxiety, nausea, vomiting, and insomnia and also by grand mal fits. The clinical picture is that of a confusional state with hallucinations and associated tremor. When untreated it has a very considerable mortality rate of 15–30 per cent (Rix, 1978).

Management (Edwards, 1967) includes the general nursing measures mentioned above. In addition attention must be paid to the physical state, searching for coexisting medical complications such as infection and keeping a careful watch on fluid, electrolyte and carbohydrate balance, temperature, and blood pressure with immediate treatment of circulatory collapse. Chlormethiazole in doses up to 2 g four times a day and chlordiazepoxide up to 100 mg four times a day, both orally in reducing regimens over 7–9 days, are the most effective and least toxic sedatives. If parenteral sedation is needed chlormethiazole can be given as an intravenous infusion but chlordiazepoxide cannot easily be administered parenterally and if a rapid response is required intravenous diazepam is more suitable. Paraldehyde is also effective but it is a more noxious drug. The phenothiazines should not be used because they may increase the risk of epileptic seizures, are more dangerous in the presence of associated liver disease (*British Medical Journal*, 1977), and are possibly less likely to be effective since they exhibit no cross-tolerance with alcohol. Vitamin supplements are only indicated in the presence of nutritional deficiency or if the Wernicke–Korsakoff syndrome is suspected.

The Wernicke–Korsakoff syndrome (*British Medical Journal*, 1979) is usually alcohol-related and due to diet-induced thiamine deficiency. Wernicke's encephalopathy is acute, subacute or chronic in onset and presents with a confusional state, ophthalmoplegia with diplopia and nystagmus, and ataxia and is associated with Korsakoff's psychosis involving marked impairment of short-term memory and confabulation. If diagnosed early and treated energetically with intravenous thiamine and parenteral injections of B vitamins the condition is often reversible.

Other psychoses

These include schizophrenia (acute and chronic), the affective psychoses (most commonly depression but occasionally mania or hypomania), and the paranoid psychoses. As opposed to patients with confusional states these psychoses classically occur in clear consciousness. They present on the general wards for three main reasons (Crown, 1972; Cutting, 1980) as follows:

1. A physical illness is present unrelated to the psychiatric illness for which the patient is currently receiving treatment
2. A physical illness occurs secondary to the psychosis or its treatment as in self-neglect in hypomania, attempted suicide in the depressed patient, or the schizophrenic who jumps off a roof to get away from his persecutory voices
3. The patient develops a symptomatic psychosis secondary to a physical illness. This is usually associated with organic features as in the toxic confusional states (see above) although it may also occur in the absence of cerebral dysfunction especially in psychosocially vulnerable individuals.

The major symptoms of schizophrenia and the paranoid states likely to lead to disturbed behaviour are paranoid delusions and associated symptoms, especially when centring on the ward staff and patients. These may lead not only to noncompliance in treatment but also to the patient becoming aggressive and violent, which may occur too in the overactive and excitable patient with hypomania. In both cases management consists of adequate sedation (see above), an attempt to establish rapport with the patient, and treatment of the underlying cause in the secondary symptomatic psychoses. When the acute situation has settled care must be directed to the ongoing treatment of the psychiatric illness itself. In some paranoid patients transfer to another medical ward may defuse the situation.

Depressive illness

Severe depression may lead to acute difficulties when the patient becomes agitated or retarded, sometimes to the point of stupor, or when he is considered to be an active suicide risk. The main symptoms are a severely depressed mood, worse in the morning, with depressive ideas sometimes delusional in intensity and associated with depressive auditory hallucinations. The classic biological symptoms of depressive illness—appetite disturbance with weight loss, sleep disturbance characterized by early morning waking, and loss of libido—may be difficult to interpret in the presence of associated physical illness. The patient should be allowed to ventilate his feelings and any reactive elements dealt with where possible. The depressive illness itself should be treated with antidepressants (Dowson, 1980) or, in the presence of delusions or hallucinations or if time is of the essence, ECT should be given. In the symptomatic psychoses the underlying cause should be found and treated. In all depressed patients suicidal ideation must be actively sought and the patient managed accordingly. Although the suicide rate has dropped since the war the number of patients admitted to hospital following an episode of deliberate self-harm—most commonly an overdose of drugs—has risen dramatically to epidemic proportions. These patients often arouse hostility in the ward staff (Patel, 1975), partly because of the self-induced nature of the "illness" and partly because of anxiety that the act might be repeated on the ward. There is a greatly increased risk of subsequent similar acts (Farmer, 1980) which may be fatal and it is thus extremely important to assess each individual properly (Davison, 1975). At present the onus for this lies with the psychiatrist (Ministry of Health, 1961, 1968) but current research suggests that others, for example physicians (Gardner et al, 1977, 1978), nurses (Hawton et al, 1979), and social workers (Newson-Smith and Hirsch, 1979), are just as capable of such assessment. This takes into account the act itself, its cause, and the planning that went into it including the means taken to avoid detection, any remaining suicidal intent, the presence of a psychiatric illness especially severe depression or of drinking problems, and the adequacy of the social support system. The patients most at risk from further fatal acts are the severely depressed, heavy drinkers, and the socially isolated especially middle-aged and elderly men (Kreitman, 1973).

Emergency management of the suicidal patient

If the patient is considered to be a high suicide risk and is suffering from a psychiatric illness he should be detained in hospital, if necessary against his wishes by putting him on a Section (see below). He should be kept under special observation around the clock preferably by a nurse with some psychiatric experience and unless his physical state prevents it this should be on a psychiatric ward. It is often helpful to sedate the patient while treating the underlying cause. The patient with severe personality difficulties often associated with heavy drinking and numerous previous acts of deliberate self-harm without any added circumscribed psychiatric illness provides one of the biggest management problems in this area. He may well be a major suicide risk but is rarely helped by inpatient treatment and few psychiatrists would consider him compulsorily detainable in hospital. It is usually necessary to tell him that he is not mentally ill but is fully responsible for his actions and that although you will try to help where possible it is ultimately his own decision as to what he does with his future.

Anxiety state

These patients often present with somatic symptoms such as palpitations, breathlessness, chest pain, paraesthesia, headache, and light-headedness which may lead to admission to a general ward for investigation. While on the ward they may have acute panic attacks with hyperventilation and many of the above symptoms. The acute state is treated by trying to relax the patient verbally or if necessary by sedation, for example diazepam intravenously. Rebreathing from a paper bag relieves the symptoms of hyperventilation. When the acute situation has subsided it is important to look into its cause. Some patients are anxious to the point of refusal about having blood taken, being given injections, or being examined. This may resolve with a sympathetic reassuring approach but if not a behavioural approach by a psychologist or psychiatrist may be useful (Lloyd and Deakin, 1975).

Hysteria (Reed, 1971; Kendell, 1974; Granville-Grossman, 1975)

Patients may be admitted with motor or sensory disturbances or disorders of memory, consciousness, or intellect which cannot be explained, on either examination or investigation, by any known organic disorder. They are often diagnosed as suffering from hysteria but this label should not be attached loosely and should only be used in the presence of positive signs of hysteria. It is important to demonstrate the existence of emotional stress prior to the onset of the illness to which it can be seen as being a reaction and it is helpful if the patient can be shown to have something to gain from his symptoms.

A useful pointer in the past history is a previous hysterical reaction to stress. Although patients with hysteria were classically said to exhibit "belle indifference", that is a lack of concern about their disabilities or the prospects of recovery, it has been shown that the vast majority are highly anxious both subjectively and objectively. Treatment is usually psychotherapeutic in nature and is aimed at resolving the underlying psychological problems, but it may also be directed at the symptoms themselves using a behavioural approach (Bird, 1979).

Affective reaction to hospital or illness

People react differently to the very real stresses of being ill and in hospital. They may become tearful and miserable and appear to have lost the will to get better or they may become anxious and fearful of investigations and treatment leading to lack of cooperation. Although understandable this often creates a feeling of hopelessness and impotence associated with anger in the staff looking after them. Help should be directed at improving communication between staff and patients, allowing them to air their feelings. In these cases it may be beneficial for an independent person such as a psychiatrist to be involved to help both parties and is particularly useful in wards where death occurs frequently.

Personality disorder

Some patients, especially those with a history of drug or alcohol abuse, may be intolerant of even minor frustrations such as not getting the nurse's attention immediately they ring for it and can become aggressive and violent. They may act impulsively and sometimes manipulate the staff, setting one off against the other. As this will obviously be disruptive it is important that the staff act consistently and set limits for the patient, if necessary with the aid of a psychiatrist (Murphy and Guze, 1960; Hackett, 1978).

The violent patient (*British Medical Journal*, 1978; Egdell, 1980)

If a patient suddenly becomes violent on the ward it is important that no member of staff is left alone with him. The staff should gather in adequate numbers as quickly as possible. They must remain calm, collected and reassuring throughout since the patient is often terrified that the situation has got out of control. If it is not possible to defuse the crisis verbally, as may occur with the confused or psychotic patient, then he should be restrained and parenterally sedated and the situation reassessed after he has settled. If the violence is considered to be part of a severe personality disturbance and not due to a psychiatric illness then the patient should be calmly told that you will be willing to listen to his problems once he has cooled off but that he is fully responsible for his actions and if he does not desist the police will be called in and he will be charged. If the patient is armed the police should be called.

When to call in a psychiatrist

A psychiatrist should be called in if either his experience is required in the diagnosis or management of the acute disorder or longer term psychiatric treatment is needed. In many cases it is more appropriate and helpful if the psychiatrist works closely with the rest of the staff, giving advice on management rather than being seen as managing the patient himself.

Transfer to a psychiatric ward

This is indicated either if inpatient psychiatric treatment is needed, for example for the suicidal depressed patient admitted following an overdose, or in general hospitals with a psychiatric ward where the patient's behaviour is unmanageable on the general ward.

Compulsory detention (Carney, 1980)

Patients can be admitted to or detained in hospital against their wishes under the Mental Health Act (1959) if they are suffering from a mental disorder that is not determined by a behavioural disturbance alone and if admission or detention is in the interests of their own health or safety and/or for the protection of others. On the general ward where one is usually concerned with compulsory detention rather than admission to hospital the order normally used is Section 30 (2). It should be filled in by the medical practitioner in charge of the patient's treatment (usually the consultant in charge) and is valid for 3 days, the day on which it is made out counting as the whole of the first day. Once such an order has been made steps should be taken as quickly as possible to make an application for the admission of the patient to hospital under the appropriate section of the Mental Health Act including, in an emergency, Section 29 (Pfeffer, 1981).

References

Barrison, I G, Viola, L, Murray-Lyon, I M (1980) *British Medical Journal*, **280**, 1040
Bird, J (1979) *British Journal of Psychiatry*, **134**, 129
British Medical Journal (1974) iii, 702
—(1977) i, 1241
—(1978) i, 1229
—(1979) ii, 291
Carney, M (1980) *Medicine, Series 3*, No.35, p.1806
Chesser, E S (1975) *Medicine, Series 2*, No. 10, p.447
Crammer, J, Barraclough, B, Heine, B (1978) Use of Drugs in Psychiatry. Gaskell, London
Crown, S (1972) *Medicine, Series 1*, No.10, p.661
Cutting, J (1980) *British Journal of Psychiatry*, **136**, 109
Davison, K (1975) *Medicine, Series 1*, No. 12, p.566
Donlon, P T, Hopkin, J, Tupin, J (1979) *American Journal of Psychiatry*, **136**, 273
Dowson, J (1980) *Medicine, Series 3*, No. 35, p.1777
Edwards, G (1967) *British Journal of Hospital Medicine*, **2**, 272

Egdell, H (1980) *Medicine, Series 3*, No. 35, p.1789
Farmer, R D T (1980) *in* The Suicide Syndrome (edited by Farmer, RDT, Hirsch, S R). Croom Helm, London. p.187
Gardner, R, Hanka, R, O'Brien, V C, Page, A J F, Rees, R (1977) *British Medical Journal*, ii, 1567
—,—, Evison, B, Mountford, P M, O'Brien, V C, Roberts, S J (1978) *ibid*. ii, 1392
Granville-Grossman, K (1975) *Medicine, Series 2*, No. 11, p. 482
Hackett, T P (1978) *in* Massachusett's General Hospital: Handbook of General Hospital Psychiatry (edited by Hackett, T P., Cassem, N H). C V Mosby, St Louis. p. 231
Hawton, K, Gath, D, Smith, E (1979) *British Medical Journal*, ii, 1040
Hore, B E (1972) *British Journal of Hospital Medicine*, **8**, 285
Jarman, C M B, Kellett, J M (1979) *British Medical Journal*, ii, 469
Kendell, R E (1974) *Medicine, Series 1*, No. 30, p. 1780
Kiloh, L G (1977) *Medicine, Series 2*, No. 10, p.460
Kreitman, (1973) *in* Companion to Psychiatric Studies, Vol 1 (edited by Forrest, A). Churchill Livingstone, Edinburgh and London. p.38
Lloyd, G G, Deakin, H G (1975) *British Medical Journal*, iv, 440
Mental Health Act (1959) Reprinted 1973. HMSO, London
Meyer, E, Mendelson, M (1961) *Psychiatry*, **24**, 197
Ministry of Health (1961) HM Circular (61) 94, HMSO, London
—(1968) Hospital Treatment of Acute Poisoning. HMSO, London
Murphy, G E, Guze, S B (1960) *American Journal of Psychotherapy*, **14**, 30
Newson-Smith, J G C, Hirsch, S R (1979) *British Journal of Psychiatry*, **134**, 335
Patel, A R (1975) *British Medical Journal*, ii, 426
Pfeffer, J M (1981) *British Journal of Hospital Medicine*, **26**, 653
Reed, J L (1971) *British Journal of Hospital Medicine*, **5**, 237
Rix, K J B (1978) *Hospital Update*, **5**, 403
Roth, M, Meyers, D II (1969) *British Journal of Hospital Medicine*, **2**, 705
Tonge, W L (1975) *Medicine, Series 2*, No. 12, p.568

Chapter 27

The endocrinology of the human pineal

P E Mullen, Otago Medical School, Dunedin, New Zealand
Ivor Smith, The Middlesex Hospital Medical School, London

The pineal in man is an endocrine organ that remains active throughout life. The calcification that occurs within the gland and is so often pointed to as indicating senescence or degeneration is, on the contrary, a byproduct of metabolic activity. Studies on human pineals obtained at postmortem indicate that the calcium-containing corpora arenacea begin to be deposited in childhood and accumulate increasingly with age (Tapp and Huxley, 1972). However, this calcification does not disrupt the integrity of the secretory pinealocytes nor does the enzymic activity within the gland decrease significantly with advancing age (Wurtman et al, 1964).

The systematic investigation of the endocrine role of the human pineal has only recently become possible with the development of sufficiently specific and sensitive methods for measuring the gland's secretions. In man our information has hitherto been largely limited to that gleaned from clinical observations and postmortem studies. Animal experimentation has generated a more formidable body of knowledge, but even here most enquiries have involved either in-vitro investigations where the enzyme activity within the gland was assumed to reflect hormonal output at the time of sacrifice or alternatively in vivo studies dependent on pinealectomy or the administration of putative pineal hormones. Considering these methodological limitations it is remarkable how much information has been acquired on pineal function and how many potentially relevant hypotheses await testing in man.

The melatonin hypothesis

In 1917 McCord and Allen published their observation that pineal extracts produced blanching of amphibian skin. Over 40 years later Lerner, a dermatologist, and his colleagues at Yale, working on an extract of a quarter of a million bovine pineals, managed to isolate and characterize the compound responsible for this effect (Lerner et al, 1960). They named it melatonin. The biosynthesis of melatonin within the pineal together with the enzymes responsible was soon elucidated (Axelrod and Weissbach, 1960; Weissbach et al, 1960). The final stage in the formation of melatonin is catalysed by hydroxyindole O-methyltransferase (HIOMT) which is effectively a pineal-specific enzyme. In the last 20 years melatonin has come to be regarded as the major, it not the sole, mediator of the endocrine role of the pineal gland. This melatonin hypothesis has acted as the

249

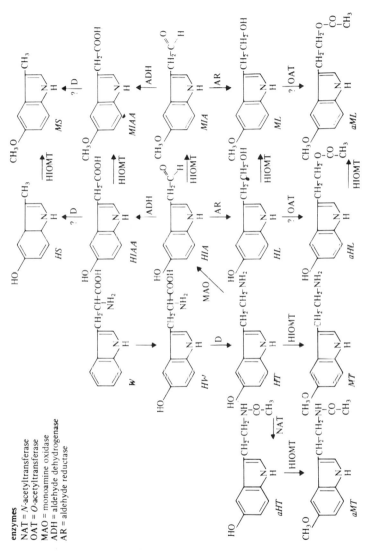

Figure 28.1 The pineal is capable of synthesizing a whole family of 5-methoxyindoles. The amino acid tryptophan (*W*) is the common precursor and is metabolized via hydroxytryptophan (*HW*) to hydroxytryptamine (*HT*). A variety of metabolic pathways is then possible leading to the production of the 5-methoxyindoles. In some cases more than one pathway is capable of producing a particular 5-methoxyindole. However, HIOMT is an essential step in the production of all of them. Melatonin (*aMT*) is produced from serotonin (*HT*) via *N*-acetyl-5-hydroxytryptamine (*aHT*). Other known pineal 5-methoxyindoles are 5-methoxytryptophol (*ML*), 5-methoxytryptamine (*MT*), 5-methoxyindole acetic acid (*MIAA*), and acetyl-methoxytryptophol (*aML*); methoxyskatole (*MS*) is a theoretically probable but not as yet finally identified addition to this family.

conceptual framework for much subsequent pineal research in both man and animals (Wurtman, 1977).

However, pineal HIOMT is now known to be capable of methylating a number of naturally occurring hydroxyindoles, thus producing a whole family of biosynthetically related methoxyindoles of which melatonin is but one member (*Figure 28.1*). Methoxytryptophol is also present in the human pineal and circulates at levels comparable to those of melatonin (Mullen et al, 1979). Methoxytryptamine has similarly been identified in human pineal tissue (Prozialeck et al, 1978) and is present at relatively high concentrations in the plasma (Hooper et al, 1980). Acetylmethoxytryptophol and methoxyindole acetic acid have been isolated from animal pineals (McIsaac et al, 1965; Smith et al, 1980) but have yet to be looked for in man. Doubtless the list of methoxyindoles secreted by the pineal gland will lengthen. The attention accorded to melatonin in pineal endocrinology may still turn out to be more an accident of history than a reflection of a true functional pre-eminence among the methoxyindoles. Furthermore, the pineal has been demonstrated to produce peptides which may also be secreted by the gland to mediate some of its endocrine functions (Pavel, 1979).

Light and pineal rhythms

Comparative anatomical studies point to the development of the pineal as a secretory organ from a phylogenetically more primitive photoreceptor, the third eye. The pineal cells of fish, amphibians and reptiles are photoreceptors; they have a structure similar to the cone cells of the retina but with clearly developed secretory granules and light stimuli may be directly converted into an endocrine response. In mammals the pineal cells develop into the exclusively secretory pinealocytes. However, they retain a neural input from the retina via the inferior accessory optic tract and the superior cervical ganglion from which the sympathetic beta-noradrenergic innervation to the pineal arises (Kappers, 1979).

Given this unique evolutionary development it is perhaps not surprising that in some animals it has been possible to demonstrate a clear relationship between photoperiodicity and both the pineal content of the methoxyindoles and the enzymes responsible for their production (Quay, 1974; Fiske, 1975). Nervous impulses from the retina conveying information about light, or more correctly the absence of light, induce the production of a hormone in the pineal. This has led to the pineal being termed a neuroendocrine transducer (Axelrod, 1974). Studies in the laboratory rat have demonstrated that in the dark the levels of noradrenaline and melatonin in the pineal increase together with the activity of the enzymes N-acetyltransferase and HIOMT. In the light this situation is reversed with the biosynthetic activity within the gland being largely suppressed. Direct studies of this type have obviously been a problem in man but there is one report of a correlation between the activity of pineal enzymes and the time of the subject's demise (Smith et al, 1977).

A diurnal rhythm in melatonin levels in human plasma and urine has been reported (Pelham et al, 1973; Arendt et al, 1977; Vaughan et al, 1978; Wetterberg, 1979). The exact nature of the fluctuations in the circulating melatonin level throughout the 24 hours is still a matter of some dispute. The result from several studies suggest a virtual absence of measurable melatonin in samples obtained during the daylight hours with a sustained elevation in those obtained at night. Other workers find peaks of melatonin present by both day and night with simply somewhat higher and more frequent surges at night. This latter finding, if correct, would indicate that the control of the metabolic activity within man's pineal is far less closely tied to changes in light and dark than that in rodents on whom the majority of animal studies have been performed. Methoxytryptophol has also been studied throughout the 24 hours (Linsell et al, 1979). This showed only a very weak diurnal rhythm with nocturnal elevation and detectable quantities were present in most subjects throughout the period. In man, unlike most other animals, changes in light and dark play little part in the control and synchronization of endocrine rhythms and it would not be all that surprising if the close link between prevailing illumination and pineal activity present in animals was lost or at least obscured in man.

It is clearly of considerable importance to establish the normal range and the basic characteristics of any significant rhythms in the circulating levels of the methoxyindoles in man. Without this information it is hardly possible to judge the relevance, if any, of the reported levels in pathological states.

The pineal and reproduction

In 1899, quite independently of each other, Ogle in England and Heubner in Germany published the first reports of the association of pineal tumours in children with precocious puberty. Heubner went further by hypothesizing that precocious sexual development was due to the removal of some kind of pineal hormone normally holding sexual maturation in check. Marburg in the first decade of this century coined the term pubertas praecox for this clinical syndrome; he suggested that hypopinealism acting via the hypothalamus was responsible for precocious sexual development and that by the reverse mechanism hyperpinealism could cause slow and incomplete development of the gonads (Marburg, 1930; Kappers, 1979). Support for this suggestion came from the clinical observation that pineal lesions that are either destructive or poorly differentiated neoplasms are associated with pubertas praecox whereas well differentiated and presumably actively secreting tumours are found in association with delayed puberty and hypogonadism (Kitay, 1954).

Animal experiments gave further support to the proposition that the pineal gland produces antigonadotrophic hormones (Reiter, 1978). Pinealectomy in rodents has a stimulatory effect on gonadal development, and the administration of pineal extract or pineal methoxyindoles such as melatonin and methoxytryptophol can produce gonadal regression. The ability of light to suppress pineal biosynthetic activity in animals such as the rat and the hamster has enabled pineal function to be manipulated by varying the length of time spent by the animal in the light. Prolongation of the daily light period suppresses pineal activity and is associated with increased size and weight of the gonads together with precocious oestrus in some species. Prolongation of the dark period or blinding results in gonadal regression or, in the immature animal, delayed sexual development. The story is unfortunately not quite straightforward since in some species at particular stages in sexual maturation the pineal and its products can act to stimulate gonadal development (Reiter and Vaughan, 1977). Thus, although the pineal would appear to exert a predominantly antigonadal influence it may also produce progonadal hormones under certain circumstances.

The levels of two pineal indoles, melatonin and methoxytryptophol, have been studied in young boys at different stages of sexual maturation (Silman et al, 1979a).

A dramatic drop in melatonin levels was observed between boys in Tanners genitalia stage 1 in which the mean morning value was 218 pg/ml and those in stages 2, 3 and 4 in whom the levels decreased to means of 30, 17 and 18 pg/ml, respectively. The drop in melatonin concentrations immediately preceded the rise in testosterone FSH and LH levels found with puberty. Silman et al (1979a) concluded that melatonin levels decrease before the first signs of puberty have become apparent and they suggested that this reduction is part of the process that initiates the physical and endocrine changes of puberty. However, it is worth remembering that melatonin can act in animals at specific stages of sexual maturation as a progonadal hormone, and it is possible that these authors have detected a prepubertal surge in melatonin rather than a drop in concentration with puberty. Unfortunately no data were provided on younger children not close to the onset of puberty. In contrast to the melatonin levels those of methoxytryptophol showed no alteration as puberty progressed. If confirmed these observations would provide an important contribution to our knowledge of the function of the human pineal.

The pineal is capable in animals of affecting ovulation, its influence being predominantly inhibitory. By means of radioimmunoassay melatonin has been measured throughout the menstrual cycle. Wetterberg et al (1976) reported that levels were highest during menstrual bleeding and fell to a mid-cycle nadir at or about the time of ovulation. These authors suggested that melatonin could act as an inhibitory influence on ovulation in man as well as in animals with the decrease in circulating levels being related to the triggering of ovulation.

Methoxytryptophol levels are also reported to vary considerably at different stages of the menstrual cycle (Hooper et al, 1979). However, they were found to be significantly higher in the first two thirds of the cycle. Women taking an oral contraceptive had consistently lower levels throughout the month. The fluctuations in methoxytryptophol levels did not appear to be related to either FSH or LH, but an inhibitory influence of progesterones on its release could explain both the changes of the cycle and the effects of the oral contraceptive.

Changes in the pattern of the daily light/dark cycle can, as already noted, influence ovulation in some experimental animals. An attempt has been made to study the effect of light on women (Dewan et al, 1978). The influence of artificial light on the menstrual cycle was looked at by exposing subjects with abnormally long or erratic periods to 3 or 4 days continuous illumination beginning 14 days after the cessation of menstruation. It was claimed that this regularized cycle lengths in a significant number of them. The effect was postulated to be due to inhibition by light of the pineal's antigonadotrophic activity and therefore ovulation occurred with the menstrual bleeding following 2 weeks later.

The changes in melatonin and methoxytryptophol levels with the menstrual cycle may have some controlling influence on the cycle itself but equally they may simply be passive responses to changes in the gonadotrophin and steroid levels. It has yet to be shown in man whether the reported changes in methoxyindole concentrations are part of the cause or merely consequent upon the rhythmic alterations in the levels of these other hormones. The pineal in animals, although it probably exerts some of its influence directly on the gonads, acts predominantly via the pituitary release of gonadotrophins.

The pineal and the pituitary

Pineal tumours in man may on occasion present as apparent pituitary dysfunction. An endocrinopathy characterized by panhypopituitarism can be the earliest manifestation of pineal neoplasia, occurring before any pressure effects from the tumour itself are evident (Puschett and Goldberg, 1968). Polyuria and polydipsia may be present consequent on the inhibition of antidiuretic hormone production together with depressed plasma cortisol and decreased urinary 17-hydroxycorticoid levels secondary to the failure of ACTH production.

The ability of the pineal to affect gonadotrophin secretion by the pituitary in laboratory animals has already been mentioned. In addition animal experiments have demonstrated an inhibitory influence of the pineal on the pituitary thyroid axis (Relkin, 1978), the pituitary adrenal axis (Ogle and Kitay, 1976), and the pituitary release of growth hormone (Ronnekleiv and McCann, 1978). The effect of the pineal on prolactin secretion is an exception since it appears to enhance the secretion in most circumstances (Reiter, 1979).

The relationship between the pineal and the pituitary is a complex one and although the pineal acts predominantly to suppress pituitary action some of its methoxyindoles can under certain conditions facilitate the release of pituitary hormones. Mess et al (1979) concluded a review of the animal literature by stating that "Generally the pineal gland plays more or less the role of a brake or attenuator in the regulation of pituitary trophic hormone secretion except for prolactin where the secretion is normally enhanced by the pineal gland".

The effects on growth hormone, FSH and LH of long-term oral administration of what must be considered pharmacological rather than physiological doses of melatonin to humans have been studied (Norland and Lerner, 1977). Only a slight depression in serum LH levels and a reduced growth hormone response to stress were noted with no effect at all on plasma cortisol, urinary 17-hydroxycorticosteroid, or T_4 levels, or on ^{131}I uptake by the thyroid. Melatonin was also reported to produce an initial transient increase in growth hormone release followed by a more extended inhibition of the hormone's response to insulin hypoglycaemia (Smythe and Lazarus, 1974). Other authors could discern no effect on human gonadotrophin secretion even after 2 weeks of injecting melatonin (Fedeleff et al, 1976).

Vaughan et al (1979) studied the effects of hypoglycaemic stress and the levodopa provocation test on melatonin release in man. While in rats hypogly caemia reportedly increased the synthesis of melatonin in the pineal, these authors failed to observe any increase in the melatonin level in man; in fact the melatonin level decreased which the authors considered to be probably due to its normal tendency to fall during the morning. They also failed to note any response in the circulating melatonin level to levodopa, although again in animals a striking elevation had been reported. In contrast the methoxytryptophol level is reported to show a significant drop in response to hypoglycaemic stress (Silman et al, 1979b). The decrease in methoxytryptophol level parallels the decrease in blood glucose concentration and precedes the increase in ACTH and growth hormone levels. This could indicate that the decrease in pineal methoxytryptophol level was implicated in the surge in pituitary hormones, which is in line with the evidence from animal experiments of the tonic inhibitory influence of the pineal on the pituitary.

In man the influence of the pineal on the pituitary still remains to be delineated. Clinical observation and animal experimentation would suggest predominantly inhibitory effects of a subtle nature.

Psychoneuroendocrinology

There is a long historical tradition of associating the pineal with abnormalities of mental function (Mullen and Silman, 1977). Even relatively recently pineal extracts have been employed as a treatment for schizophrenia although the initial enthusiasm was not borne out by later controlled trials. Melatonin crosses the blood-brain barrier with ease (Kopin et al, 1961) and its administration to humans is said to produce tranquillization, occasional mild euphoria, and with larger doses the induction of sleep (Anton Tay, 1974; Cramer et al, 1974). Melatonin-induced sleep is reportedly associated with an increase in the rapid eye movement phase, which is the opposite effect to that induced by most clinically employed hypnotics.

The mood-elevating and sleep-enhancing properties of melatonin led to its trial as an antidepressant, but unfortunately it resulted in a dramatic worsening in the patients' depressive symptomatology (Carmen et al, 1976). It was also reported that melatonin exacerbated the psychotic features in patients with schizophrenia (Altschule, 1976). The apparent induction of psychotic phenomena is of particular interest because the so-called psychotomimetic agents such as LSD and mescaline increase pineal HIOMT activity, presumably elevating methoxyindole production (Hartley and Smith, 1973). An intact pineal has even been claimed to be essential for the manifestation in animals of the behavioural effects of hallucinogens (Winters et al, 1973).

Chlorpromazine, a drug employed to treat schizophrenia, reportedly reduces HIOMT activity within the pineal and when administered over a long period to rats was found to produce atrophic changes within the pinealocytes (Horita et al, 1978).

Jimerson et al (1977) examined the urinary excretion of melatonin in a group of untreated patients with depressive illness but found no difference from a group of normal controls. Wetterberg et al (1979) also reported normal melatonin excretion but the ratio of circulating melatonin level to cortisol level sampled on four occasions during the 24 hours was altered, which was adduced as evidence for pineal dysfunction in depression. In schizophrenia these authors reported a normal diurnal pattern in melatonin, but recently a claim has been made for depressed nocturnal values in serum melatonin in a group of chronic schizophrenics. These studies are still in the early stages, but clearly pineal function deserves careful examination in the major mental illnesses.

Pinealectomy has been found to increase cerebral excitability and seizure-like discharges in some animals and melatonin administration raised the convulsive threshold. In an uncontrolled, and as yet unconfirmed, report melatonin was said to exert therapeutic benefit as an anticonvulsant (Anton Tay, 1974). Melatonin levels have been monitored in a group of epileptic subjects who showed a normal pattern of secretion (Sizonenko et al, 1979).

The pineal and cancer

There is experimental evidence that in animals both the pineal and melatonin can influence the growth of malignant tumours, although the exact influence varies for different species and different tumour types (Lapin, 1979). In man there have been several reports of pineal abnormalities in patients dying of cancer. Pineal enlargement, particularly in association with carcinoma of the breast and malignant melanoma, and degenerative changes that could reflect chronic hyperactivity of the gland have been recorded (Tapp, 1979). However, systematic studies of pineal activity in patients with various forms of malignant disease have yet to be done.

Conclusion

The human pineal which has languished for so long in relative obscurity is now under active investigation thanks to the development of measurement technologies capable of monitoring its secretions in body fluids. The currently available evidence points to the human pineal as the source of a family of methoxyindoles and suggests that these compounds have a significant endocrine role. They would appear to be involved with human reproduction, possibly in both the changes accompanying puberty and the menstrual cycle. The tonic inhibitory influence which the pineal may exert on certain aspects of pituitary function opens up possibilities for a fundamental role in endocrine dynamics. In the field of psychoneuroendocrinology the pineal secretions certainly deserve and will doubtless receive further attention.

The endocrinology of the human pineal, as with any new and rapidly developing area of research, will inevitably initially produce contradictory and sometimes grandiose claims and counterclaims. In attempting to assess the validity of work in this area over the next few years it will be important to bear in mind the limitations as well as the power of the new assay techniques. No measurement system for any of the pineal methoxyindoles is so well established as to be above question. However, with time increasingly reliable and repeatable results will no doubt accumulate, finally revealing the functions of the pineal in human physiology and pathology.

References

Altschule, M D (1976) *see* Carmen et al, 1976
Anton Tay, F (1974) *Advances in Biochemical Psychopharmacology*, **11**, 315
Arendt, J, Wetterberg, L, Heyden, T, Sizonenko, P C, Paunier, L (1977) *Hormone Research*, **8**, 65
Axelrod, J (1974) *Science*, **184**, 1341
—, Weissbach, W (1960) *Science*, **131**, 1312
Carmen, J S, Post, R M, Buswell, K, Goodwin, F K (1976) *American Journal of Psychiatry*, **133**, 1181
Cramer, H, Rudolf, J. Consbruch, U, Kendel, K (1974) *Advances in Biochemical Psychopharmacology*, **11**, 187
Dewan, E M, Menkin, M F, Rock, J (1978) *Photochemical Photobiology*, **27**, 581
Fedeleff, H, Aparicio, N J, Guitelman, A, Debeluk, L, Mancini, A, Cramer, C (1976) *Journal of Clinical Endocrinology and Metabolism*, **42**, 1014
Fiske, V M (1975) *in* Frontiers of Pineal Physiology (edited by Altschule, M D). MIT Press, Massachusetts. p.5
Hartley, R, Smith, J A (1973) *Journal of Pharmacy and Pharmacology*, **25**, 751
Heubner, O (1899) *Deutsche medizinische Wochenschrift*, **24**, 214
Hooper, R J L et al (1979) *Journal of Endocrinology*, **82**, 269
—, Silman, R E, Smith, I (1980) unpublished
Horita, N, Ischii, T, Moroji, T (1978) *Acta neuropathologica*, **42**, 49
Jimerson, D C, Lynch, H J, Post, R M, Wurtman, R J, Bunney, W E (1977) *Life Science*, **20**, 1501
Kappers, J A (1979) *Progress in Brain Research*, **52**, 3
Kitay, J I (1954) *Clinical Endocrinology*, **14**, 622
Kopin, I, Pare, C M B, Axelrod, J, Weissbach, H (1961) *Journal of Biological Chemistry*, **266**, 3027
Lapin, V (1979) *Progress in Brain Research*, **52**, 523
Lerner, A B, Case, J D, Takahashi, Y (1960) *Journal of Biological Chemistry*, **235**, 1992
Linsell, C et al (1979) *Progress in Brain Research*, **52**, 501
McCord, C P, Allen, F P (1917) *Journal of Experimental Zoology*, **23**, 207
McIsaac, W M, Farrell, G, Tarborsky, R G, Taylor, A N (1965) *Science*, **148**, 102
Marburg, O (1930) Hanbuch der Normalen und Pathologischen Physiologie. Vol. 13. Springer, Berlin
Mess, B, Trentini, G P, Ruzsas, C, De Gaetani, C (1979) *Progress in Brain Research*, **52**, 329
Mullen, P E, Silman, R E (1977) *Psychological Medicine*, **7**, 407
—et al (1979) *Psychoneuroendocrinology*, **2**, 117
Norland, J J, Lerner, A B (1977) *Journal of Clinical Endocrinology and Metabolism*, **45**, 768
Ogle, C (1899) *Transactions of the Pathological Society of London*, **1**, 4
Ogle, T F, Kitay, J (1976) *Endocrinology*, **98**, 20
Pavel, S (1979) *Progress in Brain Research*, **52**, 445

Pelham, R W, Vaughan, G M, Sandock, K L, Vaughan, M K (1973) *Journal of Clinical Endocrinology and Metabolism,* **37,** 341
Prozialeck, W C, Boehme, D H, Vogel, W H (1978) *Journal of Neurochemistry,* **30,** 1471
Puschett, J B, Goldberg, M (1968) *Annals of Internal Medicine,* **69,** 203
Quay, W B (1974) Pineal Chemistry in Cellular Physiological Mechanisms. Thomas, Springfield, Illinois
Reiter, R J (1978) Editor. The Pineal and Reproduction. Karger, Basel, p.169
—(1979) The Pineal, Vol. 4. Eden Press, Quebec
—, Vaughan, M K (1977) *Life Science,* **21,** 159
Relkin, R (1978) *Neuroendocrinology,* **25,** 310
Ronnekleiv, O K, McCann, S M (1978) *Endocrinology,* **102,** 1694
Silman, R E, Leone, R M, Hooper, R J L, Preece, M A (1979a) *Nature,* **282,** 301
—et al (1979b) *Progress in Brain Research,* **52,** 507
Sizonenko, P C, Moore, D C, Paunier, L, Beaumanair, A, Nohory, A (1979) *Progress in Brain Research,* **52,** 549
Smith, I, Francis, P E, Leone, M, Mullen, P E (1980) *Biochemical Journal,* **185,** 537
Smith, J A, Padwick, D, Mee, T J X, Minneman, K P, Bird, E D (1977) *Clinical Endocrinology,* **6,** 219
Smythe, G A, Lazarus, L (1974) *Science,* **184,** 1373
Tapp, E (1979) *Progress in Brain Research,* **52,** 481
—, Huxley, M (1972) *Journal of Pathology,* **108,** 137
Vaughan, G M, Allen, J P, Tullis, W, Siler-Khodr, T M, Pena, de la, A, Sackma, J W (1978) *Journal of Clinical Endocrinology and Metabolism,* **47,** 566
—, McDonald, S D, Jordan, R M, Allen, J P, Bell, R, Stevens, E A (1979) *Psychoneuroendocrinology,* **4,** 351
Weissbach, H, Redfield, B G, Axelrod, J (1960) *Biochemica et biophysica acta,* **43,** 352
Wetterberg, L (1979) *Progress in Brain Research,* **52,** 539
—, Arendt, J, Paunier, L, Sizonenko, P C, Van Donselaar, W, Heyden, T (1976) *Journal of Clinical Endocrinology and Metabolism,* **42,** 185
—, Friis, J, Aperia, B, Petterson, V (1979) *Lancet,* ii, 1361
Winters, W D, Alcaraz, M, Cervantes, M Y, Flores Guzman, C (1973) *Neuropharmacology,* **12,** 407
Wurtman, R J (1977) *New England Journal of Medicine,* **296,** 1329, 1383
—, Axelrod, J , Barchas, J D (1964) *Journal of Clinical Endocrinology and Metabolism,* **24,** 299

Chapter 28

Rape

Paul Bowden, The Maudsley Hospital, London

Animal studies suggest that the dominant and submissive behaviours that character-ize sexual activity are both innate and learned (Lorenz, 1966). In man the interpretation of such verbal and nonverbal language is particularly important in the selection of a partner, in courtship and copulation. In these situations consent which legalizes the activity can be disguised or withheld for reasons other than nonconsent. Who can quantify that "little force which is pleasing to a woman, which makes her grateful to the ravisher against whom she struggles" (Ovid)? Later Chaucer (*The Miller's Tale*), Shakespeare (*The Rape of Lucrece*), and Cervantes (*Don Quixote*) perpetuated the view that it is impossible to rape a woman against her will. Hemingway did not glorify such predatory male activity; indeed his sympathies lay with the victim (*For Whom the Bell Tolls*).

Differing emphasis is put on the strength of association between sexuality and violence. Thus a psychoanalyst, Melanie Klein, has stated that these behaviours have a common origin since both hostility and aggression can be felt towards a loved sexual object. Similarly, the existence of sadomasochism which is considered to be a regressive state supports the view that such subjugation is an atavistic form of sexuality. Some criminologists believe that there are essential differences between the sexes because the sexual fantasies of males frequently concern sadistic domination and humiliation whereas those of females rarely do so. Storr (1968) has argued that in the male there is a primitive necessity for pursuit and penetration that is both recognized and responded to by the yielding and submissive female. Whatever the mode of enquiry, what is said about violence in general is largely applicable to sexual violence; however, sexual behaviour has its own unique characteristics.

History

In Babylonian, Judaic and early Christian times virginity was highly prized; a maiden was of commercial value and reflected family honour. For this reason a rapist and sometimes the victim as well were executed. Although the word rape was used initially with a purely sexual connotation, it came later to imply abduction thereby reflecting its Latin origin from rapere meaning to seize, snatch, or take by force.

257

A 17th century Lord Chief Justice, Matthew Hale, voiced an opinion that was to be of considerable influence later as far as victims were concerned: "It (rape) is an accusation easily to be made and harder to be proved, and harder to be defended by the party accused tho' never so innocent". Hale's opinion was to be further consolidated by 19th century case law in which juries were directed to consider in favour of the accused any evidence of past indiscretion on the behalf of the victim.

Even today the victim continues to be disadvantaged since only the Director of Public Prosecutions can bring charges. Women alleging rape are therefore ineligible as witnesses or for legal aid and in practice they are often themselves on trial without the benefit of counsel.

Definition

The provisions of Section 1 (1) of the Sexual Offences Act 1956 were based on the view that the offence is an assault on innocence as in defloration. The Act stated that a person commited rape if he had sexual intercourse with a woman without her consent by means of force or threatening bodily harm, where apparent consent was nullified by fraud, or where individuals could not give informed consent (for example the unconscious, the mentally handicapped, the young, and those who are unable to understand the nature of the act). Emission was not necessary and any sexual penetration, however slight, was sufficient to complete the crime (compare with forcible rape in the USA).

The law was altered by the Sexual Offences (Amendment) Act 1976 which emphasizes lack of consent rather than assault. Here it is a person's wish not to engage in a particular activity that is not respected. Section 1(i) of the 1976 Act states that a man commits rape if (a) he has unlawful sexual intercourse with a woman who at the time of the intercourse does not consent to it; and (b) at the time he knows that she does not consent to the intercourse or he is reckless as to whether she consents to it. Section 1(ii) states that if at a trial for a rape offence the jury has to consider whether a man believed that a woman was consenting to sexual intercourse, the presence or absence of reasonable grounds for such a belief is a matter to which the jury is to have regard. The 1976 Amendment Act also states that no evidence and no question in cross examination shall be asked about any sexual experience of the complainant, being the woman upon whom the rape was committed, attempted or proposed, with a person other than the defendant. Section 4 makes it an offence to publish any information which might lead to the identification of any woman as the complainant.

The law

One important issue mentioned above is that the defendant used to be able to give evidence that the prosecutrix was of bad character for want of chastity or common decency. Taking Hale's lead the sexuality of the victim was of as much interest to the court as that of the attacker.

The most recent changes in the law followed the trial of Morgan whose codefendants said that he had induced them to rape his wife by telling them that her apparent nonconsent to sex was a disguise for her masochism and that she would in fact enjoy it. The jury decided that to believe the husband rather than the protestations of the wife obviously suited the defendants; it did not accept the defendants' version that Mrs Morgan showed sexual enjoyment, and they were found guilty. The Court of Appeal supported the trial judge, but the defendants appealed to the House of Lords who ruled that a man accused of rape should be acquitted if his belief in the woman's consent was genuine even if the grounds for his belief were unreasonable. The public outcry that followed was based on the last part of the Lords' ruling and the Home Secretary set up an independent group chaired by Mrs Justice Heilbron to advise whether a change in the law was necessary. The group recommended that the offence of rape should be based on lack of consent and not on violence, the previous sexual history of the prosecutrix should be inadmissible, and there should be anonymity for complainants. These recommendations were incorporated in the Sexual Offences (Amendment) Act 1976. The fact that the alleged victim now remains anonymous has been criticized by the Bar Council and the Law Society; both have asked why rape victims should be protected and other witnesses not.

A furore similar to that following the trial of Morgan and his codefendants was also provoked by the release of a guardsman who sexually assaulted a 17-year-old girl with extreme brutality. He was given a suspended sentence because of the effect imprisonment would have had on his career. The subject of rape again became a focus of publicity in 1982 when a judge gave as his reason for not imprisoning a convicted rapist the suggestion that the woman invited sex by accepting a lift. The harsh questioning of female complainants by policemen has led to the setting-up of rape squads comprising only policewomen on the grounds, presumably, that they would be more sympathetic. In the same year a refusal to bring a prosecution because of the victim's alleged mental instability led to the resignation of Scotland's Solicitor General.

A husband can only be convicted as the principal (as opposed to an accomplice) in the rape of his wife if they are legally separated. A boy of under 14 years is considered in law to be incapable of coitus and he can only be convicted of indecent assault or possibly attempted rape. Conviction for rape carries a maximum sentence of life imprisonment. In practice it is important to distinguish between the following categories.

Unlawful sexual intercourse (Section 6, Sexual Offences Act 1956)   It is an offence to have or to attempt intercourse with a girl under 13 years; her consent is immaterial (compare with statutory rape in the USA). It is similarly an offence with a girl between 13 and 16 years except where the man is under 24 years, he has not previously been charged with a like offence, and he believed her to be over 16 years.

Indecent assault (Section 15, Sexual Offences Act 1956)   It is an offence for any person to make an indecent assault on a male or female; consent is nullified if the victim is under 16 years. It is important to note that in assault it is not necessary for there to be physical contact: the victim need only apprehend unlawful force however slight.

Prevalence

Most forensic studies are limited by the fact that persons charged with an offence, and particularly those convicted, represent only a selected minority of those who exhibit a particular type of behaviour (Sparks et al, 1978). Amir (1971) suggested that the prevalence of any offence would depend on the following several factors and these are largely applicable to rape.

Reportability   This reflects the morals of the community, the injury done, the characteristics of the parties concerned (for example their relationship, age, and race), and presence of witnesses. Some victims report the rape only after they have been urged to do so while others report the incident and then refuse to prosecute further. This can be due to reluctance to give evidence, fear, or the development of some sympathy for their assailant.

Detectability   This relates to the efficiency of the police in arresting offenders.

Recordability   Misrepresentation or biased reporting may influence the recorded rates, for example in England and Wales rape followed by murder would be recorded as murder.

Organizational contingencies   These are practices related to prosecution and sentencing. Gibbens and Ahrenfeldt (1966) showed that countries with high homicide rates have few arrests for rape and they suggested that only when safety of life is guaranteed is sexual integrity of concern. Radzinowicz (1957) argued that about one fifth of sexual offenders were not detected in that they were not caught "in flagrante delicto", while one tenth of those reported were not proceeded against. Convicted rapists account for about 3 per cent of admissions to special hospitals (Gibbens et al, 1977).

Criminal statistics

In 1980, 2.7 million serious crimes were known by the police. In this context a serious crime is defined as one that can be tried at a Crown Court before a jury, although many are dealt with by magistrates, summarily.

In 1980, 21 000 sexual offences were known to the police, of which indecent assault accounted for more than half. This overall figure was the lowest annual figure for a decade and it accounted for only 0.8 per cent of all known serious crimes. Unlike other offence categories the number of sexual offences recorded annually shows a downward trend.

The number of rapes recorded annually has risen but not as much as other violent crime. In 1979 there were 1170 recorded rapes, 1225 in 1980. Part of the increase can be explained by increased reporting following the reforms introduced in the 1976 Sexual Offences (Amendment) Act. As a result of police enquiries 653 men and 4 women (accomplices) were charged with rape in magistrates' courts in 1979. Fifty one were discharged because the bench considered there was insufficient evidence to commit for trial. Forty per cent of those sent for trial were refused bail. One fifth were acquitted at trial, but of those found guilty 85 per cent were imprisoned immediately.

Types

Any labelling system is of limited value because it makes one aspect of behaviour cover a whole personality. Clinard (1963) defined deviance in relation to what is considered statistically normal at a particular time. He believed that normal sexual acts should lead to procreation and that deviant acts would include those proscribed by law.

Other systems of classification rely on the degree of consent, the characteristics of the partner (who should be of the opposite sex, a certain age, and a definite kinship distance), the nature of the act, and the setting (which is preferably private). A useful system of classification can be obtained by linking Guttmacher and Weihofen's (1952) behavioural types with the psychological profiles described by Cohen et al (1975).

Explosive

The assault is a forcible expression of pent-up sexual drives where defensive and controlling factors are overwhelmed. This group is similar to that termed "sexual" by Cohen et al (1975). Sexual behaviour has a compulsive quality that is motivated by high arousal. The act is not impulsive but is performed in fantasy beforehand and the victim is chosen as being especially sexually evocative. Rapists of this type are often shy and phobic and have minor deviations that are repressed but remain the cause of considerable guilt.

Latent homosexual

In this category rape is not the breakdown of a defence as in the explosive type but is itself a defence against homosexuality by reaction formation (that is exaggeration of the opposite tendency).

Aggressive, sadistic

These men harbour a deep-seated hatred of women. The assault is primarily destructive and typically the rapist mutilates his victim to humiliate and defile her. In this group, anger can be interpreted as a displacement of feelings towards the mother or representative (for example wife or girlfriend) onto a substitute object who is usually a stranger. Feelings towards the mother are ambivalent: on the one hand women are idealized as the source of all fulfilment, on the other—and in reality—they are seen as unfaithful, unloving and untrustworthy. These men often have a history of early sexual experiences with older women and they later become competitive masculine narcissistic types who develop socially acceptable outlets for their aggression.

Aggressive antisocial criminals

Here the assault is not a form of sexual deviance but part of a more general opportunistic hedonism.

Sex-aggression diffusion

In this type sexual arousal is linked with aggression. The individual is impotent unless there is resistance and only continuing aggression maintains arousal; there is usually no further violence after ejaculation. Typically these men have demanding, exploitative, and paranoid personalities.

West et al (1978) have produced an important study of a selected group of men convicted following serious sexual attacks. Masculine inferiority feelings were common in all types of sexual deviants but with rapists stress served to release that sexual aggression. All West's group had experienced lasting heterosexual relationships, although their social achievements often fell short of their ideals of male dominance. There was sometimes a striking gap between low career achievements and high intellectual potential. Feelings of frustration were not expressed as neurotic disorder, but were expressed as aggressive action and an obsessive preoccupation with sexual fantasies was a not uncommon precursor of crime.

MacDonald's (1971) view is that the majority of rapists have some sort of character disorder; he notes that alcoholism and homosexuality are frequently encountered and that there is a low incidence of psychosis. The Royal College of Psychiatrists' memorandum to Mrs Justice Heilbron's Advisory Group on the Law of Rape was based on MacDonald's classification. The College characterized the typical rapist: most are not mentally abnormal but they are young, vigorous, and sexually unsatisfied and inexperienced. They do not plan the attacks, although they usually receive some initial encouragement from the victims. The types of personality disorder that are most prevalent are those that normally prevent the offender from satisfactorily expressing his sexuality. There is often a history of maladjustment and delinquency, and drugs and alcohol are usually involved. Certain clinical types are associated with sexual assault: subnormality predisposes to difficulties in sexual adjustment, especially if individuals are confined in single-sex institutions where there is only occasional contact with females. A small number of rapists are found to have brain damage that diminishes self-control. Finally, if a psychosis is present (less than 5 per cent) it is most likely to be manic.

The participants

The most detailed studies of rape have been reported by MacDonald (1971) who studied the police files of 200 consecutive victims of forcible rape in Denver and by Amir (1971) who reported an analysis of 646 rapes in Philadelphia. The victim is typically a few years younger than the assailant and single. Seventy per cent of rapists fall into the 17–30 age range. Most are between 21 and 25 years old. However they tend to be older and less intelligent than other offenders including sexual offenders (Gunn, 1976) and less mentally disordered (Gibbens et al, 1977). In the USA the negro rape rate is about 12 times that for whites, but as with other crime rates racial differences are very small when groups who live under similar conditions are compared.

About one third of rapists are neighbours or acquaintances of the victims and in one fifth of offences there is some degree of victim participation. This latter group includes women who behave in a manner that constitutes a sexual invitation, those who agree to sex but later retract consent, and individuals who do not react strongly enough to the initial advance. Children can also be provocative in their sexual relationships with adults. Bender and Blau (1937) showed that children usually cooperate in the activity and sometimes they assume an active role in initiating the relationship. Similarly Gibbens and Prince (1963) found that two thirds of the child victims of sexual offenders cooperated in some manner with their assailants.

Amir (1971) distinguished between precipitative and seductive victims. The former expose themselves to risks where they are vulnerable and could legally be considered reckless or negligent. The latter can either consciously participate in the act or their involvement may be due to unconscious motives.

Rapists have fewer convictions for sexual offences than other types of sexual offenders (Gibbens et al, 1977), but they have more extensive records of nonsexual crime (Christiansen et al, 1965).

The setting

There is an increased incidence of rape between the months of May and August which probably reflects normal seasonal sexual activity. The majority of rapes take place between 8.00 pm and 1.00 am and one quarter happen on Saturdays. Alcohol is more often a factor in weekend rapes. In about 20 per cent of assaults both victim and offender have been drinking and a drunken victim is usually subjected to more violence than a sober one. The assault occurs mostly in the neighbourhood in which both participants live, usually in one or the other's place of residence.

The act

The majority of victims are intimidated physically or verbally; about one quarter are coerced by the threat of injury and a similar proportion are menaced with a weapon. By definition rape involves the use or threat of force and in Amir's (1971) study 29 per cent of victims were handled roughly, 25 per cent were beaten (20 per cent brutally), and 12 per cent choked.

The victims are mostly submissive, expressing only verbal protest or reluctance. Some resist by screaming or trying to escape and one fifth fight; understandably, submissive victims are subjected to less force. One quarter of victims are sexually humiliated in that they are forced to accept cunnilingus or fellatio or there is repeated intercourse. Occasionally a rapist uses contraceptives himself or encourages his victim to take precautions; he can also demand cooperation and shows of affection from his victim and express remorse after the act. Sometimes the victim is robbed after the assault. Murder is fortunately rare.

Gang rape

In about one third of rapes there is more than one aggressor. In the series of Gibbens et al (1977) 32.5 per cent of the 200 individuals convicted of rape in 1961 were charged along with two or more others. Amir (1971) and MacDonald (1971) found that in about 15 per cent of rapes there were two aggressors and in 25 per cent three or more. The victims of gang rapes were more often prostitutes; they tend to be treated more violently and to be unknown to the aggressors. Alcohol is a significant factor in gang rape and the rapists have more extensive histories of both sexual crime and previous violence to persons.

Follow-up

Sentence depends on the age of the victim, the relationship between offender and victim (with abuse of a position of trust being considered to be particularly bad), and indulgence in other violence or depredation. Sentence will also depend on the offender's age. Those convicted between the ages of 14 and 17 years usually receive orders for detention centre or Borstal training. Noncustodial sentences are very rare and only four probation orders and 14 suspended sentences were imposed in 1979. In contrast, 295 were sentenced to immediate imprisonment. Seventeen per cent of those imprisoned received sentences of under 2 years, 60 per cent 2–5 years and seven persons life imprisonment. Only four hospital orders were made, three of which included orders restricting discharge under Section 65, Mental Health Act 1959.

On release from prison sexual offenders tend to have fewer reconvictions than other criminals (Christiansen et al, 1965). Gibbens et al (1977) have recently reported an interesting finding in a 12-year follow-up: 12 per cent of those convicted and 14 per cent of those acquitted of rape charges in 1961 were later convicted of a sexual offence. Presumably these figures disguise a higher reconviction rate in the convicted group since they are more likely to have served sentences of imprisonment and therefore to have spent shorter periods at liberty to commit further offences. However, it is evident that many of those acquitted of rape charges are in danger of future convictions for sexual offences.

The after effects

The sequelae of any mental or physical assault are obviously related to the strength of the attack and the adequacy of pre-existing personality adjustment. Burton (1968) showed that among child victims of sexual assault only a few of the more disturbed, for whom the sexual acting-out was undoubtedly symptomatic of a general disintegration of personality, make a poor adjustment.

Among adult victims three responses to the assault have been described by Sutherland and Scherl (1970): shock, dismay, and nonspecific anxiety. Younger adults typically do not consent to their next-of-kin being informed about the attack. The next phase is of superficial adjustment with repression of anger and resentment. A period of depression frequently precedes acceptance of the event and a realistic appraisal of the victim's complicity in it. The victim must lastly resolve her feelings towards the assailant.

We are living at a time of intense enquiry into the respective roles of men and women, especially in their relationships to each other, of which the purpose seems to be to achieve social and sexual equality. In that spirit it is surprising that Mrs Justice Heilbron's recent review of rape legislation did not recommend the abolition of the offence of rape. The view that sexual violation is intrinsically different from other forms of assault and that women are uniquely vulnerable is therefore perpetuated. It is probably necessary to continue to distinguish illegal sexual activity with children, but rape could be covered by the more general laws of assault.

It is common for rapists to describe, or need to describe, their victims as women of easy virtue and this belief is used to justify the assault. This observation suggests that rape is not just a reflection of violence in society but a paradigm of men's attitudes to women. Free from social influences the sexuality of men and women is probably quite different. There are pressures on male children encouraging self-assurance, control, dominance, equating sexual experience with manhood. Men judge women in terms of their sexual attributes, they dislike qualities which are considered manly and praise docility, good naturedness and nurturing qualities. Men need to feel that they control female sexuality so that women for their part merely facilitate the male orgasm. Rape, then, is an oppressive and exploitative act, symbolic of a patriarchal society, serving to make the male valuable and important. Rape is about control; after all, men can always masturbate for orgasm!

References

Amir, M (1971) Patterns in Forcible Rape. University Press, Chicago
Bender, L, Blau, A (1937) *American Journal of Orthopsychiatry*, **7**, 500
Burton, L (1968) Vulnerable Children. Routledge and Kegan Paul, London
Christiansen, K O, Elers-Nielson, M, Le Maire, L, Stürup, G K (1965) Scandinavian Studies in Criminology. Tavistock, London
Clinard, M (1963) Sociology of Deviant Behaviour. Holt, Rinehart and Winston, New York
Cohen, M, Garofalo, R, Boucher, R, Seghorn, T (1975) *in* Violence and Victims (edited by Pasternack, S). Spectrum, New York
Gibbens, T C N, Prince, J (1963) Child Victims of Sex Offences. Institute for the Study and Treatment of Delinquency, London
—, Ahrenfeldt, R H (1966) Cultural Factors in Delinquency. Tavistock, London
—, Way, C, Soothill, K L (1977) *British Journal of Psychiatry*, **130**, 32
Gunn, J (1976) *British Journal of Hospital Medicine*, **15**, 57
Guttmacher, M S, Weihofen, H (1952) Psychiatry and the Law. Norton, New York
Home Office (1977) Criminal Statistics for England and Wales. 1976. Command Report No. 6909. HMSO, London
Lorenz, K (1966) On Aggression, Methuen, London
MacDonald, J M (1971) Rape Offenders and their Victims. Thomas, Springfield, Illinois
Radzinowicz, L (1957) Editor. English Studies in Criminal Science, Vol. 9: Sexual Offences. Macmillan, London
Sparks, R, Genn, H, Dodd, D (1978) Surveying Victims: A Study of the Measurement of Criminal Victimisation. John Wiley, London
Storr, A (1968) Human Aggression. Allen Lane, London
Sutherland, S, Scherl, D (1970) *American Journal of Orthopsychiatry*, **40**, 503
West, D J, Roy, C, Nichols, F L (1978) Understanding Sexual Attacks. Heinemann, London

Chapter 29

Incest

Robert Bluglass, Midland Centre for Forensic Psychiatry, Birmingham

Incest is one of the oldest crimes, and the numerous references to it in mythology and literature emphasize the cultural and legal prohibitions against incestuous behaviour that have existed in most countries for a very considerable period of time. However, there have been notable exceptions to this rule, and there is evidence in Greek, Roman, Egyptian and Persian mythologies that in some cultures sexual relations between members of the same family not only occurred but were sometimes required (Maisch, 1973). There are accounts of this in the Old Testament and the records of the Ptolemies who exemplify the freedom accorded by some societies to those of high rank to unite with immediate family members.

The Ptolemies (330–320 BC) allowed the marriage of close blood relatives apparently in order to preserve the purity of the royal line. Cleopatra was a notable example. She was the child of a succession of brother and sister marriages and eventually married her younger brother Ptolemy III (she was also his niece). Some early civilizations, such as the Incas, permitted brother and sister marriages for generations and some primitive societies, for example the Azande of Africa, insist that the highest chiefs enter into sexual partnerships with their own daughters (Ford and Beach, 1965).

Although rare exceptions to the incest prohibition persist in some societies, it is otherwise universally forbidden. However, there are wide variations in the degrees of relationship that are prohibited. Thus there are differences between England and Wales and Scotland (Noble and Mason, 1978). The law in California covers a wide range of relationships, while Illinois and South Australia have limited prohibition.

The laws of most countries forbid incestuous relationships, although they do not all identify incest as a specific offence. It is an offence in England and Wales, Scotland, the Australian states, Canada, New Zealand, the American states, South Africa, Austria, the Federal Republic of Germany, and Sweden. Some countries, such as the Netherlands, encompass incestuous behaviour within the definition of other offences.

There are three elements that are common to the offence in all jurisdictions (Manchester, 1978):

1. The individuals concerned must be within a specified degree of relationship
2. At least one of them must have been aware of that relationship
3. Sexual intercourse must have taken place between them.

266

Historical background

In England and Wales incest, like witchcraft, bestiality and adultery, was in earlier times considered an offence against God and for 250 years was dealt with by the ecclesiastical courts. It carried the death penalty, although Queen Elizabeth I reduced the punishment to fines and imprisonment; she was possibly influenced by the fact that her mother, Anne Boleyn, was beheaded by Henry VIII for not only adultery but also alleged incest with her brother. In Scotland too incest was a contravention of religious laws and the death penalty was in existence until 90 years ago when it was altered to life imprisonment.

In England, apart from a brief period from 1640 to 1660, incest continued to be a religious offence under the jurisdiction of the ecclesiastical courts until very recently. The first attempt to make it a crime punishable before the ordinary courts was made in 1903 but was defeated. A secondary attempt also failed in 1907. Eventually in the following year the Punishment of Incest Act, 1908, was introduced by a private member and passed by the House of Commons in an almost empty chamber at a late period on a Friday afternoon. There was considerable uncertainty about the need for this measure. Mr. Rawlinson, the Honourable Member for Cambridge University and one of the main objectors to the Bill, said that in 1908 such behaviour was "far less known than it was 20 or 30 years before" and there was no suggestion that it was on the increase. The Bishop of St Albans in the House of Lords commented on the "great frequency of incest" in the country. However, the Bill became law and received little comment in the press or elsewhere in the country.

The present law

The Punishment of Incest Act, 1908, was eventually repealed and its substance incorporated in the Sexual Offences Act, 1956. Section 10 provides that it is an offence for a man to have sexual intercourse with a woman whom he knows to be his granddaughter, daughter, sister (or half-sister), or mother. Section 11 states that it is an offence for a woman over the age of 16 years to permit a man whom she knows to be her grandfather, father, brother (or half-brother), or son to have sexual intercourse with her by her consent.

Incest is punishable by imprisonment for a period not exceeding 7 years, although if the girl is under the age of 13 years it may be for life. Attempted incest carries a maximum sentence of 2 years. Prosecution requires the sanction of the Attorney General or the Director of Public Prosecutions on his behalf.

The law in Scotland is based on Leviticus, xviii, although modification of its application is slowly taking place (Noble and Mason, 1978).

Prevalence

It is generally believed that incest is far more common than appears from the numbers known to the police, reported in various studies over the years, or convicted. Offences are frequently not reported and are more likely to be detected among lower socioeconomic groups, often as a result of investigations involving the commission of other offences. Incestuous behaviour is usually known only to social agencies, doctors, or priests.

Weinberg (1955) reported the detected rates of incest in the USA as 1–2/100 000 between 1910 and 1930 and made similar estimates for other countries. More recently it was suggested that 3.9 per cent of the average population of the USA had experienced incest (Gebhard et al, 1965) and that 13.1 per cent of the prison population had done so. However, it was rarely reported by males in Kinsey's studies (Kinsey et al, 1948), although about 4 per cent of females reported an incestuous approach by a near relative (Kinsey et al, 1953).

Noble and Mason (1978) estimate that the incidence of incest in the UK calculated from cases known to the police is 6.6/1 000 000 in England, 6.5 in Scotland, and 6.2 in Wales. The available figures are clearly approximations and, as in other criminological studies, higher figures are reported in selected groups. For instance Lukianowicz (1972) detected 26 cases of paternal incest among 650 unselected female psychiatric patients encountered in various hospital settings in Northern Ireland.

Criminal statistics

At the beginning of the century there was in England and Wales an average of 56 offences of incest reported to the police annually up to 1920. By the 1940s there was an average of 140 cases each year and the upward trend continued until the mid-1960s when there were 300–350 cases annually. The rate has not increased further and during the 1970s about 300 cases continued to be reported each year. Throughout the last 20 years only about one half of the cases known have been sent for trial. In 1974 there were 148 persons convicted of incest, 17 of them under the age of 21 years.

Relationships

Sibling relationships are probably the most frequent form of incest (Weiner, 1964), although father–daughter incest is the most commonly reported type. Stepfather–stepdaughter relationships (although not legally incest) are equally common (Maisch, 1973). Only a few reports of brother–sister and mother–son incest appear in the literature. Other possible associations (grandfather–granddaughter, uncle–niece, and aunt–nephew) are very rarely reported.

Social class

It was firmly held in the past that incest occurred mainly in remote rural areas, among individuals of limited intelligence, as a result of poverty, poor housing, or overcrowding, or in delinquent areas. Although there are elements of truth in these beliefs, more recent opinions tend to contradict them; incest occurs in all social class groups although it tends, like nonaccidental injury to children, to be more easily concealed in the higher socioeconomic categories. The reliance on court and criminal statistics tends to bias inferences about the social class of incest offenders towards the more disadvantaged groups, although the pattern of offending shows a wide variability both between one rural area and another and between one metropolitan area and another.

Father–daughter incest

It seems that on average the father is in his 40s when an incestuous relationship first begins and the daughter has reached puberty with an average age of about 12 years (with a range of 5–15 years). In some cases it is clear that the developing sexual maturity of the girl is the stimulus to the start of a sexual relationship. It often begins with the oldest girl and may continue with a change of partner to involve younger siblings. With the younger children noncoital contacts, such as masturbation and between-thigh intercourse, tend to occur. The duration of contacts differs considerably in various studies. In Lukianowicz's (1972) study in County Antrim the average length of the relationship was 8 years.

The characteristics of the fathers involved are reported with a fairly consistent level of agreement in research studies.

Intelligence

The Kinsey Institute (Gebhard et al, 1965) on the basis of comparative intelligence tests reported that incest offenders exhibit a higher level of intelligence than other sexual offenders. Only 2–9 per cent had an IQ of 70 or below.

Mental disorder

Mental illness is an unusual finding among incestuous fathers. None of the 26 fathers in Lukianowicz's (1972) survey was psychotic or frankly neurotic and none suffered from an organic illness. Only one developed a reactive depression. Similarly Maisch (1973) found only one endogenous psychosis among the 67 offenders in his study. It is significant that courts do not tend to remand men charged with incest for psychiatric reports. Of 3000 offenders referred to the Midland Centre for Forensic Psychiatry during the last 10 years approximately 30 were men charged with an offence of incest.

Abnormal personality

A statistical analysis of Maisch's (1973) material revealed the outstanding psycho-pathological behavioural traits as violent and irascible (29 per cent), maladjusted at work (23 per cent), alcoholic (24 per cent), having a previous criminal record (46 per cent), and highly sexed (14 per cent). In 50 per cent of cases these traits were expressed more or less strongly and in various combinations. They must be distinguished from a relatively "normal" group who appear in every other respect to be well adjusted individuals.

Alcohol

Like many other offenders those convicted of incest include a high proportion of alcoholics (more than for other sexual offences). Virkkunen (1974) found 22 alcoholics (48.9 per cent) among 45 cases of incest. The alcoholics had more previous criminal offences and had been more overtly aggressive at home than the nonalcoholic incest offenders and were more likely to be rejected by their wives. Similar findings have been described in other studies, for example Szabo (1962) and others reviewed in Virkkunen's (1974) paper.

Predisposing factors

Among the psychological and sociological factors that can predispose to incest are the following:

1. A man returning home after many years of separation to find an ageing wife and a young daughter who now seems almost a stranger and also a temptation

2. The loss of a wife by divorce, separation, or death, leaving a bereaved father alone with an adolescent daughter who becomes a substitute wife providing love, solace, and sexual comfort
3. Gross overcrowding, physical proximity, and alcoholism leading to sexual intimacy
4. A lack of social contact outside the family as a result of poverty and geographical remoteness
5. Anxiety associated with a lack of sexual potency
6. Marital disharmony and rejection or a decrease in marital sexual activity
7. Psychopathic characteristics of poor impulse control, aggressiveness, and lack of guilt feelings, with or without any of the above.

Wives of incestuous fathers

Weiner (1964) states that there is much evidence to suggest that the wives of incestuous fathers promote the incestuous behaviour by frustrating their husbands sexually; their unavailability as a result of illness or pregnancy may also be a factor. It has been frequently reported that they further the sexual involvement with the daughter by encouraging her to sleep in the father's bed or otherwise setting up a situation conducive to incest. Not uncommonly the wife gives tacit approval by voicing little protest or tolerating or denying obvious behaviour. Numerous examples of denial have been reported, the wife claiming complete ignorance until confronted with the situation by a turn of events or the daughter's pregnancy which is the outcome in about 20 per cent of cases.

Frequently the wife only reports the situation after a row and then tends to stand by her husband. From her point of view the diversion of his interest towards the daughter may be a relief. The wife is rarely the person who reports the matter to the police.

The daughters

The younger daughters involved are often the victims of sexual assault by violent, drunken, or psychopathic fathers.

A 30-year-old father had a previous history of violent offences, a disturbed and unhappy childhood, and an unstable marriage interrupted by separations from his wife. He began to drink increasingly heavily. Shortly after his wife's third pregnancy when sexually frustrated he demanded that his 8-year-old daughter be brought to his bed and in an alcoholic state he attempted intercourse.

Older daughters may seek affection from their fathers when both are lonely.

A 50-year-old father had been happily married for 20 years. After his wife's death he was left alone with his 16-year-old daughter. They came together when both were depressed and felt isolated and alone. Sexual intercourse occurred regularly and in a mutual spirit of affection. However, he was eventually sentenced to 18 months' imprisonment.

It is often suggested that daughters play an active and initiating role in establishing incest which may continue for a long period without protest. Frequently the daughter is rewarded with gifts and only after an argument or a fit of pique is the relationship impulsively reported to a schoolteacher or other authority. Pregnancy may result in an admission of the behaviour to a family doctor. The offspring may be brought up within the family with the other children.

Girls who have been involved in incestuous relationships with their fathers do not necessarily emerge unharmed. Lukianowicz (1972) reported that subsequently four of his 26 patients showed some frank psychiatric symptoms but 11 developed character disorders and five frigidity or aversion to sexual relations with their husbands. In six girls there were no apparent ill effects.

Brother–sister relationships

In comparison with the relatively voluminous literature on father–daughter incest there are few studies of brother–sister relationships, although Fox (1962) and Santiago (1973) both reviewed the subject in detail. Such cases appear far less commonly in statistics, but *The Observer* newspaper estimated a few years ago that the total number of incest cases known to all agencies at any one time was about 16 000 of which about one fifth (3000) would be brother–sister relationships.

The most consistent finding (Meisleman, 1978) is that the children have lacked adult supervision, particularly with regard to their sex-play activities. The youngest sister in a large family of brothers is particularly vulnerable and Weinberg (1955) has stressed that the father's absence from the family is often a key factor. When present he may be incapacitated by age or disease. In some fatherless families the brother may be elevated to a fatherly role within the family, and in other cases the sister may similarly replace the mother.

In some descriptions the siblings are said to have witnessed parental intercourse regularly and to have modelled their own behaviour on it. In other examples father–daughter incest has already occurred within the same family. The author has had more than one case of a father who had intercourse with his daughter and then later urged his son to have intercourse with her as well.

Not infrequently brother–sister relationships arise from heterosexual experimentation. Fox (1962) considered that the likelihood of sexual engagement between siblings after puberty is an inverse function of their degree of propinquity and sexual activity before puberty. Incestuous temptation in adolescence is less if the siblings have been brought up together and have indulged in preadolescent sex-play.

There are examples of brothers and sisters meeting after a prolonged separation to fall in love and live together happily in a normal relationship. They are perhaps deserving of the most sympathy when they subsequently find themselves the subjects of criminal proceedings.

Mother–son relationships

The prototype is the story of Oedipus, but the literature contains very few accounts of mother–son incest. Lukianowicz (1972) described three cases. The first mother was normal (but later developed involutional depression) with a schizophrenic son, the second was schizophrenic with an educationally subnormal son, and the third was neurotic with a normal son. Mother–son incest tends to involve at least one party of abnormal personality make-up.

Origins of the prohibition against incest

The earliest explanations of the incest taboo were rooted in magic, religion, and superstition. Towards the end of the 19th century a primitive degeneration hypothesis assumed that incest and inbreeding caused psychological harm to descendants, despite the lack of evidence to suggest that primitive peoples were aware of any possible association. The French sociologist Durkheim (1898) based his theory on the superstitions surrounding the mixing of blood between people of the same totem or clan. Others have suggested that the aversion to incest is inborn and therefore universal, but this theory fails to explain why if this is so it should be necessary to develop such strict prohibitions against it.

Westermarck (1902) advanced the alternative theory of acquired aversion, posulating that people who have grown up together and lived in close contact develop a mutual sexual indifference. This was linked with a natural selection theory suggesting that those who "bred out" survived. Others have proposed that a ban on incestuous marriages has a politicoeconomic purpose: to encourage the development of a society, secure a social structure, and pool the resources.

However, it is Freud's theory, discussed so powerfully in his *Totem and Taboo* (Freud, 1960), that has had the most influence. He viewed the incest taboo as a cultural demand made by society on the maturing child, a barrier preventing him from selecting as a sexual partner the persons (mother and father) who are the first sexual objects in his life. He also saw the repression of these impulses as a motive force in the development of neuroses in later life. Freud's incest theories were derived from the dreams, memories and fantasies of his neurotic patients as well as his own. Most were concerned with the rarely found mother–son relationship rather than the commonly encountered father–daughter form. Despite all this, towards the end of his life Freud expressed doubts about the harm that might result from incestuous unions.

Fox (1962) suggested a behavioural explanation: sexual arousal occurs among prepubertal siblings who are brought up together and this induces aversive reactions so that the children learn to avoid physical contact before they gain sexual maturity.

Genetics and incest

The risks that might result from inbreeding relate to the increased possibility of a child of closely related parents inheriting a pair of mutant recessive genes with the risk of associated congenital abnormalities or malformations. There is an equal possibility of inheriting beneficial factors.

Opinion is not uniform about the seriousness of the genetic risk which for a time was frankly dismissed as unimportant. However, there are a number of studies of the children of incestuous unions that do provide grounds for concern. Adams and Neel (1967) found that only seven of 18 children of incest were normal at 6 months. Five were stillborn or had died in early infancy, two were severely retarded and subject to seizures, three were of borderline intelligence, and one had a bilateral cleft lip.

Seemanová (1971) examined 161 Czechoslovakian children of confirmed incestuous origin and compared them with a control group. There were very few infant deaths, but in other respects the incidence of abnormalities in the incest group was similar to the group studied by Adams and Neel (1967). Carter (1967) followed-up 13 children and found eight to have serious abnormalities from which three died.

Management of reported and suspected cases

It is the duty of the Social Services Department to investigate all cases of suspected incest if it is thought that a child may be in moral danger and the circumstances might justify care proceedings to protect her. The Department is also under a duty to inform the police (Children and Young Persons Act, 1969), although it is doubtful whether it always does so.

On a complaint being made, in a typical case of father–daughter incest the primary concern is to protect the child. It is possible to remove the child fairly speedily, although more commonly the father is removed and granted bail on condition that he has no further contact with his wife and daughter before the case is heard. Much more rarely he is remanded in custody. A high proportion of fathers plead guilty and save the necessity for the child to attend court.

Sentencing

It is well recognized that there are many cases of incest known to social agencies and doctors that are not reported. Only about half the cases known to the police are prosecuted; the remainder fail because of insufficient evidence to support a charge or are not proceeded with because the circumstances of the offence make it unnecessary or inexpedient to prosecute. The allegation of an offence may prove to be fabricated, be from an unreliable source, or lack the necessary corroboration. In many cases the authorities exercise discretion.

The offences prosecuted are by an overwhelming majority those committed between father and daughter. From 1909 to 1969 there were only nine reported brother and sister cases in the Law Reports. In two of these cases the female as well as the male was prosecuted. The prosecution of females is far less frequent than that of males. The highest proportion of females tried for incest was in 1915 (12 out of a total of 64 cases). In 10 years (1960–70) 75 women and 1372 men were tried for incest.

About a half of the cases sent to trial receive a sentence of imprisonment, the most usual period being 1–3 years. A much smaller group is imprisoned for 5–7 years. Longer sentences tend to be given for offences involving daughters under the age of 16 years, when imprisonment for 6–7 years is not unusual. There have only been 14 instances of sentences exceeding 7 years since 1909.

There has been an increasing tendency to give noncustodial sentences with the recognition that rehabilitation of the family is as important as punishing the male offender or even more so. Thus suspended sentences, probation, and conditional discharge now occur more commonly. Hospital orders are rarely made, reflecting the low level of overt mental disorder found in association with this crime.

The statistics that have been outlined relate to cases known to the police or convicted of incest. There are, of course, other cases which were excluded from this eventual classification as a result of the technical nature of the sexual behaviour even though it might have been regarded as an incestuous contact from the nature of the relationship between offender and victim. Hall-Williams (1974) studied 68 cases that were considered for parole between 1970 and 1971. Of these 53 per cent were convicted of the legal offence of incest, but 3.8 per cent were convicted of indecent assault or attempted indecent assault, 22 per cent of buggery. 27 per cent of unlawful sexual intercourse, and 4 per cent of rape. Many offenders were convicted of several different legal offences simultaneously.

Effects on the family

Maisch (1973) suggested that the harmful effects on the family as a result of disclosure and the punishment of the father may be more serious than those of the incestuous behaviour alone. The economic results of the father's imprisonment may be serious. The daughter may be removed into care and the family stigmatized. In the long term, as Lukianowicz (1972) and Meisleman (1978) found, the daughter may have difficulties in sexual adjustment, become promiscuous, or occasionally develop lesbian relationships. On the other hand, it has been suggested that incest is not a cause but a symptom of family pathology and the difficulties outlined may not necessarily have been avoidable.

Mature and stable brother–sister relationships may be painfully disrupted by disclosure and the family broken without benefit to the parents, the children, or society. In a reported case involving a half-brother and half-sister who met as adults, both were put on probation and ordered never to see each other again.

Treatment

Fathers who are mentally ill are treated in hospital or on an outpatient basis, but they are a small group. The few who exhibit associated sexually deviant or hypersexual behaviour may respond to treatment with psychotherapy, hormones or antiandrogens. Some benefit from treatment directed towards their alcoholism. The majority of individuals are unsuitable for formal psychiatric treatment and do not receive it in prison.

Incest is increasingly being seen as a symptom of family pathology and treatment is more successfully directed towards casework with the family. Family therapy has been described (Cormier et al, 1962; Kennedy and Cormier, 1969) with some degree of long-term success.

Law reform

From the information available incest appears to be frequently dealt with by society outside the criminal process. As in Sweden, Australia, Canada, Scotland and other countries, the need to keep incest within the criminal law has recently been questioned in England. The Criminal Law Revision Committee has asked whether "it is necessary or desirable to retain the offence of incest as at present defined, or whether it would be sufficient for the offence to apply only where one (or both) of the parties within the specified degree of consanguinity is a young person under a prescribed age; thus ceasing to apply where both parties are consenting adults".

Incest is essentially a family offence and it has been suggested that the civil process, and particularly a family court, might more appropriately deal with it. Such a family court would have powers to authorize orders of protection, support, care, and conciliation, but as yet none exists in England and Wales. It has also been pointed out that children may be protected by the laws relating to sexual assault against children and unlawful sexual intercourse, and mature brothers and sisters should not be subject to criminal proceedings. Some, such as the South Australian committee on the subject, have suggested that it is not the place of the criminal law to penalize citizens for their moral or intellectual deficiencies. Others have said that the innate revulsion of society from incest is sufficient protection in itself.

However, another view is that the "declaratory role" of the law, as the Royal College of Psychiatrists (1976) put it, affords added protection for the family and society. Hughes (1964) considered that there is sufficient evidence of the harm that can result to justify retaining incest as a crime and felt that the law should be extended to include stepdaughters and adoptive daughters.

The Scottish Law Commission (1980) has recently reviewed the law in Scotland and has concluded that incest should be retained as a separate crime, the degrees of consanguinity required should be defined, the offence should include the illegitimate child but exclude relations by adoption, and there should be an emphasis on treatment for the family.

Most writers agree that any change in the law should retain the offence for incest involving young children. There is a substantial difference between restricting the scope of a law and abolishing it altogether. The ambivalent nature of the incest taboo in our society—the sensitive balance between revulsion and attraction—should lead us to proceed with caution.

References

Adams, M S, Neel, J V (1967) *Paediatrics*, **40**, 55

Carter, C O (1967) *Lancet*, i, 436

Cormier, B M, Kennedy, M, Sangowicz, J (1962) *Canadian Psychiatric Association Journal*, **7**, 203

Durkheim, E (1898) *L'année Sociologique*, **1**, 1

Ford, C S, Beach, F A (1965) Patterns of Sexual Behaviour. Methuen, London

Fox, J R (1962) *British Journal of Sociology*, **13**, 128

Freud, S (1960) Totem and Taboo. Routledge and Kegan Paul, London

Gebhard, P H, Gagnon, J H, Pomeroy, W B, Christenson, C V (1965) Sex Offenders. Harper and Row, New York

Hall-Williams, J E (1974) *Medicine, Science and the Law*, **14**, 64

Hughes, G (1964) *Journal of Criminal Law, Criminology and Police Science*, **55**, 322

Kennedy, M, Cormier, B M (1969) *Laval médicale*, **40**, 946

Kinsey, A C, Pomeroy, W B, Martin, C E (1948) Sexual Behaviour in the Human Male. Saunders, Philadelphia

—,—,— (1953) Sexual Behaviour in the Human Female. Saunders, Philadelphia

Lukianowicz, N (1972) *British Journal of Psychiatry*, **120**, 301

Maisch, H (1973) Incest. André Deutsch, London

Manchester, A H (1978) *in* Family Violence (edited by Eekelaar, J M, Katz, S N). Butterworths, Toronto

Meislcman, K C (1978) Incest. Jossey-Bass, San Francisco

Noble, M, Mason, J K (1978) *Journal of Medical Ethics*, **4**, 64

Royal College of Psychiatrists (1976) *British Journal of Psychiatry*. Suppl. p.8

Santiago, L P (1973) The Children of Oedipus: Brother-Sister Incest in Psychiatry, Literature, History and Mythology. Libra, New York

Scottish Law Commission (1980) The Law of Incest in Scotland. Memorandum No. 44, April 1980

Seemanová, E (1971) *Human Heredity*, **21**, 108

Szabo, D (1962) *Canadian Psychiatric Association Journal*, **7**, 235

Virkkunen, M (1974) *Medicine, Science and the Law*, **14**, 124

Weinberg, S K (1955) Incest Behaviour. Citadel, New York

Weiner, I B (1964) *Excerpta Criminologica*, **4**, 137

Westermarck, E A (1902) Geschichte der menschlichen Ehe (quoted by Maisch, 1973)

Chapter 30

Battered wives

J J Gayford, Warlingham Park Hospital, Surrey

Erin Pizzey (1974) started her campaign on behalf of battered wives in 1971 and not only exploded the myth that women liked or desired the abuse they received from violent men but also brought home the horror and gravity of the situation. It may have been more convenient to believe this falsehood in the same way as battered babies were explained in quasi-metabolic and haematological terms until Kempe et al (1962) shocked considered opinion into accepting reality. Very soon authors such as Radbill (1974) were able to look back through history and see the atrocious ways in which some adults have treated children. In the same way Gayford (1977, 1978a) and May (1978) have traced how, throughout recorded history and no doubt before, some men have abused their wives in violent ways.

At intervals throughout English history there have been notable people who have raised their voices against wife beating (Stone, 1977). Documentary evidence of marital violence is more complete from the 19th century onwards (Cobbe, 1878). There is a marked similarity between the emotive speeches in the House of Commons 100 years ago (Hansard, 1874) which resulted in a Parliamentary Commission and the more recent speeches in the House of Commons which resulted in a Select Committee on Violence in Marriage (1975).

Following the Parliamentary Commission of 1875 there was a series of law reforms such as the Women's Property Act, 1882, the Matrimonial Causes Act, 1884, and even the Summary Jurisdiction (Married Women) Act, 1895, all of which attempted in a limited way to improve the lot of the married woman. The effects of the Select Committee on Violence in Marriage (1975) are only just beginning to be seen. Gill and Coote (1975) have given a brief account of how battered wives can use the law to protect themselves and extricate themselves from their predicaments.

There is certainly a heightened awareness of marital violence with the appearance of a number of books on the subject: Gelles (1972) and Steinmetz and Strauss (1974) from the USA have contributed, as have Borland (1976), Martin (1978), Mitchell (1978) and Renvoize (1978) from the UK.

Terminology

Aggression and violence

Gunn (1973) made the point that although aggression and violence are often used as interchangeable words there is a subtle distinction. Aggression is an unprovoked

276

attack whereas violence is the exercise of physical force so as to inflict injury or damage to person or property. Thus aggression may be verbal but violence is always physical; aggression can be constructive but violence is always physically damaging. Aggressive words and physical violence may be used together in a row between two people, but words may also be used as a substitute for violence or violence may be used where words fail and control is lost. It is even possible to have a passive form of aggression, which can be provocative and may be reciprocated with violence. The role of the wife as provocateur is discussed by Snell et al (1964).

Marital or conjugal violence

In violence between spouses one party may be the attacker and the other the victim or both may attack each other. The degree of physical assualt may be trivial or serious, the duration of the attack may be short or prolonged, and weapons may be used. Usually the male is stronger and is only the victim when this physical advantage is negated by use of weapons or, more frequently if he refrains from using his full strength. Very occasionally the male may be physically disadvantaged by disease but more commonly by drugs or so much alcohol that he is nearly unconscious.

It is rare for the man to really be the victim and once the male releases his full physical force without inhibition and even resorts to weapons, few women stand a chance. Scott (1977) points out that if the victim is the weaker party he is subjected to multiple blows; if he is the stronger party he has to be felled with a single blow or the tables will be turned.

Battered

This is an emotive term that implies that repeated blows are struck in one direction with one party very much the attacker and the other the victim.

Battered wife

This term should be reserved for a women who has been subjected to severe, repeated, deliberate, and demonstrable physical injury from her marital partner (Gayford, 1975a). One blow does not make a battered wife, no matter how serious it is or even if it is fatal. It is the fact that the attacks are repeated and the blows multiple that constitutes the battering and this eventually leads to a dangerous situation.

Women may attack men and with the aid of weapons may kill them, but it is very rare indeed for them to batter men and then generally only under the circumstances discussed.

Tortured wife

This is a highly emotive term that was introduced by Cobbe (1878). If it is to be used at all it is best reserved for women who are subjected to cold calculated attacks that may have a sadistic element. This is absent in most cases of battered wives.

Family violence

This covers all types of violence within the family including child abuse (battered baby), marital violence of all the types described, and abuse of usually aged parents by their children.

Epidemiology

For every battered wife who presents for professional help or takes refuge in a hostel for battered wives, there are many others who hide their injuries or, when forced to seek medical help, give spurious reasons for their conditions. Thus epidemiology becomes virtually impossible and all estimates are extremely inaccurate. Marsden and Owens (1975) confirmed an incidence of one in 500 marriages in the Colchester area but felt that this was an underestimate because there were other known cases who were not prepared to be included in their survey. Estimates from the Samaritans and the Citizens' Advice Bureaux have been steadily rising from the meagre figure of 3 per cent of enquiries that was claimed in 1972. Politicians are bolder and prepared to claim a national incidence of 50 000 a year (Hansard, 1973) but this can only be an inspired guess or an extrapolation from other data which allows for planning.

Aetiology

Cobbe (1878) claimed that wife battering was caused by alcoholic intoxication, heteropathy, jealousy, and friction due to overcrowding and social deprivation. Heteropathy was defined as the opposite of sympathy, where the sight of pain and suffering created a desire to destroy rather than to help. Nearly 100 years later the Royal College of Psychiatrists presented to the DHSS a report on battered wives in which they suggested the same factors, minus hereropathy, and added immature or psychopathic personality, cultural factors, and drug abuse. However they thought that most psychotic disorders had little part to play (Scott, 1974). They agreed with the Royal Scottish Society for the Prevention of Cruelty to Children (1974) that there was an overlap with child abuse and a background of family violence.

Gayford (1979) reviewed the aetiological factors as seen from his study of 100 battered wives. Analytical psychodynamic hypotheses have been provided by Schultz (1960) and Snell et al (1964) which either project the blame onto the relationship between the husband and his mother or claim that the wife herself is really the instigator of the violence. Faulk (1974) concluded that men who are violent to their wives for the first time after the age of 40 are more likely to be suffering from a psychotic disorder and those in the younger age group are more likely to be psychopathic.

The following is presented as an outline of some of the aetiological factors (Gayford 1978a, 1979).

Family background

About 40 per cent of the men were exposed to violence during their childhood, compared with about a quarter of the women who witnessed violence between parents or were subjected to parental violence. More than a third of women were deprived of one or both parents before the age of 15 and over a quarter of women had to share their parents with at least five siblings. Both immigrant men and women from the Republic of Ireland and the West Indies appeared to be over-represented. All social classes were included.

Education and employment

In many cases women projected themselves as better educated than their male partners and backed this up with examination successes in a third of case histories. An overlapping third went on to further education after leaving school. Again, about a third of women had good work records, staying in a job for more than 3 years, with another overlapping third gaining satisfaction from their work; 14 per cent started training as nurses or teachers. About half the men had no employment problems, but a third were frequently out of work.

Psychiatric history

Nearly half the women had received a psychiatric consultation at some stage in their lives, but most of these were after the violence had started. Almost three quarters of battered wives had been prescribed antidepressants or tranquillizers by their GPs and over a third had made suicide attempts, again usually after the violence had started. It would appear that in only a few cases did the psychiatric disorder precede the marital violence and could truly be called an aetiological factor. An important clinical point made is that when most of the women presented to a GP, a casualty department, or a psychiatrist, the diagnosis was obscured in the majority of cases.

Alcohol and drug abuse

Heavy drinking and drunkenness appear to be major problems among the husbands of battered wives in three quarters of cases. In over 40 per cent of cases violence only occurred when the husband was drunk. Between 10 and 20 per cent of women went through a heavy-drinking phase, some with their husbands and others as a means of relieving distress caused indirectly by the violence. Alcoholism appears to be a major problem in men who batter their wives, but only a handful of women are battered because of their drinking. It would appear that women are more likely to abuse drugs than their violent husbands; most of these drugs would be obtained on prescription but in neither party did it appear to be a major cause of violence.

Morbid jealousy (Othello syndrome)

Two thirds of battered women claimed that their husbands showed signs of jealousy and this seems to be the major aetiological factor. It has to be considered together with the promiscuity of either party and excessive drinking in the man. There is no doubt that some of the men want a very close exclusive type of relationship with their wives hardly speaking to members of the opposite sex. Indeed these poor women cannot win because any relationship with their own sex is projected as a sign of lesbianism. Accounts of violence being inflicted to extract confessions were encountered.

Premarital violence

A quarter of women reported that violence started before marriage or cohabitation. It would appear that if a woman is prepared to continue a relationship with a man who is violent to her before marriage, she is in danger of this violence being repeated after marriage when some of the traditional courtship respect may have lapsed.

Sexual history, courtship, and marriage

Nearly one in 10 battered wives seemed to have been involved in an incestuous relationship. Almost a quarter of the women claimed that they had been raped (relationships with husbands and cohabitees were excluded). The conclusion from these facts is that not an insignificant number of battered wives have experienced emotionally disturbing sexual relationships, most of whom seem to tolerate this without recourse to legal proceedings.

Less than a quarter of women went through the traditional courtship including engagement, before marriage. The majority of women had regular sexual relationships before marriage or cohabitation, and only 2 per cent routinely used contraception. The mean age of marriage or cohabitation was 20.3 years (sd±3.2), with about 10 per cent doing so before their 18th birthday. Sixty per cent of women were pregnant before marriage or cohabitation and 15 per cent of these pregnancies were not by the men whom they subsequently married or with whom they cohabited.

More than a quarter of women were in their second marital relationship, over half of the first relationships having ended due to violence. More of the men (over a third) had been involved in previous relationships of which well over half had ended due to violence. Men and women who have been in previously violent relationships seem to be in danger of entering further similar relationships: this is because men have a propensity to violence and women spend their social lives in a violent subculture with exposure to the company of latently violent men, desperately seeking further relationships. Such men are prepared to accept women who have had violent marriages, along with their children who are almost inevitably disturbed.

Promiscuity with extramarital sexual relationships plays a part in precipitating jealousy and may also lead to violence directly or indirectly. Almost one woman in five admitted to extramarital affairs but nearly half the men were accused of the same activity.

It is difficult to estimate the extent to which failure in marital sexual relationships was responsible for frustration and violence. A quarter of women claimed that they had never experienced sexual enjoyment at any time during the relationship. As the violence developed, more women failed to enjoy sexual relationships, but a surprising number of women had no complaint about this aspect of their marriage.

There was no real evidence that sadism on the part of the men or masochism on the part of the women played any part in the violence. Scott (1974) also agreed with this, which suggests that the reality of marital violence destroys any enjoyment of sadomasochistic fantasy. Homosexuality of either sex did not appear to be an important factor; while absent completely in the men, only isolated cases of facultative lesbianism were found in the women at an all-female hostel.

Social conditions

The importance of poverty and poor housing conditions in the aetiology of marital violence is also difficult to estimate. Certainly a quarter of the women had their poverty made worse and more unpredictable by heavy gambling by their husbands. Few complained of poverty unless pressed, but for many social security had become a fact of life. Crowded housing conditions must have made matters worse although the converse does not appear to prevent marital violence.

Overlap with child abuse

There is now little doubt that there is an overlap between child abuse and wife battering; this was suggested by Scott (1974) and confirmed by the Royal Scottish Society for the Prevention of Cruelty to Children (1974). About a third of women admitted that in frustration, often after they themselves had been subjected to violence from their husbands, they had hit their children much harder than they should or in an uncontrolled manner. In half the cases it appeared that the husbands extended their violence to the children and this was frequently the factor that precipitated the women into leaving the marital home.

Presentation

The physical effects of men losing control and violently assaulting their wives have been studied by Fonseka (1974) who looked at radiological evidence of injuries, and by Gayford (1975a, b, 1978) who studied the injuries found on women at a refuge for battered wives. Levine (1975) and Dewsbury (1975) studied marital violence as seen in general practice. The forensic aspect of women who have been killed by their husbands is a completely different subject and is not discussed.

Injuries vary considerably from the trivial to the serious. The types that may be seen in a casualty department are described below. As with battered babies, presentation for treatment is often delayed and the story of how the injury was received may be fabricated to hide the truth. Not infrequently women try to conceal injuries, staying indoors until physical signs have subsided. Alternatively they may be accompanied by their husbands who give the account of the events, refuse to be separated from their wives, and remove them from medical care as soon as possible often against medical advice. Attempted suicides may present in the same way and alarming accounts have been given of women being kept at home for a couple of days in an unconscious or semiconscious state.

Most injuries are found on the head and the neck, with a periorbital haematoma being the commonest. When seen early (within 24 hours) the eye is swollen and closed and there may be an associated subconjunctival haemorrhage. If the blow was heavy, that is inflicted with a weapon or by the patient being kicked, the bruising extends into the malar region. Most frequently, injuries are seen late when swelling has subsided. Lacerations around the eyes are quite common, the usual mode of attack being with the fists often with rings on the fingers. Swelling of the lips with lacerations and fractures of the teeth are not infrequent. Injury to the nose with possible fracture is also fairly commonplace. Trauma below the hair-line of the scalp is said to be inflicted deliberately in the more calculated attacks that are designed to cause injury with little physical signs. Strangulation attempts are claimed by about 20 per cent of women but there are usually few signs, although the women give an alarming description of sudden loss of consciousness which suggests that they were subjected to bilateral carotid compression.

Bruising around the arms and wrists is a sign that the woman has been restrained but does not always indicate that the man was the aggressor. The appearance of much deeper bruising is thought to imply that she was kicked or hit with a weapon. Occasionally women have been thrown about a room with painful injuries to the shoulder. Ribs are frequently fractured, usually when the victim was kicked while lying on the ground, and injuries to the lumbar sacral region generally occur in the same way. As long ago as 1878 Cobbe described the horrific case of a man jumping on a pregnant woman's abdomen, and regrettably there are still similar accounts of injury to the abdomen.

Burns and scalds usually occur when the violence takes place in the kitchen and hot utensils have been used in the attack. Fractures other than those of the nose, ribs and teeth are only rarely seen, and are a sign of a more serious sustained attack.

For the most part the picture is one of a man completely losing control and hitting his wife repeatedly with his fists, kicking her, and using any available weapon as he buffets her about the room. The attack is not usually premeditated but when it is the injuries, although not necessarily more severe, have more sinister connotations and it is obvious that the woman has been subjected to a type of torture. Examples of this are women who have been burned with cigarettes, or worse still, a hot poker; also, some women have had initials carved on their breasts (Dewsbury, 1975).

After the event the man may have amnesia, or in shame may wish to blot out the memory. There is no doubt that there is a loss of control similar to that in the episodic dyscontrol syndrome (Bach-Y-Rita et al 1971). Alternatively, the events are followed by profound remorse with the husband trying to make up for the damage by exemplary conduct.

Types of battered wife

It would be untrue to say that any man can batter his wife but as Faulk (1974) found in a small sample there is a variety of types of men in prison for this offence. It would be equally untrue to say that any woman can become a battered wife although several types have been described (Gayford, 1976). Any attempt to classify people is rightly doomed to failure because human beings are too complex to be "pigeon-holed". In practice a battered wife may have various characteristics of the types described below—it is helpful to list them under headings.

Inadequate wife

It is often difficult to decide how much of the inadequacy has been precipitated by the repeated episodes of violence; an inadequate woman becomes more so under these circumstances. However, she is able to live under adversity and to tolerate difficult situations much longer than most people. She was brought up to this and her current family pattern is only a repetition of what she experienced in childhood. Social workers have despaired of helping this type of family, often labelled as "problem families" and described by Tonge et al (1975) as "families without hope".

This type of inadequate woman was probably victimized at school where she had a poor record in both attendance and achievement. One of her chances to leave home was through marriage and the only type of man who would tolerate her family background was somebody brought up in similar circumstances. Marriage tended to be early, often precipitated by pregnancy. Further children followed and accommodation was always a problem.

Her husband is unlikely to have a good work record and this may have been punctuated by prison sentences, with income further reduced by drinking and possibly gambling. An overlap with child abuse is not an infrequent complication of the family's problems. Psychiatric help has occasionally been sought but is unlikely to yield encouraging results. Treatment with antidepressants or tranquillizers can lead to suicide attempts.

It goes without saying that this type of battered wife is the most difficult to help; however, she seems to fare better in one of the Women's Aid hostels than with conventional psychiatric and social care. In other words she needs to be taken into total care with her children and to be surrounded by other women who can act as surrogate mothers to her children when required. In this way she gradually learns, but it is a lengthy process which takes many years and may be punctuated by abortive attempts at reconciliation with her husband.

There is a particular type of inadequate woman who is subjected to the most cruel and prolonged violence if she has married a bullying man. Unfortunate cases of both herself and the children being burned with cigarettes have been seen. She may be the victim of acts of sexual degradation that are sickening and have nothing to do with sex. The only thing that needs to be said about such acts is that they are not necessarily sadistic but those of a drunken man showing his disgust after he has been sexually refused. There is no doubt that this type of woman and her children need to be removed from such a situation and handled with care and consideration while legal proceedings take place. Both she and her children will need considerable rehabilitation.

Highly competent wife

At first it is difficult to see how this type of woman becomes a battered wife. She has often been brought up in a protective environment, has had a good education, and holds a responsible job. Intellectually she is frequently her husband's superior, forcing him to rely on her for help in his career. The withdrawal of this help leaves him in a vulnerable position. Her marriage may have caused a rift between her family and herself, making it difficult or embarrassing to accept help from them when there is a crisis due to violence. This type of woman with a middle-class background was studied in the USA by Snell et al (1964) when she and her husband presented for psychiatric help. They saw such women as aggressive and efficient with the husband occasionally having to assert himself, usually when his inhibitions had been removed by alcohol. Such a view was also expressed by Whitehurst (1974) who found similar middle-class families who could be taught to suppress violence for fear of public disapproval and loss of social status.

It is certainly this type of woman who presents with the hope of some psychotherapeutic intervention. If this is to be undertaken alcoholism and morbid jealousy should be excluded and a framework devised by which violence cannot bring about a rewarding situation for the husband. Most feminists would be highly critical of male-orientated psychoanalytical ideas of the woman needing to become more submissive in order to be less provocative to a male with a low frustration tolerance. Even so there are women who blame themselves for precipitating the violence, especially when they are experiencing premenstrual tension.

Provocative wife

There are many ways in which women can be provocative and so cause friction in a marital relationship. Factors such as inadequacy and overcontrol have already been discussed. Another of the more obvious causes is sexual provocation which when coupled with morbid jealousy is a most dangerous combination (Shepherd, 1961). It has been known to lead to homicide or, more accurately, uxoricide (Perdue, 1966).

This type of woman has always enjoyed the company of the opposite sex, even in childhood. Not only does she know how to seek attention but also often enjoys the game of offsetting one man against another. She is generally vivacious and energetic, with many of the qualities of the stimulus seeker who is constantly looking for excitement. This is one of the few types of women who will try to hit back in violent episodes, but she also soon learns that when a man has completely lost his temper a woman is no physical match for him. Her husband may be an exciting man in her eyes and there is a tendency towards frequent separations and reconciliations. Both she and her husband tend to have extramarital sexual relationships, but nevertheless they often have an exciting sexual relationship within the marriage in spite of the violence.

When trying to help this type of woman it is important to remember that she needs excitement. Placed in a quiet hostel when the violence has become too much, or moved to a bed-sitter, she will seek out her violent husband or at least let him know where she can be found. Alternatively she will find a new boyfriend who will have many of the qualities of her violent husband. At Chiswick Women's Aid this type of woman is invaluable in helping other women in crises and in doing this she gains the excitement she desires without endangering herself. Eventually she tires of the excitement and seeks a more peaceful domestic life.

Long-standing case

Twenty per cent of women seen by Gayford in 1973–74 had experienced violence for more than 10 years (Gayford, 1975a). This was at a time when hostels were only just becoming available and there were few places to which women could escape. Violence has become a way of life for this type of woman and she may well have experienced similar treatment from her father. There is a sad air of resignation; if she did not leave home when her children left, she stayed for the sake of possessions or pets or due to an inability to make a new way of life in middle age. If her husband is a heavy drinker, drunkenness occurs more quickly and his physical health starts to deteriorate. As a result of this the physical damage lessens and eventually he becomes a rather pathetic dependent old man.

Cases complicated by alcohol, drugs, and a psychiatric history

Occasionally, battered women who drink heavily themselves or abuse drugs join those with a psychiatric history in hospital. In all these cases it is difficult to determine which came first, the violence or the disorder, but in many the drug and alcohol abuse or the psychiatric problems continue after there has been a separation from the violent man. Battered wives who abuse alcohol frequently tend to have a family history of alcoholism or a husband with drinking problems. There is overlap between the types of women who abuse alcohol and those who abuse drugs. Both tend to suffer from other psychotic disorders such as anxiety or recurrent depression.

Violent wife

Very few women (8 per cent) regularly tried to hit back when their husbands were violent, most having learned that this only accelerated the violence and that they usually came off worse. It is strange how strong women often have even stronger husbands. Fortunately the type of woman who is frequently involved in fights with other women is rare. Less than 5 per cent of battered wives appear to be involved in a variety of problems which can end in extramarital violence. This type of woman may have a very violent husband and both may have been involved in conflicts with the law. She may be part of a drug-taking heavy-drinking set and two cases seen had lesbian tendencies.

Pseudo-battered wife

Following the publicity of the phenomenon of the battered wife there have been a few cases in which delusions of marital violence have become part of the repertoire of the paranoid schizophrenic. More commonly women claim that they have been battered because they wish to end their marriages and discredit their husbands. This type of woman does not stay long at a busy overcrowded hostel for battered wives. She can rarely present any direct evidence of the violence, but gives an account that may trap the inexperienced or the unwary.

Investigation and management

Intervention with psychotherapy should be tried only when violence has been minimal or isolated. Professional middle-class couples who value their social reputation have a behavioural restraint readily available. Cases in which there is a history of drug or alcohol abuse by either party are best treated for this disability first. Violent men are coming forward for help only gradually; this is mainly because they want to keep their wives, but generally on their own terms. Men with sudden explosive rage need to be fully investigated including EEG studies (Elliott, 1976). When violence occurs for the first time late in life, loss of control due to dementing processes must be excluded.

Periodic depressive episodes especially those with an anxiety component may cause some people to be very irritable; in the woman this can be a provocative factor and in the man it may precipitate violence. Claims of schizophrenia in the man are far more common than cases actually substantiated. Anxiety and especially agoraphobia in battered wives are not uncommonly seen and some behavioural treatment of the agoraphobia may be beneficial. Cases in which there is an element of morbid jealousy need to be handled with great care and most would see this as a sign that the parties should seek separation. Even this may not be an end of the problem because not infrequently this type of jealous man may keep his former wife under surveillance after divorce. He may take exception to her attempting new relationships and even demand what he still considers to be his conjugal rights.

It is extremely common for children of battered wives to suffer from behavioural disturbances including bed-wetting, school refusal, theft, and vandalism. Few battered wives are able to cope with these disorders. Some of the temper tantrums seen in these children are quite frightening to behold and may exclude them from most organizations for children. Children from these families often need to be taken into care, but their mothers may resent this and compensate their loss by initiating a further pregnancy.

When a woman has decided to take legal action (either criminal or civil) against her husband, she will find it an almost impossible task to continue living under the same roof while the legal proceedings reach their conclusion. The threat of further violence has deterred many women from going ahead. More commonly there is a genuine ambivalence over the whole matter which may swing each way a number of times before a final decision is reached.

Hostels for battered wives have only recently become available (Harrison, 1975). These are run by voluntary organizations under the general term of Women's Aid and can provide more than just shelter. Most offer a counselling service that includes access to a solicitor who has the necessary skills and is prepared to represent the women under legal aid.

There are two main types of hostel, the open door and the restricted admission. The open-door hostels, of which the most famous is Chiswick Women's Aid founded by Erin Pizzey, take women and children who present no matter where they originate from or what time of day or night they arrive. These hostels tend to be crowded and attract the most severe cases with their disturbed children. There is a central crisis refuge that takes all new cases, which is supported by facilities for children, and secondary hostels where women and children may reside on a long-term basis. The restricted-admission hostels tend not to publicize their addresses and admission has to be made through specific and rather secret channels. Most are small houses where only a given number of women and children can be accommodated in family rooms. They tend to be more comfortable and occasionally house women who would not fit the definition of a battered wife. The Select Committee on Violence in Marriage (1975) requested the Department of the Environment to encourage local authorities or voluntary organizations to provide refuges on the basis of one family place per 10 000 of the population.

The rehabilitation of women and children is a long and complicated process which may be hindered if the battered wife seeks a new relationship with another man of a similar type. At a mean age of 31 with, on average, two disturbed children, most battered wives have difficulty in finding stable partners. It is a sad fact that many of their children will take marital violence into the next generation. Cases have been seen where this condition has passed through three generations.

The dynamics of violence in marriage

Behavioural theory suggests that violence is a learned pattern of behaviour (Scott, 1958). Analytical theory tends to equate aggression and violence and postulates that this is always preceded by frustration (Dollard et al, 1944). Marital violence, like most real violent situations, substantiates some elements of both theories but raises questions about others. Gorney (1971) argued that with increased intensity of emotional feeling there is a greater liability of eruption into violence. The psychodynamics of marital violence are postulated and discussed fairly fully by Snell et al (1964), Faulk (1974), and Gayford (1978a, b).

The relationship between battered wives and their husbands is intense, with both parties striving to keep it alive in spite of the obvious failings. If this were not so, there would simply be a separation between the two parties. Both have made some investment in the relationship and see themselves losing if they are the ones to pull out, even if that loss will only be material. Gayford (1975b) showed that only a third of women had no positive feelings for their husbands.

Both parties need to be considered in terms of their frustration tolerance which can be lowered by external social factors or internal psychological and physical factors. The focus falls on the husband's frustration tolerance which, when exhausted, will be the critical factor. Some men will never be violent; this is not their way of dealing with situations. Others have learned from experience, which may include the example of their parents, that violence appears to solve problems where other ways fail. This has to be associated with some blunting of the perception of what happens to general relationships when violence erupts.

Both parties can be provocative, but in this article the focus is on the wife as the victim. Women vary a great deal in their provocative qualities and these may be affected by physical, psychological, and social situations. If a woman of low provocation is paired with a man of high frustration tolerance, violence is highly unlikely; even if a highly provocative woman is paired with this same type of man with high frustration tolerance, violence is unlikely but divorce is quite possible. The problem of violence starts when a man with low frustration tolerance is paired with a highly provocative woman; this is what happens in violent marriages.

Many women report the feeling of tension rising before violence erupts. In some cases this may take only minutes, but others have described this feeling building up for days. Alcohol is very important in this equation because it removes inhibitions and allows violence to erupt.

Less than 20 per cent of battered wives are not legally married but they are trapped in the relationship by the same factors as the wedded women, namely the difficulty in leaving because of children. It is rare for childless women to present because they somehow manage to escape the full severity of the attack. All ages of adult women present; usually battered wives are in their late 20s and early 30s, although older women are not immune. By the time women have found it necessary to take refuge in a hostel for battered wives they have generally been in the marital relationship for some years.

References

Bach-Y-Rita, G, Lion, J R, Climent, C E, Ervin, F R (1971) *American Journal of Psychiatry*, **127**, 1473
Borland, M (1976) Editor. Violence in the Family. Manchester University Press, Manchester
Cobbe, F P (1878) *The Contemporary Review*, **32**, 57
Dewsbury, A R (1975) *Royal Society of Health Journal*, **96**, 290
Dollard, J, Miller, N E, Doob, L W, Mowrer, O H, Sears, R R (1944) Frustration and Aggression. Institute of Human Relationships, Yale University
Elliott, F A (1976) *Practitioner*, **217**, 51
Faulk, M (1974) *Medicine, Science and the Law*, **14**, 180
Fonseka, S (1974) *British Journal of Clinical Practice*, **28**, 400
Gayford, J J (1975a) *British Medical Journal*, i, 194
—(1975b) *Medicine, Science and the Law*, **15**, 237
—(1976) *Welfare Officer*, **25**, 5

—(1977) *Practitioner*, **219**, 122
—(1978a) Battered Wives: The Study of the Aetiology and Psychosocial Effects among One Hundred Women. MD Thesis, University of London
—(1978b) *in* Violence and the Family (edited by Martin, J P). John Wiley, Chichester, p.19
—(1979) *Medicine, Science and the Law*, **19**, 19
Gelles, R J (1972) The Violent Home: A Study of Physical Aggression between Husbands and Wives. Saga Publications, London
Gill, T, Coote, A (1975) Battered Women: How to use the Law. Cobden Trust, London
Gorney, R (1971) *American Journal of Psychiatry*, **128**, 436
Gunn, J C (1973) Violence in Human Society. David and Charles, Newton Abbott
Hansard (1874) Criminal Law; Assaults on Women. Resolution 219, 18 May. p.396
—(1973) Speech by Jack Ashley MP, 17 July. p.218
Harrison, P (1975) *New Society*, **34**, 361
Kempe, C H, Silverman, F N, Steele, B S, Droegemuller, W, Silver, H K (1962) *Journal of the American Medical Association*, **181**, 17
Levine, M B (1975) *Medicine, Science and the Law*, **15**, 172
Marsden, D, Owens, D (1975) *New Society*, **32**, 333
Martin, J P (1978) Editor. Violence and the Family. John Wiley, Chichester
May, M (1978) *in* Violence and the Family (edited by Martin, J P). John Wiley, Chichester. p.135
Mitchell, A R K (1978) Violence in the Family. Wayland Publishers, Hove
Perdue, W C (1966) *Diseases of the Nervous System*, **27**, 808
Pizzey, E (1974) Scream Quietly or the Neighbours Will Hear. Penguin, Harmondsworth
Radbill, S X (1974) *in* The Battered Child, 2nd edn (edited by Helfer, R E, Kempe, C H). University of Chicago Press, USA
Renvoize, J (1978) Web of Violence: A Study of Family Violence. Routledge and Kegan Paul, London
Royal Scottish Society for Prevention of Cruelty to Children (1974) Battered Wives Survey
Schultz, L G (1960) *Journal of Social Therapy*, **6**, 103
Scott, J P (1958) Aggression. University of Chicago Press, USA
Scott, P D (1974) *British Journal of Psychiatry*, **125**, 433
— (1977) *ibid.* **131**, 127
Select Committee on Violence in Marriage (1975) HC55311. HMSO, London
Shepherd, M (1961) *Journal of Mental Science*, **107**, 687
Snell, J E, Rosenwald, R J, Robey, A (1964) *Archives of General Psychiatry*, **11**, 107
Steinmetz, S K, Strauss, M A (1974) Editors. Violence in the Family. Dodd, Mead and Company, New York
Stone, L (1977) The Family, Sex and Marriage in England 1500–1800. Weidenfeld and Nicolson, London
Tonge, W L, James, D S, Hillam, S M (1975) *British Journal of Psychiatry*, Special Publication No. 11
Whitehurst, R N (1974) *in* Violence in the Family (edited by Steinmetz, S K, Strauss, M A), Dodd, Mead and Company, New York

Chapter 31

Fitness to plead

Marion Swan, Winterton Hospital, Cleveland

In recent years only a few defendants have been found unfit to plead—about 100 cases per annum. It is, however, an issue that is likely to confront most psychiatrists at some point in their careers and to be encountered by the forensic psychiatrist quite frequently. Because a working knowledge of the subject involves the grasp of some complex legal points, the issue of fitness to plead is often misunderstood and, indeed, avoided by some doctors.

Fitness to plead is such a fundamental concept in the British legal system that any doctor preparing medical reports (and particularly psychiatric reports) for the courts should be aware of the basic issues involved. The criteria for unfitness to plead should always be considered in the defendant's assessment.

Definitions and terminology

The following terms may be found confusing and need definition.

Fitness for trial

This covers all the issues that may affect whether or not an accused person is fit to stand trial and may include such temporary incapacity as appendicitis or other physical illness. It is usually possible to deal with the latter by postponing the trial. However, where the incapacity is of a psychiatric nature and is prolonged it may be dealt with in one of the two following ways:

1. Transfer from prison to hospital under Section 73 of the Mental Health Act, 1959 (see below)
2. The accused may be considered to be unfit to plead and therefore "under disability".

Fitness to plead

Normally a man is held to be responsible for any criminal act or omission and liable to punishment for it. Equally it is a fundamental rule of law (with the exception of absolute offences) that a person cannot be guilty of a crime if he has not the wit to form criminal intent. This absolves children and many mentally disordered people from guilt. Furthermore it has been accepted as inhumane to subject to trial someone who is unable to defend himself and is, therefore, unfit to plead (Forrest, 1978).

Fitness to plead is the term used by many doctors and lawyers that relates to the ability of the defendant to enter a plea in a court of law. If the jury finds the accused person unable to enter a plea he is considered to be under disability. The Report of the Committee on Mentally Abnormal Offenders, known as the Butler Report (Home Office and DHSS, 1975), recommends replacement of the term "unfit to plead" by "under disability in relation to trial" (under disability, for short), although the term under disability was introduced in the Criminal Procedure (Insanity) Act, 1964.

Historical perspective

The decision as to whether an insane offender could be tried has for centuries been complicated by the way in which such people have been linked in the courts with two other awkward cases—the deaf mute and the man who refuses to plead.

For mediaeval and Tudor judges the alleged offender who seemed too insane to try was a minor part of a more complex problem. A common difficulty was the man who refused to plead. Unless an offender pleaded he could not be convicted or executed and his property could not be forfeited to the Exchequer. However, the penalty was still high—the man who refused to plead was slowly pressed to death under a heavy weight unless his endurance gave out and he consented to plead. This penalty was not officially abolished until 1772 (Walker, 1968).

The evidence of the Old Bailey sessions papers suggests that it was not until the middle of the 18th century that the insane prisoner had any chance of being found unfit for trial. The usual outcome when this occurred was for the accused to be remanded indefinitely.

From about 1830 onwards judges became more precise in explaining to juries exactly how insane the prisoner must be in order to be found unfit to plead. Judge Alderson stated that the jury should consider whether the accused was "of sufficient intellect to comprehend the course of proceedings in the trial so as to make a proper defence—to know that he might challenge any of you to whom he may object, and to comprehend the details of the evidence". These words became the most authoritative definition of the test of fitness to plead.

In theory it remains true that if the accused has been transferred to a mental hospital under Section 73 of the Mental Health Act, 1959, before his trial, or is found unfit to plead by a jury, then the trial is merely deferred until he is in a fit state to be tried. In practice the trial only takes place if the accused is suspected of having feigned the disorder or makes a quick recovery.

Present legal position (Smith and Hogan, 1975, 1978)

An accused person's sanity may become relevant before the trial. In these preliminary proceedings the effect of finding that the accused is mentally dis-ordered may prevent him from being tried at all. He may be transferred from prison to hospital under Section 73 of the Mental Health Act, 1959 (see below) or he may be presented for trial.

If the accused is brought for trial he may be found to be under disability as defined by Section 4 of the Criminal Procedure (Insanity) Act, 1964.

Criteria

The question at this stage is whether the accused is able to understand the charge, possible consequences, and difference between pleas of guilty and not guilty, to challenge jurors, to instruct counsel, and to follow the evidence in court. If he is able to do these things he has a right to be tried if he wishes, even though he may not be capable of acting in his best interests (R v Robertson, 1968).

The same criteria are theoretically applicable where the prosecution contends that the accused is fit to plead and he denies it, but legal sources indicate that they might be more leniently applied in such a case.

Interpretation

It was held in the case of Podola (see Walker, 1968) that a man is fit to plead where a hysterical amnesia prevents him from remembering events during the whole of the period material to the commission of the crime alleged but whose mind is, at the time of the trial, completely normal. The same court was prepared to concede that a deaf mute was "insane"—the word used in the Criminal Lunatics Act, 1884—but declined "to extend the meaning of the word to include persons who are mentally normal at the time of the hearing of the proceedings against them and are perfectly capable of instructing their solicitors as to what submission their counsel is to put forward with regard to the commission of the crime".

Although the word insane is not used in the current legislation about fitness to plead, the law is unchanged.

Who raises the issue?

The issue of fitness to plead cannot be dealt with in the magistrates' court. In the crown court it may be raised by the judge on his own initiative or at the request of the prosecution or the defence. Where neither party raises the issue, the judge should do so if he has doubts about the fitness of the accused (Poole, 1966). The judge may resolve his doubts about this by reading the medical reports but it is considered undesirable for him to hear medical evidence at this stage in the proceedings.

Procedure

If the question of fitness to plead is raised by counsel for the prosecution or the defence or if the judge has doubts, the issue must be tried by a jury especially empanelled for the purpose (Section 4[4] of the Criminal Procedure (Insanity) Act, 1964). If the accused is found unfit to plead the court makes an order to admit him to a hospital specified by the Home Secretary (Section 5[1] [c] of the Criminal Procedure (Insanity) Act, 1964) where he may be detained without limit of time, the power to discharge him being exercisable only by the Home Secretary (Sections 47 and 65 of the Mental Health Act, 1959).

Burden of proof

Where the defence raises the issue of fitness to plead, the onus of proving that the accused is unfit is on the defence. The defence is required to prove the case on a balance of probabilities. If the issue is raised by the prosecution and disputed by the defence, the burden of proof is on the prosecution and the matter must be proved beyond reasonable doubt. If the issue is raised by the judge and disputed by the defence, the onus is again on the prosecution.

At what point in the trial?

A difficult problem may arise when there is evidence of both a substantive defence to the charge and unfitness to plead. Until recently the issue of fitness to plead was tried before the trial of the general issue. This meant that if the defendant was found to be unfit, he was deprived of his right to raise the issues of his defence. He might then be detained indefinitely even though a defence witness could have proved that he could not have committed the offence.

This has been resolved by Section 4 of the Criminal Procedure (Insanity) Act, 1964. The general rule remains that the question of fitness to plead should be determined as soon as it arises (Section 4[3]) but the judge is now given the discretion to postpone it until any time up to the opening of the case for the defence, where having regard to the defendant's supposed disability he considers it expedient and in the defendant's interest to do so (Section 4[2]). If at the end of the case for the prosecution there is insufficient evidence to justify a conviction then the jury should be directed to acquit. However, if there is a substantial case against the accused the issue of fitness to plead is determined at this point in the trial by another jury especially empanelled for the purpose.

Where the defence depends on positive evidence (for example, a witness in court who can prove that the defendant was 10 miles away at the time of the alleged crime) rather than on the weakness of the prosecution's case, it is possible to request the judge to call the defence witness before the end of the prosecution's case.

Right of appeal

It is possible to appeal against a verdict of unfitness to plead. This is done through a court of law, that is the Court of Criminal Appeal, and not through the Mental Health Review Tribunal.

Psychiatric examination of the accused

In order to reach a decision about whether or not the accused is under disability it is necessary for the psychiatrist to satisfy himself regarding the ability of the accused to meet the legal criteria outlined above (Gunn, 1979).

The psychiatrist must ask himself the following questions. (It must be remembered that it is the mental state of the accused at the time of the trial and not at the time of the alleged offence that is relevant.)

1. Does the accused understand the nature and possible consequence of the charge?
2. Does he understand the difference between a plea of guilty and one of not guilty?
3. Can he instruct his legal representatives?

4. Can he follow the evidence in court?
5. Can he challenge a juror?

If the answer to any one of these questions is "no", then the accused should be considered under disability. It is important, on assessment of the accused, not to coach him in the answers to the questions since this will invalidate independent examinations by other psychiatrists. It should also be remembered that the accused might have been coached already by his solicitor or parents or by the police and one must consider this. This is particularly relevant when a mentally handicapped person is being examined.

While the ultimate decision about this matter is taken by a jury, the members will almost certainly be asked to consider psychiatric evidence in reaching a decision. It is therefore important that the doctor writing his report or giving oral evidence in court expresses himself on this point clearly and in simple language, using terms that can be understood by the judge, the lawyers, and the jury, all of whom must be assumed to lack knowledge of both medicine and medical terminology.

If an accused is considered to be under disability by a psychiatrist, it is likely that he is suffering from either severe subnormality or mental illness. In the former case treatment is unlikely to improve his mental state. However, in the case of mental illness psychiatric treatment can result in considerable improvement (Whitlock, 1966).

Related issues

Transfer from prison to hospital under Section 73 of the Mental Health Act, 1959

Where the accused has been committed in custody for trial and the Home Secretary is satisfied by reports from at least two medical practitioners that he is suffering from mental illness or severe subnormality, he may order the accused to be detained in a hospital provided that he is of the opinion, having regard to the public interest, that it is expedient to do so (Section 73 of the Mental Health Act, 1959).

Under the Criminal Lunatics Act, 1884, the Home Secretary exercised this power only, "Where the prisoner's condition is such that immediate removal to a mental hospital is necessary, that it would not be practicable to bring him before a Court, or that the trial is likely to have an injurious effect on his mental state".

The basis for this practice is presumably still applicable, that is "that the issue of insanity should be determined by the jury whenever possible and the power should be exercised only when there is likely to be a scandal if the prisoner is brought up for trial" (Criminal Lunatics Act, 1884).

It is also possible, when a person is remanded and requires medical treatment, for a magistrate or a judge, as a condition of bail, to remand him to a hospital for the specific purpose of assessment and/or treatment if a hospital is willing to accept him.

Whether this method of transfer or Section 73 of the Mental Health Act, 1959, is used depends on the circumstances of the individual case. It is generally better for all concerned if it is possible to arrange medical treatment for the offender before the trial, so that he is fit to plead. He may still be dealt with by an order under Section 60 of the Mental Health Act, 1959, if further hospital treatment is indicated and he is found guilty (see below).

A verdict of "not guilty by reason of insanity"

This is likely to be relevant only where the accused is charged with a serious offence, but may apply to any charge tried in the crown court.

It is difficult initially to comprehend a case where the accused is considered fit to plead but is insane. However when the criteria for fitness to plead are considered it is clearly possible and it is a reflection of the legal rather than a medical definition of insanity which causes this apparent anomaly.

The Royal Commission on Capital Punishment (1953) states: "Someone who is certifiably insane may often, nevertheless, be fit to plead to the indictment and follow the proceedings at the trial and that, if he is, he should ordinarily be allowed to do so, because it is, in principle, desirable that a person charged with a criminal offence should, whenever possible, be tried, so that the question whether he committed the crime may be determined by a jury".

The use of Section 60 of the Mental Health Act, 1959

1. Where the accused is found fit to plead and is then found guilty by the jury he may still be admitted to a psychiatric hospital using Part V of the Mental Health Act, 1959, the judge making an order under Section 60 with or without a restriction order under Section 65 of this Act.
2. Under Section 60, Subsection 2, it is possible in the magistrates' court, but in no higher court, to make a hospital order *without conviction* if the court is satisfied "that the accused did the act or made the omission charged". The usual medical oral or written evidence is required by the court.

This subsection is not often used. Many psychiatrists think that it should be used more frequently because in their opinion someone who has a recoverable mental illness should not have a conviction recorded against him since it may have far-reaching consequences for the rest of his life. It only applies to those offences that can be tried in the magistrates' court and those punishable by imprisonment, but its more widespread use would prevent the issue of fitness to plead being raised in connection with minor offences.

The mute offender

Where a person is found to be mute by "visitation of God" and therefore unfit for trial, he is dealt with in the same way as someone who is found to be under disability. He must be committed to a hospital named by the Home Secretary. This does not necessarily mean a mental hospital, but could for example be a home for the deaf.

Current criticisms of the present legislation

There is much criticism of the present legislation in relation to fitness to plead.

The question of fitness to plead generally arises when the accused pleads not guilty. If a man pleads guilty he can be dealt with under Section 60 of the Mental Health Act, 1959, in the normal way. As such, he will not be subject to the restrictions imposed on him if he is found unfit to plead unless a judge in the crown court considers that he should impose a restriction "without limit of time" under Section 65 of the Mental Health Act, 1959. This means that the patient who is unfit to plead usually has to be treated under greater restrictions, although he has not been convicted, than a similar patient who commits the same offence but who is fit to plead. (This is particularly so with minor offences.)

There is also a danger that an innocent man may be branded as a "criminal lunatic" because of his disability at the time he should have been tried. Although a patient who is unfit to plead is not formally found guilty it is generally, but erroneously, assumed that he committed the offence with which he was charged.

It is also possible that a man who has been detained in hospital for a considerable period of time will have to be returned to court for trial when he is well. If he is then found guilty he will be sentenced to a further period of detention, possibly in prison. The man who is mentally disordered may therefore receive, in effect, two "sentences" for the same crime and so is given unequal treatment under the law (Whitehead, 1973). It should be noted that unfitness to plead is not a sentence in the sense of a conviction being recorded.

A number of replies can be made to these criticisms and it is possible that the law may be revised in the not too distant future. Some further criticisms and also some suggested reforms are outlined in the Report by the Butler Committee. Because of their importance these are discussed at some length below.

The Butler Report

The following general points are made in the Report:

1. The term unfit to plead should be replaced by under disability in relation to trial.
2. The present tests determining whether a defendant is under disability should be modified by omission of the reference to challenging a juror. The accused should, in addition, be able to plead with understanding to the indictment.
3. The present situation regarding amnesia should stand unaltered.
4. The importance of establishing the facts should be recognized;
a. If a person is under disability there are strong arguments for establishing this at the earliest possible moment. The sooner the defendant can be relieved of the stress of appearance in court and begin treatment the better for him, the better for the dignity of the legal process, and the greater the saving of public time and money.
b. There must be safeguards, however, against the possibility that it might become easy for people to be put away, perhaps for long periods of time, without proper justification. There must also be no suspicion that arbitrary committals to hospital might take place, perhaps to suit the convenience of the authorities.
c. Equally, the public may look for reassurance that criminal offences are not being glossed over on a pretext that the defendant is not fit to stand trial.

The Criminal Law Revision Committee (1963) has noted this dilemma that a person may be entitled to an acquittal on the facts and yet it may be impossible to try him properly because of his disability.

There are powerful arguments in favour of trying to establish the facts in such cases, before accepting that the defendant should be indefinitely detained. If he did not commit the offence there may be no justification for putting him in hospital. He may, for example, be a mentally handicapped person living peaceably with his mother, and a grievous wrong would be done to him if he were committed to hospital on a charge that could not be substantiated. If he goes to hospital the responsible medical officer and the adviser to the Home Secretary must act on the assumption that the offence was committed, and this may affect their estimations of when he is safe to be released.

The following shortcomings are identified in the crown court:

1. The magistrates cannot deal with the defendant who is unfit to plead and he must be automatically sent to the crown court.
2. Once it has been determined by the court that the defendant is under disability there is no provision for an investigation of the facts by the court. Even where the prosecution evidence is heard, there is no provision for any evidence by the defence. Unless an acquittal is returned on the evidence of the prosecution alone, the person under disability must be committed to hospital under an indefinite order.
3. A person so committed remains untried until the Home Secretary decides otherwise, and this may mean a very long period of detention, even detention for life.
4. At present it is not in the interests of the defendant to seek the protection of a disability plea unless the charge is very serious. If the trial went ahead he might be acquitted altogether, but even if he is convicted he can hope to receive a finite sentence.

The following shortcomings are identified in the magistrates' court:

1. There is no explicit power for magistrates to remand the accused for medical examination before a finding of guilt. There is also no statutory authority enabling the magistrates to hear evidence on the issue of fitness to plead or to stand trial.
2. The magistrates cannot deal with the offender who appears unfit to plead and have to commit him to the crown court.

Several proposals are made as follows.

Determination of disability

The issue of disability should be decided at the outset of the trial or as soon as it is raised.

If disability is found but the medical evidence indicates recovery within a few months, the judge may adjourn the proceedings for a minimum of 6 months. At the adjourned proceedings the question of disability is reopened. The defendant may now be fit to plead.

If he has not recovered or the medical advice indicates initially that recovery is unlikely (for example, in the case of severe subnormality), a trial of the facts should take place.

The judge should decide the question of disability if the medical evidence is unanimous or even if it is disputed, unless the defence in the latter case desires the decision to be made by a jury.

Trial of the facts

Even if the defendant is found to be under disability there should be a trial of the facts to the fullest extent possible. This is to enable the jury to return a verdict of not guilty where the evidence is insufficient for a conviction. The normal rules of evidence should apply and if the members of the jury are not satisfied beyond reasonable doubt that the defendant did the act, or had the necessary mental state at the time, they should return a verdict of not guilty. If they are satisfied that he did the act they should state that "the defendant should be dealt with as a person under disability". The verdict of guilty is not appropriate because of the defendant's disability. There is, of course, the possibility that the defendant might have been able to expound on the evidence to convince the jury of his innocence had he been mentally fit and it is for this reason that neither a conviction nor a sentence is appropriate.

Disposal

The present law should be changed to give the court some discretion about the disposal of the defendant under disability. Evidence presented by the judges (to the Butler Committee) suggests that mandatory disposal is undesirable.

The following orders are suggested:

1. An order for inpatient treatment with or without a restriction order
2. An order for hospital outpatient treatment
3. An order for forfeiture of any firearm, motor vehicle, and so on, used in the crime
4. A guardianship order
5. Any disqualification (for example, from driving) normally open to the court to make on conviction
6. Discharge without any order.

The usual criteria for making orders under 1, 2 and 4 should be observed.

Appeal

This should remain as at present, that is through the Court of Appeal. In the event of the recovery of the defendant after the return of a disability verdict following a trial of the facts, he should be allowed to apply to the Court of Appeal for a normal trial.

Jurisdiction

Jurisdiction to determine the issue of disability in relation to trial should be given to magistrates' courts.

Magistrates should also be empowered to call for reports on the mental condition of the defendant at any stage in the proceedings if he is thought to be under disability. Such reports should be in the form required for orders under Section 60 of the Mental Health Act, 1959.

The same magistrates' court that hears evidence on disability should not proceed to a trial of the facts or a full trial. This should occur before a differently constituted court (that is, a different bench of magistrates—analogous to the second jury in the crown court).

In cases of disability the procedure should be the same as that suggested for the crown court, except for the making of orders restricting discharge from hospital. This should be dealt with by the crown court.

Appeals against disability verdicts reached in magistrates' courts should be made to the Queen's Bench.

Medical evidence

There should be a statutory requirement for the supporting evidence of two doctors to be presented to the court before the accused can be found to be under disability in relation to trial. This would bring the medical evidence required in line with that necessary to implement Section 60 of the Mental Health Act, 1959. In the same way one (but not both) of the doctors should be approved under Section 28 of this Act.

These proposals put forward in the Butler Report are generally accepted in chapter 5 of the *White Paper on the Review of the Mental Health Act, 1959* (HMSO, 1978).

Conclusion

The present legislation about fitness to plead has been reviewed and placed in its historical perspective. The current state of affairs is unacceptable to many psychiatrists and to the concept of British justice because it denies the accused the right to prove that he did not commit the offence with which he is charged. It is to be hoped that the proposals and recommendations of the Butler Report and the White Paper (HMSO, 1978) will be implemented speedily so that this situation is rectified.

In the meantime if the mentally ill can be treated prior to the trial, when possible, to ensure their fitness for it, they will be entitled to all the advantages of a proper hearing of their case by the court. They can still be dealt with under the Mental Health Act, 1959, if they were ill at the time of the offence.

My gratitude is expressed to Dr D G A Westbury, Consultant in Forensic Psychiatry, Northern Regional Health Authority and the Home Office, for his patient appraisal of the manuscript of this article and the many helpful comments he made about it.

References

Criminal Law Revision Committee (1963) Third Report. Command Report No.2149. HMSO, London
Criminal Lunatics Act (1884) HMSO, London
Criminal Procedure (Insanity) Act (1964) HMSO, London
Forrest, A (1978) A Companion to Psychiatric Studies, 2nd edn. Churchill Livingstone, London
Gunn, J (1979) *in* Recent Advances in Clinical Psychiatry, Vol 3 (edited by Granville-Grossman, K L). Churchill Livingstone, London. p.289
HMSO (1978) White Paper on the Review of the Mental Health Act, 1959. HMSO, London
Home Office, DHSS (1975) Report of the Committee on Mentally Abnormal Offenders. Command Report No.6244. HMSO, London
Mental Health Act (1959) Reprinted 1973. HMSO, London
Poole, A R (1966) *Criminal Law Review*, **6**
R v Robertson (1968)3 A11.ER557, CA

Royal Commission on Capital Punishment (1953) Command Report No. 8932. HMSO, London
Smith, J C, Hogan, B (1975) Criminal Law: Cases and Materials. Butterworths, London. p.162
—,—(1978) Criminal Law, 4th edn. Butterworths, London. p.159
Walker, N (1968) Crime and Insanity in England, Vol. 1. Edinburgh University Press, Edinburgh
Whitehead, J A (1973) *International Journal of Offender Therapy and Comparative Criminology*, **17**, 2
Whitlock, F A (1966) Criminal Responsibility and Mental Illness. Butterworths, London

Index